CHRONIC KIDNEY DISEASE - FROM PATHOPHYSIOLOGY TO CLINICAL IMPROVEMENTS

Edited by **Thomas Rath**

Chronic Kidney Disease - from Pathophysiology to Clinical Improvements
http://dx.doi.org/10.5772/66239
Edited by Thomas Rath

Contributors

P Veeramuthumari, Ali Malik, Chowdhury Ahsan, Arhama Malik, Sumit Sehgal, Hashim Hussnain Ahmed, Subodh Devabhaktuni, Edward Co, Syed Shah, Ane Claudia Fernandes Nunes, Camilla Fanelli, Ayman Noreddin, Yuriy Milovanov, Svetlana Milovanova, Nikolay Mukhin, Marina Taranova, Ludmila Urievna Milovanova, Victor Fomin, Aigul Usubalieva, Ana Paula Silva, Anabela Malho Guedes, Pedro Leão Neves, Damir Rebić, Aida Hamzić-Mehmedbašić, David Johnson, Melissa Nataatmadja, Yeoungjee Cho, Katrina Campbell, Alejandra Guillermina Miranda-Diaz, Leonardo Pazarín-Villaseñor, Francisco Yanowski-Escatell, Jorge Andrade-Sierra, Luis Miguel Roman-Pintos, Rishila Ghosh, Pawan Kumar Kare, Manushi Siddarth, Om Prakash Kalra, Ashok Kumar Tripathi, Simona Mihai, Elena Codrici, Ionela Daniela Popescu, Ana-Maria Enciu, Laura Georgiana Necula, Gabriela Anton, Cristiana Pistol-Tanase, Luís Manuel Mota Sousa, Ana Vanessa Antunes, Sandy S P Severino, Cristina M. A. Marques-Vieira, Cristina R. S. L. Baixinho, Helena M. G. José, Cristina Capusa, Daria Popescu

Published by InTech
Janeza Trdine 9, 51000 Rijeka, Croatia

Publishing Process Manager Romina Skomersic
Technical Editor SPi Global
Cover InTech Design team

First published February, 2018
Printed in Croatia
Legal deposit, Croatia: National and University Library in Zagreb

Additional hard copies can be obtained from orders@intechopen.com

Chronic Kidney Disease - from Pathophysiology to Clinical Improvements, Edited by Thomas Rath
p. cm.
Print ISBN 978-953-51-3843-3
Online ISBN 978-953-51-3844-0

For EU product safety concerns :
IN TECH d . o . o . , Prolaz Marije Krucifikse Kozulić 3 , 51000 Rijeka , Croatia ,
info@intechopen . com or visit our website at intechopen . com .

Meet the editor

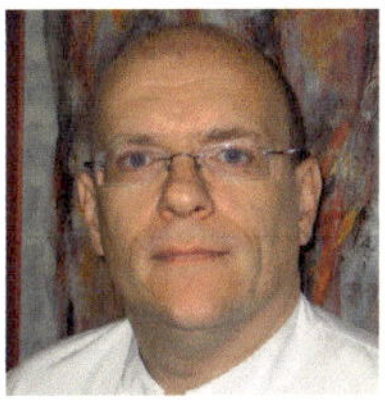

Thomas Rath is a doctor in Medicine and specialist in Internal Medicine, Nephrology and Infectious Diseases. He lives in Kaiserslautern, a city of 100,000 inhabitants in the southwest part of Germany. After completing his studies at the University of Mainz, he became a resident at the Westpfalz-Klinikum in Kaiserslautern, a tertiary care hospital with 1300 hospital beds. There, he is the head of the Department of Nephrology and Transplantation Medicine and also for the outpatient clinic for patients with infectious diseases. He is an active member of many national and international societies. In his scientific career, he has published more than 25 papers in peer-reviewed journals and more than 150 abstracts and posters on national and international congresses. He gives lectures at the Technical University of Kaiserslautern on "artificial organ support".

Contents

Preface

Known worldwide, chronic kidney disease (CKD) is a disease that affects up to 4% of the population with increasing figures also in the developing countries. Life expectancy of patients affected by CKD is shortened compared to the overall population, and only a minority of patients reach end-stage renal disease (ESRD) with the need for dialysis or renal transplantation; death overtakes dialysis.

Most of the patients with CKD will die because of cardiovascular complications. Interestingly, the traditional risk factors for cardiovascular diseases (hypertension, diabetes mellitus, smoking, etc.) seem to have less influence on the fate of the patients. However, the role of uremic toxins in the development of cardiovascular complications is not fully understood.

The progression of renal disease and the occurrence of complications are associated with alterations in inflammation processes. More and more data are added to shed light on the pathophysiological mechanisms involved in the progression of CKD and development of complications leading to substantial clinical and socioeconomic effects.

One of the earliest changes related to CKD are the disorders of the phosphorus-calcium metabolism. There is a well-known link between high serum phosphate levels and the occurrence of cardiovascular complications in patients on dialysis but also in the general population. New biological markers like fibroblast growth factor 23 (FGF-23) and Klotho give us insight into the interplay of hormones, functional aspects of the renal tubulus system and endothelial function.

The interaction of the products of gut microbiota like indoxyl sulphate (IS) and p-cresyl sulphate (PCS) with renal function and cardiovascular risk is very interesting. Both show increasing serum concentrations in patients with CKD. Therefore, a "gut-kidney-axis" is postulated, and IS and PCS are seen as therapeutic targets to slow the progression of kidney disease and improve cardiovascular outcome.

Besides new pathophysiological insights and pharmacologically based therapies, established dietary restrictions, especially a low-protein diet, have beneficial effects on the progression of CKD. But also environmental aspects have gained more attention. Organochlorine pesticides used in farming and agriculture are suspected to increase the incidence and severity of CKD.

All these fascinating aspects of scientific medicine are presented in this book. In addition, chapters dealing with the genetic aspects of polycystic kidney disease and also the clinical handling of patients with CKD and peritoneal dialysis will be beneficial for the open-minded reader.

This book comprises a total of 13 chapters from authors and researches from different countries and continents, thus reflecting worldwide importance of CKD.

We are grateful to all the contributors and experts for the preparation and submission of their stimulating manuscripts. And, last but not least, many thanks go to the team of InTech for giving us the opportunity to publish all these very interesting papers and thoughts in a peer-reviewed open access book.

Dr. Thomas Rath
Department of Nephrology and Transplantation Medicine
Westpfalz-Klinikum
Kaiserslautern, Germany

Section 1

Cardiovascular Aspects in CKD

Chapter 1

Traditional, Nontraditional, and Uremia-Related Threats for Cardiovascular Disease in Chronic Kidney Disease

Damir Rebić and Aida Hamzić-Mehmedbašić

Additional information is available at the end of the chapter

http://dx.doi.org/10.5772/intechopen.69574

Abstract

As many as 40–50% of all patients suffering from chronic kidney disease (CKD) die from reasons related to cardiovascular disease (CVD). The severity of the illness is directly connected to higher mortality caused by cardiovascular factors, with the cause of the CKD not as significant for the relationship. This risk of high cardiovascular mortality and morbidity is actually so high that it surpasses the risk of the patients reaching end-stage renal disease. Within the context of CKD, CVD has certain distinct characteristics. Left ventricular hypertrophy (LVH) is commonly used as a predictor of cardiovascular (CV) mortality. The striking cardiac interstitial fibrosis, a crucial part of uremic cardiomyopathy, and nonobstructive vascular diseases are highly prevalent CV pathology in CKD patients. Traditional risk factors appear to be of less importance in the CKD population compared to the general population but have been hypothesized as uremic toxins as a risk factor of cardiorenal syndrome. In this chapter, we discuss the importance of renal function in the pathophysiology of heart failure. We also elaborate on the novel understanding of chronic kidney disease and its role in cardiovascular disease progression.

Keywords: chronic kidney disease, cardiovascular disease risk factors, traditional risk factors, nontraditional risk factors, uremia-related risk factors, cardiorenal syndrome, renocardiac syndrome

1. Introduction

Patients suffering from chronic kidney disease (CKD) have the higher risk of facing complications or mortality from causes related to cardiovascular disease (CVD) than reaching its end-stage renal disease (ESRD) [1]. In fact, 9 out of 10 patients face cardiovascular issues and/or die due to these causes before they ever progress to ESRD [2]. A number of epidemiologic studies and research concluded that a strong relationship exists between CKD and morbidity and mortality related to CVD. Taking better care of cardiovascular (CV) risk factors during the past 10 years has led to a drop of 40% in mortality caused by coronary artery disease [3]. This, however, has not spilled over to patients suffering from CKD or those that have progression to ESRD [4, 5]. This has an effect of increasing issues caused by CVD in CKD patients, as well as highlighting further those risk factors that go alongside old age, primarily arterial hypertension, vascular calcification, dyslipidemia, oxidative stress and inflammation [6]. An aging population and increasing incidence of hypertension, diabetes mellitus, obesity and other comorbid factors are associated with an increasing incidence of cardiorenal disorders [7]. Risk factors are usually intertwined, making it difficult to separate the traditional and newly discovered risk factors, which actually have very strong ties.

2. Main body

2.1. Reverse epidemiology

Reverse epidemiology is the paradoxical observation that the well-documented associations in the general population between dyslipidemia, hypertension, obesity and poor outcomes does not exist or even may be reversed in dialysis patients. It should be mentioned that this phenomenon is not only observed in dialysis patients but also in geriatric populations and chronic heart failure (CHF). Studies have suggested that this confounded epidemiology is due to the overriding effect of malnutrition and persistent inflammation [8].

CVD in the setting of CKD has its own specific characteristics. First, despite the high incidence of accelerated atherosclerosis and high fatality following myocardial infarction (MI) in patients suffering from chronic kidney disease, a very small number of heart disease-related deaths are caused by ischemic heart disease—between 15 and 25% [9]. CVD-caused mortality is predicted by left ventricular hypertrophy (LVH), which is typically used as a forecaster. The mortality usually happens in the form of heart failure, myocardial infarction and sudden cardiac failure. Regardless of hypertension, a common cardiovascular pathology in patients with CKD is striking cardiac interstitial fibrosis, which occurs within uremic cardiomyopathy and nonobstructive vascular disease. Most common examples would be vascular stiffness, calcification and ossification [10]. These causes are predictive of negative cardiovascular events and can be used in explaining why sudden cardiac death and ischemic heart disease occur so often when there is no significant atherosclerosis. Importantly, traditional risk factors of CVD that we know are not as important in patients suffering from CKD as they are in the general population. Primarily, this is in reference to hypertension, diabetes mellitus, smoking and hyperlipidemia [9]. This can be seen through a stubbornly high CV mortality in CKD patients who control these factors. Evidence appearing right now indicates that uremic toxins and abnormal calcium-phosphate metabolism, which belong to novel CKD risk factors, directly add to the development and evolution of cardiovascular disease. Chronic kidney disease is already by nature a progressive kind of disease, which is further augmented through these factors, which, in turn, increase the risk for the "cardiorenal syndrome".

Also, it has been hypothesized that uremic toxins as a risk factor of cardiorenal syndrome. Despite tremendous advances in the development of dialysis technology, CV mortality is still unacceptably high in dialysis patients. Rates of all-cause mortality for dialysis patients are 8.2 times greater than the general population. After CVD has started off, the probability of survival after a five-year period reduce to 18% and 47% for patients on dialysis and following transplantation, respectively. This is quite low compared to 64% survival chance of general population. Patients in long-term dialysis must take special care of their left ventricular hypertrophy development [11] that develops even if the blood pressure level is normalized and is no longer anemic. Three-quarters of patients on dialysis for more than 10 years have left ventricular hypertrophy (LVH). Cardiac fibrosis gets worse with time in these patients but its effect are reversed after transplantation has been performed [12]. An interesting finding is the negative correlation between duration of renal replacement therapy (RRT) prior to the transplantation and the recovery of cardiac functions after a successful procedure. Dialysis performed now fails to discard a large quantity of organic matter completely, which under normal conditions be excreted by the kidneys. This is because of its high molecular size and high protein affinity [12]. Due to pathophysiological actions of this matter, these uremic compounds can add to the overall CV risk in patients with chronic renal disease. According to their physicochemical determinants, there are three groups of uremic-retention compounds: small compounds soluble in water, middle molecules and small protein-bound compounds [13]. These uremic-retention solutes with negative biological effects are called uremic toxins.

In the past few years, we have reached some understanding to their cardiovascular adverse effect, but we still need to reach conclusions regarding the mechanisms through which this occurs [13].

2.2. Pathophysiologic mechanisms

It is unclear as to what causes this high risk of cardiovascular disease in CKD patients. Uremia and ESRD-related risk factors, some of which are older age, hypertension, dyslipidemia, diabetes mellitus and LVH, are highly prevalent in CKD. However, these factors do not fully account for the extent of CVD in CKD. Several cross-sectional studies have suggested that other factors that are not included in the Framingham risk profile may play an independent and important role in promoting vascular disease in these patients. Unique risk factors related to ESRD and uremia such as hemodynamic and metabolic alterations, hyperhomocysteinaemia, oxidative stress, inflammation and anemia have been identified and also likely contribute to the excess CVD risk [14]. Several mechanisms are involved in the pathophysiology of CVD in CKD interrelated and complex ways. In CKD, several clinical pathologic entities underlie CVD, including endothelial dysfunction, accelerated atherosclerosis, arteriosclerosis, and cardiomyopathy [15].

2.3. Neurohumoral activation and hemodynamic alterations

Hemodynamic changes and neurohumoral factors such as renin-angiotensin-aldosterone system (RAAS) and sympathetic nervous system (SNS) activation play an important role in the interactions between the heart and the kidneys in patients with CKD and CVD (**Figure 1**). RAAS and SNS are both key regulatory systems for the maintenance of cardiovascular and renal function. Loss of renal mass in CKD leads to the accumulation of sodium and water resulting in hypertension and fluid overload in patients with Cardiorenal syndrome (CRS). In the setting of CKD, elevated concentration of angiotensin II increases sodium retention, regulates glomerular filtration rate (GFR), potentiates the renal effects of SNS stimulation and increases release of arginine vasopressin (AVP) from the posterior pituitary gland and aldosterone from the adrenal cortex [16].

Sympathetic stimulation results in several physiologic changes that under normal circumstances serve to maintain cardiac output and vascular integrity. In the setting of heart failure, overactivity of SNS worsens cardiac performance. Sympathetic hyperactivity is present in early and advanced stages of CKD, with levels that increase with worsening renal function [17]. Overdrive of renal adrenergic receptors promotes release of renin from juxtaglomerular cells and reabsorption of sodium from tubular cells. Angiotensin II and aldosterone

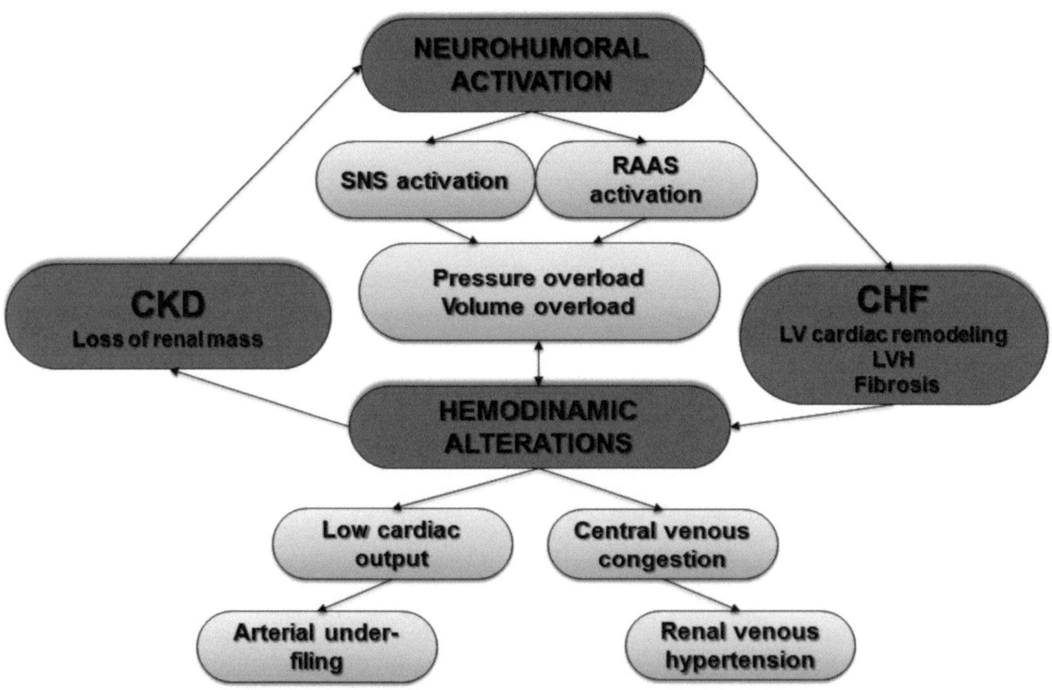

Figure 1. Neurohumoral activation and hemodynamic alterations in CKD and CHF. *Note*: CKD, chronic kidney disease; CHF, chronic heart failure; SNS, sympathetic nervous system; RAAS, renin-angiotensin-aldosterone system; LV, left ventricular; LVH, left ventricular hypertrophy.

both causes systemic arterial vasoconstriction and directly promote cardiac remodeling. AVP exerts its physiologic effects via activation of V1 and V2 receptors. Activation of V1a receptors on vascular smooth muscle cells results in vasoconstriction, while activation of V2 receptors on the collecting duct increases reabsorption of hypotonic water. Patients with CKD and CHF suffer from elevated afterload occurring after an increase in systemic vascular resistance, which arises from vasoconstriction mediated by the V1a receptor, as well as from increased preload due to water retention that occurs following the anti-diuretic effect mediated by the V2 receptor. AVP also has direct promoting effect of fibrosis and myocardial hypertrophy [18].

Volume overload occurs, due to expansion of extracellular fluid arising from aldosterone, which is responsible for the rising reabsorption of sodium and water. Ventricular filling pressures increase, caused by retention of fluids, resulting in symptoms connected with HF such as dyspnea, jugular venous distension, hepatic congestion, peripheral edema and orthopnea. Preload, or higher ventricular filling pressures, increase the workload of heart and cause dilatation of the damaged ventricle. Other conditions along with chronic kidney disease increase the cardiac output demand, leading to volume overload; chronic anemia is one among them. It is the condition where the oxygen-transporting capacity of blood has gone down. Another is when the patient has an arteriovenous fistula for the hemodialysis (HD) access, which requires some cardiac output, leaving less to systemic circulation [19].

Regulation of sodium balance is important for the maintenance of appropriate blood pressure and body fluid volume. Increased blood pressure resulting from a normal cardiac response to increasing fluid volume and pressure natriuresis and which is required for excretion of excess sodium and body fluid. Abnormal pressure natriuresis in heart failure due to low cardiac output has been described in low-flow theory. In patients with CKD who have insufficient sodium excretion because of reduced GFR due to reduced numbers of functional nephrons, there is an insufficient pressure natriuresis. Pressure natriuresis is also affected by neurohumoral factors such as RAAS and SNS. The combination of pump failure and low cardiac output leads to vascular congestion and edema that are worsened through a nonsensical renal reaction where water and sodium retention occurs, even though extracellular volume is expanded. Vascular congestion and edema become worse, under these conditions [20].

Low cardiac output and arterial underfilling are previously thought to be main causes of impaired renal function in heart failure. However, some evidence suggests that renal venous hypertension due to venous congestion, rather than arterial underfilling, may cause renal dysfunction. Central venous congestion is clinically evident as increased jugular venous pressure and peripheral edema. Increased central venous is transmitted downstream to the capillary beds of other organ systems including the kidneys. Recent clinical trials showed the relationship between increase in central venous pressure and decrease in estimated GFR [21]. GFR is considered to decrease in response to reduction in the net filtration pressure caused by increased hydrostatic pressure in Bowman's capsule secondary to increased interstitial pressure. These factors suggest that abnormal pressure natriuresis due to decreased GFR, exacerbation of venous congestion and worsening of heart failure due to low cardiac output create a positive-feedback cycle [16].

2.4. Uremic cardiomyopathy

In the general population, pathological LVH is connected to poor survival prognosis, the development of diastolic dysfunction, arrhythmias and cardiac failure progression. A similar state is present with predialysis, as well as dialysis patients. Although the terms used to describe this condition overlap, uremic cardiomyopathy marks the influence of reduced renal function on functional cardiac capability [22]. Epidemiological studies show that the primary manifestation of uremic cardiomyopathy is LVH. Reduced renal function in different stages of arrest, combined with cardiac diseases, most often causes the development of uremic cardiomyopathy. Go et al. in a study on a large number of examinees determined that the reduction of GFR by 50%, increases the overall risk of death by five times [23]. The treatment of ESRD by kidney transplantation severely reduces the risk of cardiovascular death, but with persistence of some mortality risks. The study conducted by Zoccali et al. shows that short-term dialysis patients have a better prognosis and survival concerning cardiovascular diseases post kidney transplantation. The same authors determined that LVH is an independent factor of cardiovascular risk, connected to significant survival rate reduction [24]. LVH pathogenesis in uremic cardiomyopathy remains uncertain. Taking into account the high frequency of hypertension in patients with a difficult chronic renal disease, one of the hypotheses is that LVH occurs as a product of blood pressure encumbrance. In patients with diabetic nephropathy, blood pressure, as an independent risk factor, leads to the increase of left ventricular mass (LVM), as well as the LV mass index (LVMI). The application of blood pressure drugs, as well as dialysis treatment successfully reduces ventricular mass [25], and so, this treatment is used in normotensive patients. The application of angiotensin-converting enzyme (ACE) inhibitors reduces LVM in dialysis patients, previously normotensive. Larsen et al. have shown that left ventricular wall size is reduced in patients on intensive, continuous and daily dialysis, over the course of a year, unlike those patients who had intermittent dialysis three times a week, despite similar systolic blood pressure values. Another potential cause of uremic cardiomyopathy is volume encumbrance, which can cause the development of eccentric LVH, by increasing left ventricular end diastolic diameter (LVEDD). The reduction of interdialytic mass correlates with LVMI reduction, but LVH can persist, irrelevant of LVMI normalization. Another hypothesis on the etiology of uremic cardiomyopathy is that the accumulation of hypertrophic growth factor, connecter to ESRD, initiates signal activation independent of mechanical stress, which leads to cardiac pathology progression. Several matters can modulate cardiac growth and function, which are accumulated in ESRD patients, primarily endothelin-1, parathyroid hormone (PTH), tumor necrosis factor alpha (TNF-α), leptin, interleukin1 alpha (IL-1α) and interleukin 6 (IL-6) [26].

2.5. Left ventricular hypertrophy

The prevalence of LVH is high among patients suffering from ESRD. Structural changes appear in the early stages of kidney function damage. In prospective research, just prior to the start of RRT, 74% of patients had LVH, with a high LVMI, as an independent mortality predictor after 2 years of dialysis treatment. Up to 80% of dialysis patients have increased LVM [27]. The increase of LVM in ESRD patients can be caused by an increase of LVEDD as a result of volume encumbrance, the increase of LV wall thickening, and the combination of characteristics of both eccentric and concentric LVH. The precise distinction of LVH between eccentric and concentric is sometimes difficult in hemodialysis patients, because of cyclical variations of extracellular fluid and humoral balance. The internal dimensions of LV are under the influence of the volume status, and the decrease of blood volume during dialysis reduces LV diameter, causing "acute" changes in the relative thickness of the left ventricular wall. In stable patients with compensated hypertrophy, the systolic function remains within normal boundaries, while diastolic charging often varies. The LVH is an adaptive response to increased heart rate. LVH is both damaging and beneficial at the same time. The benefits are tied to the number of sarcomeres and the increase of heart function capability, which allows for energy conservation. Such an effect sustains normal systolic function during the initial, compensated, or "adaptive" phase of LVH development. Continued stress gradually leads to an "inappropriate" hypertrophic response. In this phase of LVH, a loss of balance between energy consumption and production occurs in the activated myocardial cells, which eventually results in chronic energy deficiency and accelerated myocyte death [28]. The increase of extracellular matrix and collagen content makes the functional competence of heart contractions sustainable, however, at the expense of weakened diastolic charging. LVH usually occurs as a response to initiated mechanical stress. Pressure encumbrance results in the parallel addition of new sarcomeres, with a disproportionate increase in LV wall thickness and a normal ventricular diameter (concentric hypertrophy). Volume encumbrance primarily results in the addition of new sarcomeres in series, and a secondary order of new sarcomeres parallel, which again leads to the increase of LV diameter, with an increase of wall thickness (eccentric hypertrophy). The development and markings of LVH are under the influence of several factors such as age, gender and race, a co-existing disease such as diabetes, systemic disease or kidney failure [29] (**Figure 3**).

2.6. Vascular remodeling and CKD

The changes in the vascular system of uremic patients are attributed to a synergistic effect of numerous factors such as dyslipidemia, prothrombotic factors, anemia, hypertension, increased oxidative stress, hyperparathyroidism, synthesis disorder homocysteine and nitric oxide, endothelial dysfunction as well as LV remodeling, which leads to the modification of structural and functional cardiac and vascular characteristics.

Accelerated atherosclerosis and more frequent and generally higher intensity cardiovascular events go alongside CKD. Atherosclerosis is an intimal disease where vascular lesions and plaques develop. A specific morphology can be noticed in lesions in patients with CKD. They can be calcified, with media thickness. In contrast, the atherosclerotic lesions are fibro atheromatous in the general population.

In CKD, as in the general population, the accumulation of conventional risk factors initiates the atherosclerotic process. Among these risk factors, dyslipidemia is a major determinant.

More than one CKD uremia-related factor leads to renal function which is substantially reduced. Despite multiple pathobiological factors being involved, vascular disease is aggravated by the calcification of the intimal atheromatous lesions and vascular wall media, which are representations of mineral metabolism disturbances.

Older populations suffering from CKD have a higher prevalence of occlusive atherosclerotic disease. Clinically, this is mirrored as ischemic heart disease (myocardial infarction, angina and sudden cardiac death), heart failure, peripheral and cerebrovascular vascular disease [30].

Arteriosclerosis must be taken into consideration when discussing CKD patients with CV risk. It is a process of remodeling, diffuse and nonocclusive by nature, involving the central arteries. Its determinants are an increased luminal diameter, medial calcification, destruction of the elastic lamellae, and an extracellular matrix increase. The arterial wall shows signs of stiffness due to these changes, meaning it is not as elastic. We still do not exactly know the link between this arterial stiffness and CKD. Altered mineral homeostasis is a suspect in this connection, due to the high medial calcification. In the ESRD, hyperphosphatemia, a higher level of calcium-phosphate product, hyperparathyroidism and lower 1.25-dyhydroxyvitamin D levels are characteristics of mineral imbalance metabolism [31].

Diffuse nonocclusive medial calcification and increased arterial stiffnesses are the more dominant forms of vascular pathology in adolescents and young adults with CKD. These morphologic changes are associated with systolic hypertension, wide pulse pressure, LVH, coronary hypoperfusion, further renal damage, congestive heart failure and sudden death (**Figure 2**).

Impaired endothelial function is a characteristic of early stages of chronic kidney disease, and multiple possible causes have been identified: (1) reduced clearance of endothelial NO

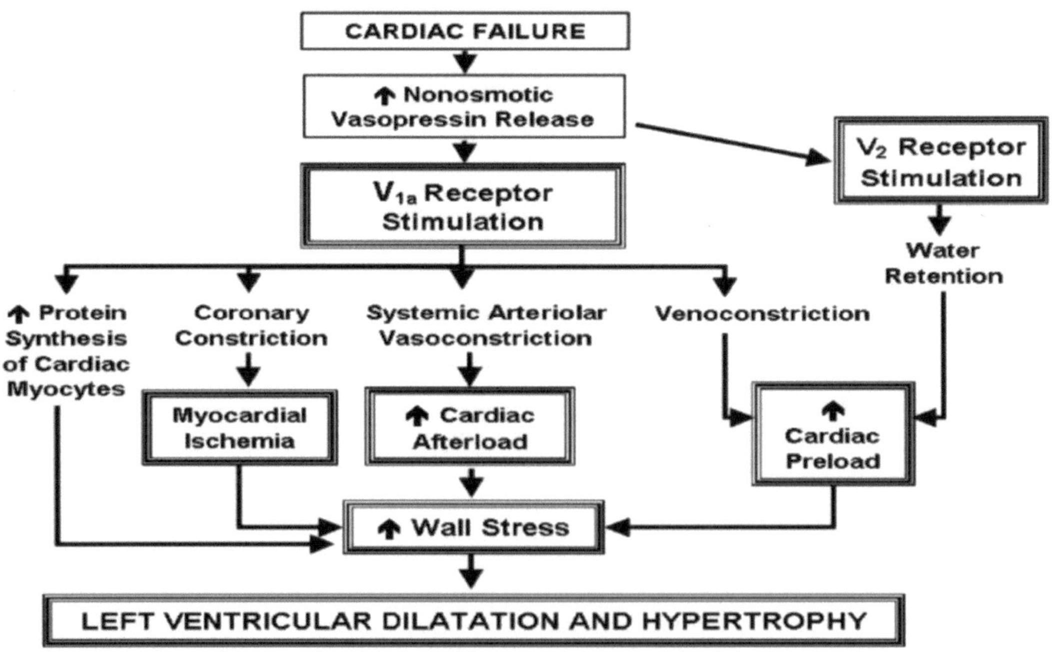

Figure 2. Mechanisms left ventricular remodeling.

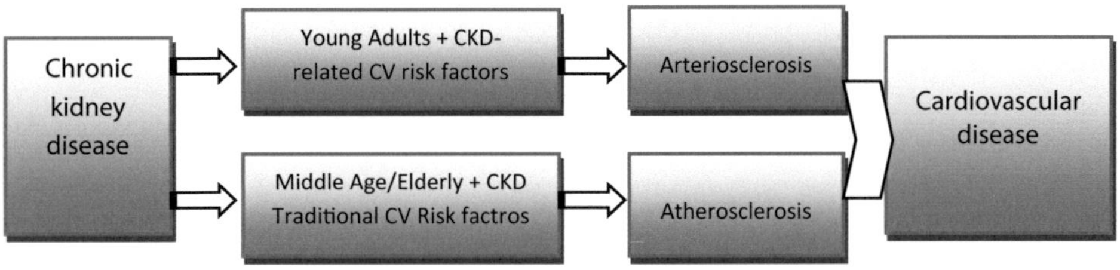

Figure 3. Pathogenesis of atherosclerosis and arteriosclerosis.

synthase (e-NOS) inhibitor asymmetric dimethylarginine (ADMA), which leads to reduced bioavailability of endothelial NO; (2) activation of angiotensin II, which induces oxidative stress; (3) high levels of homocysteine; (4) chronic inflammation; (5) dyslipidemia and (6) endothelial progenitor cell deficiency [32]. Endothelial dysfunction contributes significantly to the initiation and progression of CVD in CKD. It exacerbates arterial luminal narrowing and arterial wall stiffening by allowing development of intima-media thickening, medial hypertrophy and calcification [30].

2.7. Uremia-related CVD

A significant number of patients with uremia that are in the late stage of their renal disease show the following: (1) symptoms of myocardial ischemia without coronary artery disease by coronary angiography and (2) difficult or impossible to treat congestive heart failure. Functional and morphological characteristics of uremia are to blame for the existence of these clinical conditions [33]. As they are expected to enter ESRD, and as their kidney function is worsened, patients suffering from uremia generally have hypertension, anemia, hyperactive circulation caused by arteriovenous fistulae, increased stiffness of the arteries, and LVH and cardiac dilatation caused by overload of pressure and volume and a metabolic profile that does not fit normal characteristics. The myocardium structure is also changed due to intra-myocardial thickening of the coronary artery, reduced density of myocardial capillary and higher levels of interstitial myocardial fibrosis. These factors put together lead to cardiomyopathy. Chemical anomalies in patients suffering from CKD or ESRD, including hyperkalemia, uremia, acidosis and calcium/phosphorus dysregulation, lead to higher rates of cardiac arrhythmia [33]. Primary cardiac arrhythmias account for 50% of CV deaths in patients with ESRD. Structural heart disease secondary to CKD/ESRD such as LVH, valvular abnormalities, conduction system calcification and heart failure can independently worsen the outcome of arrhythmias in this population [34].

CVD progression in CKD a higher and burden is undoubtedly connected with the late stages of CKD. In comparison with individuals of the same gender and age from the general population, ESRD patients face 100 times higher morbidity and mortality rates. Accelerated CVD is promoted by chronic kidney disease, which is one of its most significant risk factors. The relationship is an exponential one between CKD and CVD. It is already in the first stages of kidney damage that the risk starts growing and continues all the way through to the late stage disease, where ESRD patients face 20–30 times higher risk than the general population. The risk can be seen when eGFR levels are below 50–60 ml/min/1.73 m^2, and it becomes extremely high once eGFR drops <45 ml/min/1.73 m^2 [33].

2.8. CVD in kidney transplant recipients

Although kidney transplant recipients recover adequate renal function, CVD remains an important cause of morbidity and mortality: mortality rates are twice as high as in mortality rates are twice as high as in the general population, adjusted for age and gender. The most likely explanation is the high prevalence of conventional risk factors such as hypertension, diabetes mellitus, LVH, and dyslipidemia, as well as risk factors that do not belong to the traditional spectrum, that are connected to transplantation such as the effect of immunosuppressive medication or organ rejection. In comparison with the population in dialysis, patients that conducted a kidney transplant have a lower rate of CVD mortality. This is most likely caused by the removal of kidney-specific risk factors following the transplantation [35].

3. Traditional risk factors

Hypertension, smoking, hyperlipidemia, obesity and diabetes are all risk factors which are connected to CVD in general populations, but also in PD patients, and are categorized into so-called traditional risk factors.

3.1. Age and gender

Male gender is another well-known risk factor for CVD in the general population, and the frequency of acute myocardial infarction is as much as 2.5 times higher than in the female population suffering from CKD, adjusted for age. However, due to menopause caused by age or comorbidity, the senior female population will also be at higher risk of CVD. Research has shown that about 70% of women on hemodialysis (HD) were menopausal before or after starting RRT, and the incidence of Acute Myocardial Infarction (AMI) was 3–5 times higher in female patients suffering from chronic kidney disease, compared to the age-adjusted general population [36, 37].

3.2. Tobacco smoking

Smoking is not only a risk factor for the development of CVD but is also connected to the risk of developing CKD, defined as the reduction GFR at <45 ml/min/1.73 m^2. In a large study from Norway, long-term smoking of over 20 cigarettes a day is connected to 1.52 times increased the relative risk of CKD occurrence [38]. However, it is relatively unknown whether smoking increases the risk of CV death in dialysis patients. A small study on diabetic dialysis patients found no effects of smoking on the risk of CV death, although a series of studies showed that smoking, or a history of smoking, is an independent risk factor for increased morbidity and mortality [39]. These apparent differences can be framed through the presence of other risk factors in some populations, which can supersede the effects of smoking in various multivariable analyses.

3.3. Diabetes mellitus

North-American registry data show that the number of diabetic patients annually admitted to RRT more than doubled from 1995 to 2000. Diabetes mellitus has become the single most important cause of ESRD. Renal replacement therapy continues showing unsatisfactory results for diabetic patients, as survival rates are low. Compared to dialysis patients with other underlying kidney conditions, those with diabetes have the lowest chance of survival. The main cause of death is coronary heart disease—myocardial infarction (MI), angina, history of bypass surgery, PTCA and pathology on coronary angiography. Cardiovascular issues, primarily coronary atheroma, add up before the diabetic patient enters renal replacement therapy programs. Therefore, it is crucial to improving care for the patient with diabetes before he enters the end-stage of the disease. Diabetic patients with underlying CKD face an increased cardiac risk after developing acute MI, which is mirrored through atrial and ventricular arrhythmia, atrioventricular (AV) block, asystole, pulmonary congestion and cardiogenic shock [40].

3.4. Arterial hypertension

Arterial hypertension is very common in CKD patients and is connected to increased risk of CV death [41]. Hypertension is often present in dialysis patients. According to the results of an Italian multicentric study, 88% of 504 patients treated with RRT suffer from arterial hypertension, with anti-hypertensive therapy included. Arterial hypertension in dialysis patients is usually connected to volume encumbrance. In a report by the UK renal registry in 2008, it is stated that in a larger number of patients treated with HD the targeted blood pressure was achieved, as opposed to peritoneal dialysis (PD) patients (45–33%) [42]. However, unlike the general population of dialysis-treated patients, the connection between high blood pressure and mortality is not so pronounced. Hypertension strongly correlates with LVH, which is often found in CKD. Almost 70% of patients at the beginning of dialysis therapy suffer from an echocardiography recognizable LVH. According to research done by Coen et al., LVH is more potent in long-term dialysis patients than in HD patients, most likely because of inadequate volume control [43].

Low blood pressure has a negative effect on the rates of survival of dialysis patients. However, hypertension is used as a predictor of mortality in patients with CKD before or at the initiation of dialysis. To be able to comprehend this paradox, a separation of blood pressure must be made into systolic, diastolic, mean arterial pressure (MAP) and pulse pressure. Isolated systolic hypertension combined with a high pulse pressure is the most common anomaly regarding blood pressure in patients on dialysis. This occurs due to medial sclerosis of arteries with secondary arterial stiffening. This, in turn, leads to higher pulse-wave velocity, creating an increased peak systolic pressure thanks to a pulse wave reflected too early. LV dysfunction and congestive heart failure occur as a result. A consequence, afterward, could be a lower MAP and diastolic pressure, combined with high CVD risk. Altogether, this points to a U-shaped relationship between blood pressure and mortality: isolated systolic hypertension and increased pulse pressure probably point to high risk, in the long-run, in dialysis patients, whereas low mean and diastolic blood pressure predict a high change of early death. The danger that is not obvious, when it comes to hypertension, is that a large percentage of CKD patients are "nondippers", that is, do not have their blood pressure levels drop during the night. Sleep apnea has been shown to be a condition in CKD which has not attracted as much attention as necessary, considering it is associated with no dipping blood pressure, SNS activation and increased CVD risk [44].

3.5. Atherosclerosis

It has been proven that arterial rigidity, which is usually estimated by pulse-wave velocity on the aorta, the quantity of common carotid artery (CCA) intima-media thickness (IMT), and also by peak systolic velocity in the systole on the CCA, is a useful predictor of CV morbidity and mortality in the general population, and as such, in patients suffering from CKD.

Zoccali et al. [38], through their research, have determined that in a large group of patients suffering from CKD, the rigidity of large arteries was independently connected with age, blood pressure, as well as other risk factors for the development of CVD. The presence of vascular calcifications has shown itself to be one of the most prominent factors connected to arterial rigidity. However, relevant studies in dialysis patients are relatively small and have numerous limitations [45].

3.6. Obesity

Obesity is a risk factor for the development of CV diseases in the general population but is also connected to an increased risk factor for the development of CKD. The results of studies performed on dialysis patients have not been consistent about the influence of obesity on survival rates. The results of some studies showed that obesity is connected to better survival rates, while other studies have discovered that there is a connection between obesity and increased mortality risk. A prospective, time limited analysis in 688 dialysis patients showed that only those with a BMI <18.5 have an increased risk of CV death. High BMI had no protective effective but was also not connected to reduced survival risk [46].

3.7. Dyslipidemia

Dyslipidemia is known as a traditional risk factor for CVD in the general population, as well as in dialysis patients. Several observational studies have shown that the values of cholesterol and low-density lipoprotein (LDL) are among the most significant independent CV morbidity and mortality factors. Patients with damaged renal function suffer from significant changes in lipoprotein metabolism, which has a precise role in atherosclerotic pathogenesis. This is still controversial [47]. Renal dyslipidemia is characterized by an atherogenic apolipoprotein profile. This means there are lower levels of apolipoprotein A (apoA)-containing lipoproteins and higher levels of apoB-containing lipoproteins. CKD, as a progressive disease, is connected with high levels of apoCIII. Whereas total serum cholesterol levels, in general, are normal, or even low, high-density lipoprotein (HDL)-cholesterol is reduced; and low-density lipoprotein (LDL), intermediate-density lipoprotein (IDL), very low-density lipoprotein (VLDL)-cholesterol, plasma triglycerides, and lipoprotein(a) (Lp(a)) levels are increased. Compared to HD patients, patients treated with PD more often have both hypercholesterolemia and hypertriglyceridemia. Elevated Lp(a) levels have been reported to be associated with increased CVD mortality both in HD and PD patients. Two randomized controlled trials showed no benefit of statin treatment in dialysis patients [48].

3.8. Insulin resistance (IR)

A number of issues found in metabolic syndrome patients such as insulin resistance (IR), can be found in chronic kidney disease as well, a so-called uremic-metabolic syndrome. The etiology of resistance to insulin in CKD is multifactorial, with factors such as fat accumulation, lack of vitamin D, metabolic acidosis, inflammation, and uremic toxins accumulation all contributing. These factors create adverse changes in the pathway for the insulin receptor signal. Available data shows that IR is present in CKD patients starting from the early stages of renal failure. The potential of IR to promote blood vessel damage, regardless of the coexistence of other vascular risk factors, is large [49]. In several studies, the role of IR in patients on dialysis was analyzed, and a connection between IR and a disturbed fatty acid metabolism has been discovered, which further contributed to left ventricular dysfunction. Also, more and more evidence points to the fact that the application of ACE inhibitors (ACEIs) can modulate IR. In PD, IR of the tissue can be worsened by the intake of glucose through dialysis solutions. However, these studies are controversial as well: in patients on cycler PD, IR is greater than HD patients, while in PD patients, IR is normalized, similar to HD patients. By using icodextrin dialysis solutions, insulin levels in serum could potentially be reduced, and insulin sensitivity increased [50].

4. Nontraditional and/or uremia-specific risk factors

A known risk factor for the genesis of CV disease is GFR < 60 ml/min/1.73 m^2. A further drop in GFR values, below 45 ml/min/1.73 m^2, increases the risk of CV death. Potential factors tied to CKD and uremia, as well as the development of CV morbidity, includes inflammation, malnutrition, endothelial dysfunction, oxidative stress, vascular calcifications, vitamin D deficiency and hyperhomocysteinemia [51].

4.1. Renal failure per se

Newly acquired evidence points to a strong, independent relationship between low eGFR and mortality risk, CV events and hospitalization [52]. The mechanisms behind the process of progressive renal function deterioration's acceleration of the atherogenic process are not well known. However, the presence and severity of multiple novel CKD risk factors, including inflammation, oxidative stress, vascular calcification and accumulation of advanced glycation end products (AGEs) increases. Many other accumulating solutes for uremic retention, for example, ADMA, guanidine, homocysteine, indoxyl sulfate and p-cresol, could have a pro-atherogenic effect. Kidneys may also produce substances like renalase which should control and limit CVD, but a renal function deterioration leads to vascular disease through separate mechanisms and not retention.

4.2. Inflammation

Chronic inflammation is characterized by the persistent effect of a causative stimulus, destroying cells and tissue and having a deteriorating effect on the body. In later stages of CKD, the systemic concentrations of both pro- and anti-inflammatory cytokines are significantly higher as production has increased, coupled with decreased renal clearance. Aside from this, there are plenty of dialysis-related issues (such as membrane biocompatibility and thrombosed AV fistula) and nondialysis factors (e.g. infection, comorbidity, poor oral health, failed kidney transplants, genetic factors, diet) that may contribute to a continuous inflammation.

Inflammation, the effects of local inflammatory stimuli such as oxidation products, end advanced glycosylation products and chronic infective processes modify blood vessels in the sense of atherosclerosis development. These changes benefit proatherogenic adhesion molecule production, for example, intercellular adhesion molecule1 (ICAM-1) and vascular cell adhesion molecule 1 (VCAM-1), growth factor, as well as chemokine (such as IL-6, long pentraxin 3 (PTX3), S-albumin, TNF and white blood cell count). Such inflammatory intermediates encourage the synthesis of acute phase proteins such as C-reactive protein (CRP), reduction of albumin synthesis in the liver of dialysis-treated patients [53], which leads to endothelial dysfunction, which is usually defined as reduced vasodilatation capability, which again creates early atherosclerosis occurrence predisposition. However, the question, whether inflammation is a reflection of vascular damage, or actually supports factors that cause vascular injury, remains unanswered. The precise link between inflammation, endothelial dysfunction, oxidative stress, CVD and mortality in dialysis patients remains unknown. In a prospective study of dialysis patients, CRP level of >6 mg/L was an independent predictive mark of possible myocardial infarction. Aside from that, the proinflammatory IL-6 mark is increased in ESRD patients but is also an independent mortality predictor in patients on dialysis [54].

However, as many features are known to mediate atherosclerosis such as endothelial dysfunction, vascular calcification, IR, and increased oxidative stress, all are more or less associated with inflammation biomarkers, the association between chronic inflammation and CVD may also be indirect.

4.3. Endothelial dysfunction

In dialysis patients, endothelial function is reduced, the same as in hemodialysis patients, most likely because of a reduced bioavailability of NO. In a study conducted in 2009, flow-mediated vasodilatation is significantly lower in PD patients than in the healthy population, which negatively correlates with inflammation markers such as CRP or IL-6 [55]. There is evidence that suggests that the endogenic inhibitor of NO, ADMA, has a significant role in the origin and occurrence of CVD and mortality in dialysis patients. NO deficit and ADMA accumulation promote endothelial dysfunction, vasoconstriction, and arterial thrombosis. The remaining factors of endothelial dysfunction such as soluble adhesive molecules are predictors of all causes of CV in ESRD patients. The levels of VCAM-1 negatively correlate with LVH in patients undergoing RRT.

Evidence from newer studies shows that detached circulating endothelial cells (CEC) are suitable markers for endothelial damage [56]. They can be used for predicting purposes in order to prevent future CV events in HD patients. As a feedback to ischemic insult and cytokine stimulation, endothelial progenitor cells (EPC) are mobilized from the bone marrow to act as "repair" cells in response to the endothelial injury. As to reduced numbers of and/or a functional impairment of EPC due to inflammation and/or toxic effects of retained uremic solutes, there seems to be a disparity between EPC and CEC, which could eventually cause endothelial dysfunction in CKD patients.

4.4. Malnutrition and protein-energy wasting (PEW)

A marked connection between malnutrition, increased levels of CRP and atherosclerosis is well known, although the precise mechanisms of their synergistic effects on the organism are not known. This relationship was first described by Stenvinkel et al. in a study on CKD patients [57]. Patients with CRP levels >10 mg/L have significantly lesser values of serum albumin and a higher prevalence of atherosclerosis than patients with a lower CKD level. The combination of malnutrition, inflammation and atherosclerosis presence has been described by Stenvinkel as MIA (Malnutrition Inflammation Atherosclerosis) syndrome. A 2008 study has shown that MIA syndrome is connected to increased mortality risks [58]. In a Korean study, comorbidity cardiovascular diseases were present in 78% of patients on dialysis with signs of malnutrition. These patients have a 3.3 times greater risk of mortality than patients suffering from malnutrition with no comorbidity conditions [59]. Taking malnutrition, protein deficits, and inflammation into account, the recommendation for the description of this entity in CKD patients is protein-energy wasting (PEW). PEW is characterized by reduced protein and initiation energy accumulation. Several studies have shown that there are two types of malnutrition: the first is connected to poor food intake, and the second to inflammation and present comorbidity. Low levels of serum albumin can only be found in the second type of malnutrition, but the exact contribution of malnutrition or inflammation in the development of risk of CV mortality in dialysis patients remains uncertain [58]. A large number of studies have dealt in hypoalbuminemia and the outcome of treating patients on dialysis. It has been determined that serum albumin levels below 40 g/L are combined with 4–20 times increased mortality. In addition, 45% of PD patients die during the first year of dialysis treatment in cases where albumin levels drop below 25 g/L. A CANUSA study has shown an 8% survival rate increase in cases of serum albumin growth of only 1% [60].

4.5. Oxidative stress

Oxidative stress is defined as the damage of tissue which stems from the disturbed balance between excessive oxidation compound production and insufficient anti-oxidant defensive function. CKD patients have a deficiency in the anti-oxidant defensive mechanism (because of e.g., reduced vitamin levels, or hypoalbuminemia) and increased pro-oxidant compound activity (e.g. accumulation of solvent materials such as AGEs and β2-microglobulin). Oxidative stress leads to the production of free radicals, highly reactive compounds that can oxidize proteins lipids and nucleic acids. High concentrations of these molecules are present in CKD patients. Oxidation products of proteins and oxidized DNA have been discovered in leukocytes with residual renal function (RRF). The underlying connection between increased levels of oxidation stress and the risk of CV death in ESRD patients is still unknown, even though the results of several prospective studies point to the conclusion that oxidation stress can be a risk factor for CV morbidity and mortality in ESRD patients [14]. Four pathways of oxidative stress exist in CKD (carbonyl stress, nitrosative stress, chlorinated stress and classical oxidative stress). Evidence suggests that oxidative stress plays a major role. The relation between accumulation of AGE and the cardiovascular disease's outcome is not as transparent and obvious. Studies focusing on Chronic Myelogenous Leukemia (CML) and pentosidine found no significant effect on mortality. However, one study pointed to the conclusion that skin autofluorescence predicted death in HD patients [61].

One of the most important toxins connected to the uremic environment and connected to oxidative stress and inflammation stage and the presence of inflammation biomarkers is β2-microglobulin. Increased levels of β2-microglobulin in plasma are a known marker of chronic renal function failure and are among the most important toxins tied to uremia. In PD patients, the level of β2-microglobulin is primarily tied to amyloidosis. In recent times it has been suggested that β2-microglobulin could be a new biomarker of peripheral arterial disease and an independent predictor of aortic rigidity in the atherosclerotic process, in both the general population and ESRD patients [62]. Additionally, increased levels of β2-microglobulin present a new marker for differentiating the levels of acute cardiac arrest creation risk in patients with creatinine levels $\leq$265 μmol/L [54]. All of these results point to an important role of β2-microglobulin in CV risk prediction in dialysis patients.

4.6. Hyperparathyroidism

In ESRD patients, the ability of the diseased kidney to produce 1.25-dihydroxycalciferol is reduced, which significantly contributes to the development of osteodystrophy, secondary hyperparathyroidism and the disturbed metabolism of divalent ions. PTH is considered a potent uremic toxin that harmfully affects myocardial cells. The improvement of left ventricular dysfunction after parathyroidectomy in uremic patients with increased PTH points to a connection between left ventricular function and hyperparathyroidism. All this confirms the assumption about the role of parathormone as a risk factor in the development of uremic cardiomyopathy. Significant research results point to the conclusion that a small level of vitamin D is connected to CVD in the general population, and that a greater concentration of that vitamin can have a positive influence on survival. Similar results were discovered in predialysis patients. Wang et al. have determined that low concentrations of serum 25-hydroxyvitamin D in dialysis patients are connected to increased risk of fatal or nonfatal CV incidents. It seems that the effects of vitamin D on the CV system are connected to residual renal function, LVH and cardiac dysfunction [54].

4.7. Cardiovascular calcification

The arterial media, atherosclerotic plaques and heart valves are affected through this cardiovascular process. One of the main signs of medial calcification is arterial stiffness, which is shown clinically through an increased pulse pressure. The pathophysiological role of plaque calcification is less clear, as it is mostly soft plaques, which rupture and cause AMI. It is now evident that the burden caused by atherosclerotic calcification is a suitable risk marker for cardiovascular events. In patients in dialysis, valvular calcification leads to a developing stenosis and morbidity that goes with it, after targeting and affecting the aortic and mitral valves [63].

In the general population, coronary artery calcification is infrequently observed in younger age groups. It is a phenomenon that increases with age, and the majority of people affected by vascular calcification are >65 years. In ESRD patients, on the other hand, extensive vascular calcification can be commonly observed in much younger age groups as well. The calcification process frequently starts before the initiation of dialysis treatment. The prevalence and extent of vascular calcification, arterial media calcification and arterial stiffness have recently been shown to be strong predictors of CVD and all-cause mortality in dialysis patients.

Besides diabetes mellitus, CV calcification can, with the presence of uremia, be caused by abnormal calcium and phosphate metabolism and an enduring inflammation as it may by several mechanisms mediate untimely atherosclerosis and premature CVD.

Fetuin-A, an important inhibitor of vascular calcification, is down-regulated during the inflammation process, and low levels are linked to poor survival in dialysis patients. However, fetuin-A is certainly not the only modifier of extraosseous calcification. Phosphate, calcium and some proinflammatory mediators have the capacity to induce osteogenic differentiation, which is a transition of vascular smooth muscle cells toward osteoblast behavior. A system of calcification inhibitors (and inducers) is of major importance, as the extracellular calcium and phosphate environment must be formally considered as being "supersaturated" regarding the chemical solubility product of these ions in an aqueous solution. Among them, leptin, matrix GLA protein, TNF-α, pyrophosphates, bone morphogenetic proteins and osteoprotegerin, may be related to a process of accelerated vascular calcification in ESRD [64].

4.8. Hyperhomocysteinemia

Homocysteine (Hcy) is a nonprotein sulfur-containing amino acid that has attracted considerable interest by vascular researchers, as it may by several mechanisms mediate premature atherosclerosis and CVD. The prevalence of hyperhomocysteinemia in patients with advanced CKD is >90%. In contrast to the well-documented association between total Hcy (tHcy) and vascular disease in the general population, the relationship between tHcy and CVD is not that clear and strong assuming renal function is reduced, with studies and reports demonstrating low levels of tHcy in patients with chronic kidney disease with CVD [13]. Although there are several reasons that may explain this paradoxical relationship, one of the most significant relationships is the strong association between tHcy and hypoalbuminemia, PEW and inflammation. S-albumin and tHcy have an established strong positive correlation, and hypoalbuminemia is an established predictor of adverse outcomes that this relationship may confound the impact of tHcy on vascular disease [65].

4.9. Autonomic dysfunction

Decreased baroreflex sensitivity is significant for CKD and one of its main attributes, which can, together with inflammation and wasting, lead to an increased risk of sudden death. Increased sympathetic nerve activity can be seen in CKD patients quite frequently, and it is a predictor of an adverse result [66]. Sympathetic overactivity is probably partial due to sleep apnea, which is considered a contributor to the condition in patients with moderate and severe-stage CKD.

4.10. Anemia

In ESRD, the condition causes LVH and LV dilatation. Normalizing hemoglobin has not shown any CV outcome improvement, despite a partial correction of anemia using erythropoietin causing a regression in LVH. The appropriate target hematocrit to minimize LVH or other CVD has not been defined. However, briefly summarizing guideline recommendations favors target hemoglobin of about 11 g/dl [66].

4.11. Hormonal disorder

The loss of kidney function and the altered metabolic milieu in CKD affects hormone secretion and response of target tissues, causing a number of endocrine dysfunctions that may affect both PEW prevalence and future CVD risk. Changes in the GH-IGF-1 axis lead to many important CKD complications such as growth retardation, PEW, atherosclerosis and disease progression. Other common hormonal disturbances in chronic kidney disease are subclinical hypothyroidism and the low-T3 syndrome, which occurs in one-fifth of CKD patients. However, chance of CV events increases in the general population with thyroid changes, and thyroid production is substantially reduced by inflammation. Therefore, the hypothesis exists saying these factors create a connection between stress caused by inflammation and a negative cardiovascular event in CKD patients [66]. Finally, during the chronic kidney disease, the sex hormone profile does not stay the same. In as many as 50–70% of males in ESRD, male hypogonadism occurs. Testosterone decline occurs for multiple reasons such as low synthesis of muscle protein and hemoglobin, as well as atherosclerosis development and arterial vasoconstriction and/or hardening. This relationship between male hypogonadism and increased risk of death caused by CV factors in dialysis patients has been brought to attention, which will hopefully put some focus on this issue. New studies conducted on nonCKD patients using low testosterone dosage showed satisfactory outcomes such as muscle gain and improved metabolism (no studies have been conducted regarding interventions targeting the adverse outcomes of CV) [67].

4.12. Residual renal function (RRF)

The residual renal function is important for dialysis patients because it contributes to total daily clearance of 20% or more. It is thought that a dialysis patient has preserved RRF if his clearance of creatinine is greater than 1.5 mL/min. In PD and HD patients, RRF is connected to all causes of mortality, and so it is connected with the risk of CV death. The vital role of RRF in the survival of PD patients was determined in large prospective studies such as the CANUSA and ADEMEX studies. In the ADEMEX study, by a prospective, randomized examination of 965 dialysis patients with a weekly diuresis of 10 L/m^2, a relative mortality risk drop of 11% was noted [68]. These results were also confirmed by the NECOSAD study, where the rate of reduction of RRF was a stronger predictor of mortality and technical insufficiency of long-term PD treatment, in relation to basic RRF [58].

4.13. Volume overload and ultrafiltration insufficiency

Ultrafiltration insufficiency occurs in around a third of dialysis patients and can lead to arterial hypertension and volume encumbrance. Volume overload promoted the development of LVH and leads to increased serum concentrations of natriuretic peptide, because of their increased myocardial production. These peptides are used as a prognostic marker for the general mortality of ESRD patients [69].

The connection between the lack of peritoneal ultrafiltration and mortality has been proven in anuric patients. When fluid intake is not adjusted to peritoneal ultrafiltration, the patient will develop volume overload, which increases the risk of CVD.

4.14. Genetic and epigenetic factors

Genetic factors can influence the appearance and frequency of vascular complications in dialysis patients. Thus, polymorphism of a single nucleotide in the IL-6 gene is connected to increased levels of IL-6 in plasma, and comorbidity in HD patients, greater diastolic pressure values and left ventricular mass [70]. Polymorphism of the enzyme, which transforms angiotensin I to angiotensin II, can determine the degree of the function of recombined human erythropoietin in PD patients, which presents a significant prescreening for the assessment of erythropoietin resistance. Polymorphism on the human receptor of vitamin D is combined with an increased risk of the development of hypercalcemia, modulation of NO activity via the polymorphism of endothelial NOS, as well as functionally relevant polymorphism of the IL-6, which together can have a significant effect on basic peritoneal permeability [71]. In the future, research in this field could enable a more precise approach for the identification of risk groups of patients treated by PD, and the development of personalized treatment strategies.

A new approach in the research of atherosclerosis focuses on the role of epigenetics, which change studies in gene expression that are not coded in the DNA sequence itself but are instead a consequence of post-translatory changes in the DNA-protein. These epigenetic changes can be lost in several sequential cellular generations. Changes in the genome methylation of DNA have important regulatory functions in normal and pathological cellular processes. A persistent inflammatory reaction is most likely connected to DNA hypermethylation [72]. Further research is necessary to determine whether epigenetic DNA changes are connected to accelerated atherosclerosis in uremia.

5. Chronic cardiorenal and renocardiac syndrome interaction

The interplay between cardiac and renal disease is complex and the term CRS has been introduced recently as an attempt to describe the close interaction between CV and renal systems, especially in the chronic disease settings. Division of CRS into five categories is proposed by Ronco et al. [73]. This classification is based on etiologic and chronologic factors [74]. The temporal relationship between the heart and kidney disease as well as the coexistence of CVD and CKD represent important aspects of chronic cardiorenal and renocardiac syndromes definition. CRS type 2, or chronic cardiorenal syndrome, is characterized by chronic abnormalities in cardiac function leading to kidney injury or dysfunction. CHF causally underlies the occurrence and progression of CKD [75]. CRS type 4, or chronic renocardiac syndrome, has been defined as "chronic abnormalities in renal function leading to cardiac disease" and recognizes the extreme burden of CVD in patients with CKD such as chronic glomerular disease and autosomal dominant polycystic kidney disease (ADPKD). This is the condition where primary CKD contributes a reduction in cardiac function such as cardiac remodeling, left ventricular diastolic dysfunction or hypertrophy, and/or an increased risk for CV events such as MI, heart failure or stroke [76].

Coexistence of the chronic heart and kidney disease was clearly described in large observational studies. However, this type of data cannot establish whether the primary process is the kidney disease (CRS type 4) or the heart disease (CRS type 2). For these situations, it has been suggested to use term CRS "type 2/4". For example, large database studies have shown the prevalence of CKD of 26–63% in the population of CHF patients. Likewise, retrospective and/or secondary post hoc analyses from large clinical registries have evaluated the CV event rates and outcomes in selected CKD-specific populations [77]. The severity of CKD in those studies ranged from near normal kidney function to End stage kidney disease (ESKD). Furthermore, in a secondary analysis of the HEMO Study, cardiac disease was found in 80% of ESKD patients at enrollment [78]. During 12 months follow-up, 39.8% patients had cardiac-related hospitalizations with angina and acute myocardial infarction accounting for 42.7% of these hospitalizations. There were 39.4% of cardiac deaths. Baseline cardiac disease was highly predictive of cardiac-related death during follow-up (relative risk 2.57). Moreover, other authors have suggested that chronic maintenance hemodialysis induces repetitive myocardial injury and can accelerate systolic dysfunction [79].

6. Biomarkers of adverse cardiovascular events in CKD patients

Biomarkers must be determined in situations where we have renal and cardiac issues and dysfunctions, as it is crucial to know if any functional and structural damage occurred in the beginning stages of the disease. They are then used to separate the patients according to the risk level by considering established renal and cardiac parameters, in order to establish individual treatment and prognosis. These biomarkers may help with early diagnosis, prognosis, treatment and monitoring of CRS. There can be any measurable parameter, like components of serum or urine. In patients with CRS, a group of multiple biomarkers, rather than a single test, may improve diagnosis and better define prognosis [80].

Recent studies have evaluated the utility of biomarkers in the assessment of the CV risk in CKD population. Several cardiac biomarkers such as natriuretic peptides, troponins, CRP, homocysteine, plasminogen activator inhibitor 1 (PAI-1), ADMA, adiponectin (APN) and AGEs have been demonstrated to correlate with CV outcomes in CKD patients. Renal biomarkers such as cystatin C, neutrophil gelatinase-associated lipocalin (NGAL), kidney injury molecule-1 (KIM-1), N-acetyl-beta-D-glucosaminidase (NAG), fibroblast growth factor-23 (FGF23), matrix metalloproteinases (MMPs) and interleukin-18 (IL-18) have been recently found to be diagnostic and prognostic markers of CV outcomes in CKD (**Table 1**) [81].

6.1. Cardiac biomarkers

The natriuretic peptides are family of hormones that share a common 17 amino acid ring structure and have actions targeted to protect the CV system from the effects of volume overload.

Cardiac biomarkers	Renal biomarkers
Natriuretic peptides	Cystatin C
Troponins	Neutrophil gelatinase-associated lipocalin (NGAL)
C-reactive protein (CRP)	N-acetyl-beta-D-glucosaminidase (NAG)
Homocysteine	Kidney injury molecule-1 (KIM-1)
Plasminogen activator inhibitor 1(PAI-1)	Interleukin-18 (IL-18)
Asymmetric dimethylarginine (ADMA)	Fibroblast growth factor-23 (FGF23)
Adiponectin (APN)	Matrix metalloproteinases (MMPs)
Advanced glycation end products (AGEs)	

Table 1. Biomarkers of adverse cardiovascular events in chronic kidney disease.

B-type natiuretic peptide (BNP) produced by ventricular myocardium in response to ventricular stretching, and its inactive fragment N-terminal proBNP (NT-proBNP) are well-known diagnostic and prognostic markers in patients with heart failure. BNP and NT-proBNP are also useful markers of adverse CV events and overall mortality in CKD patients. They correlate with severity of heart failure and left ventricular dysfunction and can be used in guiding the management of heart failure in CKD patients. Some evidence suggests that NT-proBNP and high-sensitivity CRP (hs-CRP) are independent predictors of overall mortality in a nondialysis CKD population and their role in risk stratification can be useful in this specific patient population [82]. Similar results were found in the dialysis-dependent ESKD patients. High levels of NT-proBNP and cardiac troponin T showed to be strongly associated with adverse CV morbidity and mortality in HD patients [83]. In chronic PD patients, NT-pro-BNP is prognostic marker of congestive heart failure, mortality or combined end point including death and other adverse CV outcomes [84].

Plasminogen activator inhibitor 1 (PAI-1), a specific inhibitor of tissue-type and urokinase-type plasminogen activators (t-PA and u-PA), plays a critical role in regulating the fibrinolysis. PAI-1 is classified as an endothelial dysfunction marker. The activated or injured endothelial cells synthesize higher rates of PAI-1 and endothelial dysfunction was recognized as an initial event of atherosclerosis. Elevated PAI-1 levels are associated with increased CV risk in the general population. Plasma levels of PAI-1 are also associated with the occurrence of a first AMI in a population with high prevalence of coronary heart disease. In addition, high plasma PAI-1 concentration was found to be independent predictor of CV in patients ongoing PD [85].

Adiponectin (APN) is a protein secreted by adipocytes with activities focusing on anti-inflammatory and anti-atherogenic goals. It also increases the body's insulin sensitivity. The way it assumed its functions are by suppressing proinflammatory cytokines such as TNF-a and IL-6 from being released and promoting the release of anti-inflammatory cytokines such as IL-10, as well as through increasing sensitivity to insulin. Through these roles, it controls anti-atherosclerotic activities. Low levels of APN can be seen in obese patients, those with metabolic syndrome, diabetes mellitus, coronary artery disease and essential hypertension. On the other hand, APN plasma levels are three times higher than regular levels in patients with

CKD, probably due to catabolism or reduced clearance. Some observational studies linked APN to adverse CV outcomes in patients with CKD. Low plasma APN levels were predictive of CV events among nondiabetic patients with mild to moderate CKD. Furthermore, low APN levels were found among the dialysis patients who developed CV complications [86].

6.2. Renal biomarkers

Cystatin C is 13-kDa protein synthesized at a constant rate in all nucleated cells. It is freely filtered by the glomerulus and is reabsorbed and catabolized completely in the proximal tubule with a lack of tubular secretion. It is considered to be a better marker of early kidney dysfunction and more reliable marker of kidney function than serum creatinine. Cystatin C is very useful biomarker in CKD and used for CVD assessment. Cystatin C seems to be better predictor of mortality and CV events than serum creatinine [87]. High cystatin C concentrations predict substantial increased risks of all-cause mortality, CV events and incident heart failure [88] and are associated with increased LVM and a concentric LVH phenotype independent of renal function [89].

Across the CVD spectrum, including peripheral arterial disease, stroke, abdominal aortic aneurysm, heart failure and coronary artery disease, a connection has been established between high plasma levels of cystatin C and negative outcomes and risk stratification, without any particular explanations behind the mechanisms of the connection. Possible ties between negative CV outcomes and high cystatin C levels could stem from deteriorated renal function, atherogenesis and inflammatory mediators, myocardial tissue remodeling as well as other factors such as genetic determinants, age and aging and social habits [90].

NGAL is 25-kDa protein with 178 amino acids belonging to the lipocalin family [91]. It is highly expressed in kidney following ischemic and nephrotoxic injury. Plasma/serum and urine NGAL is used as an early marker of acute kidney injury (AKI) in several renal diseases. NGAL has also been investigated as a prognostic marker in CKD patients. Plasma and urine NGAL levels predict progression of CKD and reflected the severity of renal disease in the study performed by Bolignano et al. [92]. However, although urine NGAL was an independent risk factor for progression among patients with established CKD of diverse etiology in Chronic Renal Insufficiency Cohort (CRIC) study, it did not substantially improve prediction of outcome events in this patient population [93]. Nevertheless, NGAL has also shown promising results as a marker of CV risk in dialysis patients. In the study by Furuya et al., elevated levels of serum NGAL were independent risk factors for de novo CVD in HD patients [94]. Furthermore, hemodialysis patients with high NGAL levels in combination with high BNP levels had the greatest risk of CVD [86].

KIM-1 is a transmembrane glycoprotein with immunoglobulin-like features. Within 24–48 h after kidney injury, KIM-1 expression is dramatically increased in proximal tubular epithelial cells. It is increased in the urine in AKI. Experimental studies suggest that KIM-1 may be an indicator of AKI to CKD transition. In the setting of patients with CHF, urinary KIM-1 outperformed NGAL and NAG in predicting a combined CV outcome of death, heart transplantation, MI, coronary angioplasty or heart failure hospitalization. However, when compared to patients with heart failure without CKD, urinary KIM-1 levels were not statistically elevated in heart failure patients with CKD [95, 96].

NAG is an enzyme of hydrolase class that is abundant in the kidney, predominantly in the lysosomes of proximal tubular cells. The increased excretion of NAG is thought to be a specific marker of functional tubular impairment in many renal pathologies. Likewise KIM-1, NAG has been a useful marker of acute kidney injury (AKI) [97]. A recent study in type 1 diabetes mellitus found that lower levels of urinary NAG were associated with the regression of microalbuminuria [98]. It has not been assessed longitudinally in CKD [95]. In patients with CHF, urinary NAG was associated with an increased risk of death, heart failure hospitalizations and heart transplantation, independent of GFR [99].

IL-18 is a proinflammatory cytokine that is released by the epithelial cells of the proximal tubule within hours of renal injury. It is significantly increased in AKI in comparison to urinary tract infection and nephrotic syndrome [96]. The destabilization of human coronary plaques can be connected to IL-18, which was originally thought to be a factor that promotes interferon-γ synthesis. In addition, in one study it was confirmed that young and middle-aged patients with a recent AMI have higher IL-18 concentration in serum than age- and sex-matched control subjects, showing that concentration of this cytokine is associated with severity of coronary atherosclerosis [100]. In addition, recent evidence suggests that serum IL-18 is an important indicator and predictor of CV death in two-year follow-up among non-diabetic patients suffering from CKD, with history of AMI in the previous year [101].

Fibroblast growth factor-23 (FGF23) is a newly discovered hormone produced in the bone that regulates phosphate and vitamin D metabolism by the kidneys. The main physiological functions of FGF23 are mediated by FGF receptors, generally in the presence of Klotho coreceptors. Decreased phosphorus excretion triggers FGF23 production, which in turn stimulates Klotho coreceptors in the kidneys [102]. CKD progression leads to compensatory elevation of FGF23 levels, resulting in typical CKD manifestations such as hyperphosphatemia, secondary hyperparathyroidism and bone disease, and progression to ESRD [80]. Elevated FGF23 has been associated with LVH, and it has been suggested that FGF23 may induce myocardial hypertrophy through a direct effect on cardiac myocytes [102]. FGF-23 has been independently associated with risk of all-cause death in dialysis and CKD patients, heart failure, CV events and death in the general population [86].

Matrix metalloproteinases (MMPs) are a large family of endopeptidases capable of degrading all components of the extracellular matrix and are therefore responsible for controlling the pathophysiological remodeling of tissues, including CV and renal systems. MMPs are classified according to their structure and substrate specificity, so MMP-2 and MMP-9 belong to the family of gelatinases that can cleave denatured collagen (gelatin), elastin and type IV collagen. Traditionally, MMPs were conceived of as exclusively anti-fibrotic tissue components; however, in the last few years, new paradigms have emerged in which inadequate extracellular matrix turnover governed by MMPs is also the hallmark of many pathological and generalized states such as inflammation, deleterious remodeling, oxidative stress and apoptosis [103]. Previous studies have demonstrated that increase in circulating levels of MMP-2 or MMP-9 are associated with arterial stiffness, hypertension and kidney disease progression in diabetic nephropathy. Recent data have proposed an important role of MMPs as markers of deleterious remodeling in the progression of renal disease and CVD [104]. Deleterious remodeling at the glomerular basement membrane, governed by pathological MMP activity, could contribute to glomerular hyperfiltration, albuminuria and loss of renal function [103]. The vascular changes observed in CKD patients not only consist of atherosclerosis but also arteriosclerosis associated with both medial and intimal vascular calcifications. The degree of arterial stiffening and the extent of calcification are closely related, and both of these variables are strong and independent prognostic markers of all-cause and CV mortality in patients on HD. Over the last few years, matrix metalloproteinases (MMPs) have been increasingly implicated in connective tissue remodeling during atherogenesis. MMPs are involved in plaque rupture, which is the main pathological cause of myocardial infarction. Interstitial collagenase (MMP-1) is the only MMP that can cleave native collagen types I and III, which are major structural components of the fibrous plaque cap. MMP-1 might play a significant role in fibrous plaque disruption by contributing to the degradation of interstitial collagens and thinning of the fibrous cap [105].

7. Strategies to improve cardiovascular outcome in CKD

7.1. Medical therapies to improve cardiovascular outcome

Risk modification is very important in CKD patient in order to improve outcomes. Strategies to reduce CV risk in CKD patients should target traditional, nontraditional and uremia-related factors. Recent opinions suggest a potential benefit from a more individualized perspective, that takes into account patient-specific trends and distinctive dynamic features of the actual clinical situation [106].

Blood pressure management has been advocated for both reducing cardiovascular risk and for slowing the renal progression of CKD. In all CKD patients, blood pressure should be <140/90 mm Hg and in patients with CKD and diabetes or those with significant proteinuria, target values should be <130/80 mm Hg. Agents acting via the RAAS, including ACE inhibitors (ACEIs) and angiotensin receptor blockers (ARBs), are often recommended as first-line treatment particularly in patients with diabetes and/or proteinuria. ACEIs have positive effects on neurohormonal activity and ventricular remodeling, while ARBs seem to reduce oxidative stress and inflammation [107]. In a randomized trial performed on ESKD patients, fosinopril was found to reduce CV death, heart failure, myocardial infarction and nonfatal stroke. Beta-blockers were found to reduce the cardiac risk in coronary artery disease patients with or without CKD in the Bezafibrate Infarction Prevention study. A significant reduction of CV mortality and occurrence of sudden death was demonstrated in dialysis patients treated with carvedilol. However, new dialysis patients not previously treated with beta-blockers were more likely to develop new-onset heart failure [107].

One most neglected aspect is the effect of sodium intake on blood pressure. Only a minority of renal patients reduce sodium chloride intake to the recommended target of 7 g/day. Apart from reduced salt intake, co-administration of diuretics is mandatory (in early stages, mostly thiazides). Loop diuretics are required in advanced stages of CKD.

Anemia is considered to be one of the most important factors along with hypertension for the development of LVH in CKD patients. In terms of erythropoiesis-stimulating agents, despite a strong suggestion of benefit to anemia management in observational studies, a number of studies in predialysis patients yielded disappointing results. The TREAT study involved diabetic CKD patients with moderate anemia treated with darbepoetin alfa [108]. Correction of anemia to hemoglobin level of 13 g/dL was associated with increased risk of stroke. Recent systematization and meta-analysis of erythropoiesis-stimulating agent therapy showed that this type of therapy has 1.5 times higher risk of stroke, as well as promotes hypertension and even increases the mortality risk, risk of severe CV events and ESRD with higher hemoglobin targets [109]. These studies have not been in vain, as they have led to changes in the usage of the medication for the purpose of correction of anemia in CKD patients to a target quantity of 11–12 g/dL [107]. Increased homocysteine has been associated with adverse CV outcomes CKD population. Folic acid, vitamin B6 and vitamin B12 in combination are an effective and inexpensive strategy to decrease homocysteine in most populations. However, trials of multivitamins in ESRD patients have been disappointing with negative results from a number of well-conducted clinical trials. This could be explained partly by the fact that vitamins fail to normalize homocysteine in ESRD patients, and toxicity from the vitamins themselves potentially could offset any theoretical benefit [110].

CKD-mineral and bone disorder (CKD-MBD) has been linked to the progression of cardiac disease, and investigators have shown a link between even mild degrees of renal injury and vascular calcification. Therefore, strategies to control phosphate, control PTH and vitamin D analogs have been mainstays of therapy in this regard [111]. In terms of phosphate binding, a Cochrane systematic review discovered that the effect of sevelamer hydrochloride and lanthanum carbonate were not as beneficial as calcium salts for the purpose of phosphate control. Some of the studies appeared to show improvements in the surrogate outcome of vascular calcification, which subsequently did not add to any reduction in CV morbidity or mortality [111].

Statins play a central role in the primary and secondary management of the CVD risk. Results of SHARP (Study of Heart and Renal Protection) study showed a significant benefit of the combination of simvastatin and ezetimibe in lowering the risk of major atherosclerotic events. This study included both ESRD patients and CKD patients not on dialysis. However, the subgroup of ESRD patients in SHARP seemed to experience less benefit compared to lesser degrees of CKD, and all-cause mortality was unaffected. Consistent with this negative findings, the initiation of treatment with rosuvastatin in the AURORA study had no significant effect on the composite primary end point of death from CV causes, nonfatal MI or nonfatal stroke in ESRD patient undergoing HD. It seems that CKD patients could benefit from statins but pragmatic approach is to recommend therapy with statins in CKD stages I–IV with increased risk of CVD [107].

7.2. Dialytic strategies to improve cardiovascular outcome

Dialytic strategies are used to improve cardiovascular outcome. Dialysis technology improvements should lead to improvements in hemodynamic stability, oxidative and inflammatory stress and increase the efficiency of removing low and middle toxins, which leads to 'cardioprotective dialysis'. Both the use of modern machines that fit safety, quality of therapy, performance and monitoring standards and the use of new biomaterials designed to mitigate inflammation and enhance membrane performance represent the application of new technologies [81]. In HD synthetic membranes are regarded as being more "biocompatible" in that they incite less of an immune response than cellulose-based membranes. However, Cochrane meta-analysis found no evidence of benefit when synthetic (high-flux) membranes were compared to cellulose/modified cellulose membranes in terms of reduced mortality in HD patients. This meta-analysis also showed that synthetic membranes achieved significantly higher Kt/V values when compared to modified cellulose membranes [112]. Results that are shown in the study of House et al. were compared the use of high-flux and low-flux hemodialysis on homocysteine and lipid profiles. The larger intradialytic effect of high-flux dialysis on homocysteine did not significantly affect predialysis levels after 3 months of study [113]. In contrast to this finding, high-flux membranes were associated with improved 2-year survival in the study of Chauveau et al. [114]. Other authors have reported that 'hemofiltration' or 'hemodiafiltration' treatment was associated with better blood pressure control, lower incidence of intradialytic hypotension or arrhythmia, better β2-microglobulin, phosphate clearance, reduced inflammation and oxidative stress as well as reduced hospitalization rate [81]. Ultrapure dialysate might also contribute to improvements in the morbidity and mortality of HD patients. Honda et al. found that serum myeloperoxidase and hs-CRP levels were significantly decreased in the patients treated with ultrapure dialysate compared to the patients undergoing HD using conventional dialysate. Ultrapure dialysate can improve the chronic inflammatory status, oxidative stress, and lipid abnormalities, suggesting a possible contribution to reduced CVD risk [115].

PD might circumvent the hemodynamic instability of frequent and rapid ultrafiltration associated with conventional HD. Previous randomized controlled trials and many other observational studies have produced conflicting results as to which therapy may have a CV advantage. Some registry data suggests PD is associated with a lower mortality than HD in the first 1–2 years but thereafter may be higher on PD than HD. Other registry data do not support this. The decision to undergo either PD or HD is based on many factors which include the differential damage the RRT may have on the CV system [116].

8. Post-translational modifications (PTMs) in CKD and CVD

Post-translational modifications (PTMs) of proteins and peptides have recently gained much attention, as they are involved in the pathogenesis of CVD and also play a role in the progression of CKD. PTMs are covalent changes of proteins or peptides that are altered either by proteolytic cleavage or by adding moieties to one or more amino acids. The most commonly reported PTMs are carbamoylation, glycation and oxidation [117].

8.1. Carbamylation

Carbamylation is a nonenzymatic spontaneous reaction of a primary amine or a free sulfhydryl group of proteins with isocyanate. This process is increased during CKD because of hyperuricemia, and in other pathologies like atherosclerosis, where isocyanic may be formed from thiocyanate by myeloperoxidase in atheroma plates [118]. As kidney function declines, metabolic substances such as urea and its derivates, cyanate and ammonia, dramatically increase thus leading to a significant amount of carbamylated proteins. Carbamylation of caeruloplasmin increases oxidative stress by decreasing the ferroxidase activity; carbamylated HDL reduces the lecithin-cholesterol acyltransferase thus inducing cholesterol accumulation; carbamylated LDL induces endothelial apoptosis and proliferation [76]. Amino acid therapy is applicable for reduction of protein carbonylation in CKD patients. The United States Food and Drug Administration (FDA) recently approved intravenous amino acid solution for this purpose (clinical trials.gov Identifier: NCT01612429). It was reported that uremic patients are deficient of free amino acids so that an infusion of free amino acids protects the proteins from carbamoylation due to the fact that both free amino acids and proteins compete with cyanate [117].

8.2. Glycation

Glycation is a nonenzymatic reaction of reducing sugars with the amino group of amino acids, nucleic acids, lipids and proteins. AGEs are considered extremely significant in determining the development of CVD in diabetic patients by changing the structure, function and characteristics of tissue through crosslinking inter- and extracellular matrix proteins and modulation of cellular processes through binding to receptors located on the cell's surface [119]. As CKD develops, the kidney is unable to successfully excrete AGE, leading to high concentrations. AGEs can be considered as uremic toxins, as they increase CV morbidity in patients suffering from CKD by altering their vascular matrix, thus increasing arterial stiffening, vascular calcifications and left ventricular hypertrophy. The pathophysiological effects of AGEs can be blocked by using inhibitors of AGE synthesis (aminoguanidine, pyridoxamine, benfotiamine, ALT-946, OBP-9195 and pimagedine); AGE cross-link breakers (alagebrium, N-phenacetyl thiazollium, TRC4186 and C-36) and anti-RAGE, which serve as a receptor blocker [120].

8.3. Oxidation/carbonylation

Oxidation generally refers to the loss of electrons or gain of oxygen or loss of hydrogen by a molecule. The addition of reactive carbonyl functional groups on proteins is generally termed as protein carbonylation. Oxidation mechanism is also involved in carbonylation. There is a close relationship between oxidative stress and carbonyl stress and these are enhanced in correlation with the progression of CKD among predialysis CKD patients. Proteins are the major targets for these reactive oxygen and nitrogen species, leading to peptide-bound cleavage or oxidation of side chains of amino acids resulting in the structural and functional changes of oxidized proteins. Almost all amino acids are vulnerable to radical attacks of reactive oxygen and nitrogen species. Oxidized forms of phenylalanine and tyrosine, markers for the oxidative damage, are all together termed as advanced oxidation protein products (AOPP). Clinical studies revealed that LDL oxidation, AOPP and protein carbonyls can be used as biomarkers of oxidative stress in CKD patients. AOPP levels independently predict atherosclerotic CV events in patients with CKD in the predialysis phase and might directly contribute to the uremia-associated accelerated atherogenesis [117]. Oxidized LDL could be involved in the stiffening of vascular wall which contributes to structural changes in the artery that may lead to CVD [121]. Anti-oxidant therapy could be beneficial in uremic patients with oxidative stress since the oxidative metabolites accumulate in CKD. Treatment with N-acetylcysteine in dialysis patients reduced the levels of oxidized LDL and partly improved anemia [122]. Vitamin E and C as well as ACEIs reduce ROS production, thereby decreasing oxidative stress in CKD patients [123]. Coenzyme Q10 (CoQ10) administration was effective in protecting against oxidative stress in dialysis patients in a phase IV clinical trial (ClinicalTrials.gov Identifier: NCT00307996).

Author details

Damir Rebić* and Aida Hamzić-Mehmedbašić†

*Address all correspondence to: damir.rebic@gmail.com

Clinic for Nephrology, Clinical Center University of Sarajevo, Sarajevo, Bosnia and Herzegovina

†Contributed equally to the paper.

References

[1] Foley RN, Collins AJ. The USRDS: What you need to know about what it can and can't tell us about ESRD. Clinical Journal of the American Society of Nephrology. 2013;**8**(5):845-851. DOI: 10.2215/CJN.06840712

[2] Levey AS, Atkins R, Coresh J, Cohen EP, Collins AJ, Eckardt KU, Nahas ME, Jaber BL, Jadoul M, Levin A, Powe NR, Rossert J, Wheeler DC, Lameire N, Eknoyan G. Chronic kidney disease as a global public health problem: Approaches and initiatives—A position statement from Kidney Disease Improving Global Outcomes. Kidney International. 2007;**72**(3):247-259.

[3] Schocken DD, Benjamin EJ, Fonarow GC, Krumholz HM, Levy D, Mensah GA, Narula J, Shor ES, Young JB, Hong Y; American Heart Association Council on Epidemiology and Prevention; American Heart Association Council on Clinical Cardiology; American Heart Association Council on Cardiovascular Nursing; American Heart Association Council on High Blood Pressure Research; Quality of Care and Outcomes Research Interdisciplinary Working Group; Functional Genomics and Translational Biology Interdisciplinary Working Group. Prevention of heart failure: A scientific statement from the American Heart Association Councils on Epidemiology and Prevention, Clinical Cardiology, Cardiovascular Nursing, and High Blood Pressure Research; Quality of Care and Outcomes Research Interdisciplinary Working Group; and Functional Genomics and Translational Biology Interdisciplinary Working Group. Circulation. 2008;**117**(19):2544-2565. DOI: 10.1161/CIRCULATIONAHA.107.188965

[4] Schrier RW. Cardiorenal versus renocardiac syndrome: Is there a difference? Nature Clinical Practice Nephrology. 2007;**3**:637

[5] Virzì GM, Clementi A, Brocca A, de Cal M, Marcante S, Ronco C. Cardiorenal syndrome type 5 in sepsis: Role of endotoxin in cell death pathways and inflammation. Kidney and Blood Pressure Research. 2016;**41**(6):1008-1015. DOI: 10.1159/000452602

[6] Ronco C, Di Lullo L. Cardiorenal syndrome in western countries: Epidemiology, diagnosis and management approaches. Kidney Diseases (Basel). 2017;**2**(4):151-163

[7] Di Lullo L, Bellasi A, Russo D, Cozzolino M, Ronco C. Cardiorenal acute kidney injury: Epidemiology, presentation, causes, pathophysiology and treatment. International Journal of Cardiology. 2017;**227**:143-150. DOI: 10.1016/j.ijcard.2016.11.156

[8] Choong Hou K, Sin Yoong Kong K, Kee Yi Shern T, Tan Wei Chieh J. Impact of chronic kidney insufficiency on cardiovascular outcomes in patients that undergo coronary revascularization: A historical review. ASEAN Heart Journal. 2016;**24**:8. eCollection 2016. DOI: 10.7603/s40602-016-0008-1

[9] U.S. Renal Data System, USRDS. Annual Data Report: Atlas of Chronic Kidney Disease and End-stage Renal Disease in the United States. Bethesda: National Institutes of Health, National Institute of Diabetes and Digestive and Kidney Diseases; 2012.

[10] Glassock RJ, Pecoits-Filho R, Barberato SH. Left ventricular mass in chronic kidney disease and ESRD. Clinical Journal of the American Society of Nephrology. 2009;**4**(Suppl 1): S79-S91. DOI: 10.2215/CJN.04860709

[11] Gross ML, Ritz E. Hypertrophy and fibrosis in the cardiomyopathy of uremia—Beyond coronary heart disease. Seminars in Dialysis. 2008;**21**:308-318. DOI: 10.1111/j.1525-139X.2008.00454.x

[12] An JN, Kim YH, Park JB, Hwang JH, Yoo KD, Park JY, Kim CT, Kim HL, Kim YJ, Han DJ, Lim CS, Kim YS, Lee JP. Heart. 2015;**101**(22):1826-1833. DOI: 10.1136/heartjnl-2015-308142

[13] Ikegaya K, Nokihara K, Yasuhara T. Characterization of sulfhydryl heterogeneity in human serum albumin and recombinant human serum albumin for clinical use. Bioscience Biotechnology and Biochemistry. 2010;**74**:2232-2236

[14] Ilori TO, Wang X, Huang M, Gutierrez OM, Narayan KM, Goodman M, McClellan W, Plantinga L, Ojo AO. Oxidative balance score and the risk of end-stage renal disease and cardiovascular disease. American Journal of Nephrology. 2017;**45**(4):338-345. DOI: 10.1159/000464257

[15] Hs Bsa, Moger V, Swamy M. Cardiorenal syndrome type 4: A study of cardiovascular diseases in chronic kidney disease. Indian Heart Journal. 2017;**69**(1):11-16. DOI: 10.1016/j.ihj.2016.07.006

[16] Tsuruya K, Eriguchi M. Cardiorenal syndrome in chronic kidney disease. Current Opinion in Nephrology and Hypertension. 2015;**24**(2):154-162. DOI: 10.1097/MNH.0000000000000099

[17] Grassi G, Quarti-Trevano F, Seravalle G, Arenare F, Volpe M, Furiani S, Dell'Oro R, Mancia G. Early sympathetic activation in the initial clinical stages of chronic renal failure. Hypertension. 2011;**57**(4):846-851. DOI: 10.1161/HYPERTENSIONAHA.110.164780

[18] Larsen T, Narala K, McCullough PA. Type 4 cardiorenal syndrome: Myocardial dysfunction, fibrosis, and heart failure in patients with chronic kidney disease. Journal of Clinical & Experimental Cardiology. 2012;**3**:186. DOI: 10.4172/2155-9880.1000186

[19] McCullough PA, Lepor NE. The deadly triangle of anemia, renal insufficiency, and cardiovascular disease: Implications for prognosis and treatment. Reviews in Cardiovascular Medicine. 2005;**6**(1):1-10. DOI: 10.1016/j.carrev.2005.06.002

[20] Herzog CA, Asinger RW, Berger AK, Charytan DM, Díez J, Hart RG, Eckardt KU, Kasiske BL, McCullough PA, Passman RS, DeLoach SS, Pun PH, Ritz E. Cardiovascular disease in chronic kidney disease. A clinical update from Kidney Disease: Improving Global Outcomes (KDIGO). Kidney International. 2011;**80**:572-586. DOI: 10.1038/ki.2011.223

[21] Damman K, van Deursen VM, Navis G, Voors AA, van Veldhuisen DJ, Hillege HL. Increased central venous pressure is associated with impaired renal function and mortality in a broad spectrum of patients with cardiovascular disease. Journal of the American College of Cardiology. 2009;**53**(7):582-588. DOI: 10.1016/j.jacc.2008.08.080.

[22] Bouillon G, Carmeliet L, Verlinden E, van Etten A, Verstuyf HF, Luderer L, Lieben C, Demay M. Endocrine Reviews. Vitamin D and human health: lessons from vitamin D receptor null mice. Endocr Rev. 2008;**29**(6):726-76. DOI: 10.1210/er.2008-0004.

[23] Verstuyf A, Carmeliet G, Bouillon R, Mathieu C. Vitamin D: A pleiotropic hormone. Kidney International. 2010;**78**:140. DOI: 10.1038/ki.2010.17

[24] Lai YH, Fang TC. The pleiotropic effect of vitamin D. ISRN Nephrology. 2013;**2013**:898125. DOI: 10.5402/2013/898125. eCollection 2013.

[25] Bendik I, Friedel A, Roos FF, Weber P, Eggersdorfer M. Vitamin D: a critical and essential micronutrient for human health. Front Physiol. 2014;**5**:248. doi: 10.3389/fphys.2014.00248

[26] Jones G, Prosser DE, Kaufmann M. Cytochrome P450-mediated metabolism of vitamin D. J Lipid Res. 2014;**55**(1):13-31. doi: 10.1194/jlr.R031534

[27] Zerwekh JE. Blood biomarkers of vitamin D status. Am J Clin Nutr. 2008;**87**(4):1087S-91S

[28] Morris HA, Anderson PH. Autocrine and paracrine actions of vitamin d. Clin Biochem Rev. 2010;**31**(4):129-38

[29] Lieben L, Carmeliet G, Masuyama R. Calcemic actions of vitamin D: effects on the intestine, kidney and bone. Best Pract Res Clin Endocrinol Metab. 2011;**25**(4):561-72. doi: 10.1016/j.beem.2011.05.008. Review

[30] de Pádua Netto MV, Bonfim TC, Costa EN, de Lima HV, Netto LC. Cardiovascular risk estimated in renal transplant recipients with the Framingham score. Transplantation Proceedings. 2012;**44**(8):2337-2340. DOI: 10.1016/j.transproceed.2012.07.054

[31] Wanner C, Amann K, Shoji T. The heart and vascular system in dialysis. Lancet. 2016; **388**(10041):276-284. DOI: 10.1016/S0140-6736(16)30508-6

[32] Lee HJ, Kim W, Kim WS, Woo JS, Kim YG, Moon JY, Lee SH, Ihm CG, Lee TW, Jeong KH. Circulating endothelial progenitor cell levels predict cardiovascular events in end-stage renal disease patients on maintenance hemodialysis. Nephron. 2015;**130**(3):151-158. DOI: 10.1159/000430471

[33] Park M, Hsu CY, Go AS, Feldman HI, Xie D, Zhang X, Mifflin T, Waikar SS, Sabbisetti VS, Bonventre JV, Coresh J, Nelson RG, Kimmel PL, Kusek JW, Rahman M, Schelling JR, Vasan RS, Liu KD; Chronic Renal Insufficiency Cohort (CRIC) Study Investigators; CKD Biomarkers Consortium. Urine kidney injury biomarkers and risks of cardiovascular disease events and all-cause death: The CRIC study. Clinical Journal of the American Society of Nephrology. 2017. pii: CJN.08560816. DOI: 10.2215/CJN.08560816

[34] Tumlin JA, Costanzo MR, Chawla LS, Herzog CA, Kellum JA, McCullough PA, Ronco C. Cardiorenal syndrome type 4: Insights on clinical presentationpathophysiology from the eleventh consensus conference of the Acute Dialysis Quality Initiative (ADQI). Contributions to Nephrology. 2013;**182:**158-173. DOI: 10.1159/000349972

[35] Seoane-Pillado MT, Pita-Fernández S, Valdés-Cañedo F, Seijo-Bestilleiro R, Pértega-Díaz S, Fernández-Rivera C, Alonso-Hernández Á, González-Martín C, Balboa-Barreiro V. Incidence of cardiovascular events and associated risk factors in kidney transplant patients: A competing risks survival analysis. BMC Cardiovascular Disorders. 2017;**17**(1):72. DOI: 10.1186/s12872-017-0505-6

[36] Vishram JK, Borglykke A, Andreasen AH, Jeppesen J, Ibsen H, Jørgensen T, Palmieri L, Giampaoli S, Donfrancesco C, Kee F, et al. Impact of age and gender on the prevalence and prognostic importance of the metabolic syndrome and its components in Europeans. The MORGAM Prospective Cohort Project. PLoS One. 2014;**9**(9):e107294

[37] Wang IK, Kung PT, Kuo WY, Tsai WC, Chang YC, Liang CC, Chang CT, Yeh HC, Wang SM, Chuang FR, Wang KY, Lin CY, Huang CC. Impact of dialysis modality on the survival of end-stage renal disease patients with or without cardiovascular disease. Journal of Nephrology. 2013;**26**(2):331-341. DOI: 10.5301/jn.5000149

[38] Zoccali C. Traditional and emerging cardiovascular and renal risk factors: An epidemiological perspective. Kidney International. 2006;**70**(1):26-33

[39] Krediet, RT; Balafa, O. Cardiovascular risk in the peritoneal dialysis patient. Nature Reviews Nephrology. 2010;**6**:451-460. DOI: 10.1038/nrneph.2010.68

[40] Salama FE, Anass QA, Abdelrahman AA, Saeed EB. Chemerin: A biomarker for cardiovascular disease in diabetic chronic kidney disease patients. Saudi Journal of Kidney Diseases and Transplantation. 2016;**27**(5):977-984. DOI: 10.4103/1319-2442.190867

[41] Heerspink HJ, Ninomiya T, Zoungas S, de Zeeuw D, Grobbee DE, Jardine MJ. Effect of lowering blood pressure on cardiovascular events and mortality in patients on

dialysis: A systematic review and meta- analysis of randomized controlled trials. Lancet. 2009;**373**:1009-1015. DOI: 10.1016/S0140-6736(09)60212-9

[42] Weiner DE, Tighiouart H, Amin MG, Griffith JL, Stark PC, MacLeod BD. Chronic kidney disease as a risk factor for cardiovascular disease and all-cause mortality: A pooled analysis of community-based studies. Journal of the American Society of Nephrology. 2004;**15**:1307-1315

[43] Coen G, Manni M, Mantella D, Pierantozzi A, Balducci A, Condo S. Are PTH serum levels predictive of coronary calcifications in haemodialysis patients? Nephrology, Dialysis, Transplantation. 2007;**22**(11):3262-3267

[44] Velasquez MT, Beddhu S, Nobakht E, Rahman M, Raj DS. Ambulatory blood pressure in chronic kidney disease: Ready for prime time? Kidney International Reports. 2016;**1**(2):94-104. DOI: 10.1016/j.ekir.2016.05.001

[45] Subbiah AK, Chhabra YK, Mahajan S. Cardiovascular disease in patients with chronic kidney disease: A neglected subgroup. Heart Asia. 2016;**8**(2):56-61

[46] de Mutsert, R; Grootendorst, DC; Boeschoten, EW; Dekker, FW; Krediet, RT. Is obesity associated with a survival advantage in patients starting peritoneal dialysis? Contributions to Nephrology. 2009;**163**:124-131

[47] Vishram JK. Prognostic interactions between cardiovascular risk factors. Danish Medical Journal. 2014;**61**(7):B4892

[48] Fellstrom BC, Jardine AG, Schmieder RE, et al. Rosuvastatin and cardiovascular events in patients undergoing hemodialysis. New England Journal of Medicine. 2009;**360**:1395-1407. DOI: 10.1056/NEJMoa0810177

[49] Chen NC, Hsu CY, Chen CL. The strategy to prevent and regress the vascular calcification in dialysis patients. BioMed Research International. 2017;**2017**:9035193. DOI: 10.1155/2017/9035193

[50] Fortes PC, de Moraes TP, Mendes JG, Stinghen AE, Ribeiro SC, Pecoits-Filho R. Insulin resistance and glucose homeostasis in peritoneal dialysis. Peritoneal Dialysis International. 2009;**29:**S145-S148

[51] Marcos EG, Geelhoed B, Van Der Harst P, Bakker SJ, Gansevoort RT, Hillege HL, Van Gelder IC, Rienstra M. Relation of renal dysfunction with incident atrial fibrillation and cardiovascular morbidity and mortality: The PREVEND study. Europace. 2017 Jan 20. pii: euw373. DOI: 10.1093/europace/euw373

[52] Tonelli M, Pfeffer MA. Kidney disease and cardiovascular risk. Annual Review of Medicine. 2007;**58**:123-139

[53] Tseng JR, Lin CW, Chen SH, Yen TH, Lin PY, Lee MH, Yen TC. Clinical usefulness of ^{18}F-FDG PET/CT for the detection of infections of unknown origin in patients undergoing maintenance hemodialysis. Journal of Nuclear Medicine. 2015;**56**(5):681-687. DOI: 10.2967/jnumed.114.151696

[54] Pisetkul C, Chanchairujira K, Chotipanvittayakul N, Ong-Ajyooth L, Chanchairujira T. Malnutrition-inflammation score associated with atherosclerosis, inflammation and short-term outcome in hemodialysis patients. Journal of the Medical Association of Thailand. 2010;**93**(Suppl. 1):S147-S156

[55] Choi HY, Lee JE, Han SH, Yoo TH, Kim BS, Park HC. Association of inflammation and protein-energy wasting with endothelial dysfunction in peritoneal dialysis patients. Nephrology, Dialysis, Transplantation. 2010;**25**:1266-1271

[56] Scialla JJ, Wolf M. Roles of phosphate and fibroblast growth factor 23 in cardiovascular disease. Nature Reviews Nephrology. 2014;**10**(5):268-278. DOI: 10.1038/nrneph.2014.49

[57] Stenvinkel P, Heimbürger O, Paultre F, Diczfalusy U, Wang T, Berglund L. Strong association between malnutrition, inflammation, and atherosclerosis in chronic renal failure. Kidney International. 1999;**55**:1899-1911

[58] de Mutsert R, Grootendorst DC, Axelsson J, Boeschoten EW, Krediet RT, Dekker FW, NECOSAD Study Group. Excess mortality due to interaction between protein-energy wasting, inflammation and cardiovascular disease in chronic dialysis patients. Nephrology, Dialysis, Transplantation. 2008;**23**:2957-2964

[59] Chung SH, Lindholm B, Lee HB. Is malnutrition an independent predictor of mortality in peritoneal dialysis patients? Nephrology, Dialysis, Transplantation. 2003;**18**:2134-2140

[60] Canada-USA (CANUSA) Peritoneal dialysis Study Group. Adequacy of dialysis and nutrition in continuous peritoneal dialysis: Association with clinical outcomes. Journal of the American Society of Nephrology.1996;**7**:196-207

[61] Small DM, Beetham KS, Howden EJ, Briskey DR, Johnson DW, Isbel NM, Gobe GC, Coombes JS. Effects of exercise and lifestyle intervention on oxidative stress in chronic kidney disease. Redox Report. 2017;**11**:1-10. DOI: 10.1080/13510002.2016.1276314

[62] Boudouris G, Verginadis II, Simos YS, Zouridakis A, Ragos V, Karkabounas SC. Oxidative stress in patients treated with continuous ambulatory peritoneal dialysis (CAPD) and the significant role of vitamin C and E supplementation. International Urology and Nephrology. 2012;**21**:212-216

[63] Custódio MR, Koike MK, Neves KR, dos Reis LM, Graciolli FG, Neves CL, Batista DG, Magalhães AO, Hawlitschek P, Oliveira IB, Dominguez WV, Moysés RM, Jorgetti V. Parathyroid hormone and phosphorus overload in uremia: Impact on cardiovascular system. Nephrology, Dialysis, Transplantation. 2012;**27**(4):1437-1445. DOI: 10.1093/ndt/gfr447

[64] Jung S, Querfeld U, Müller D, Rudolph B, Peters H, Krämer S. Submaximal suppression of parathyroid hormone ameliorates calcitriol-induced aortic calcification and remodeling and myocardial fibrosis in uremic rats. Journal of Hypertension. 2012;**30**(11):2182-2191. DOI: 10.1097/HJH.0b013e328357c049

[65] Ye Z, Zhang Q, Li Y, Wang C, Zhang J, Ma X, Peng H, Lou T. High prevalence of hyper-homocysteinemia and its association with target organ damage in chinese patients with chronic kidney disease. Nutrients. 2016;**8**(10):645

[66] Parekh RS, Plantinga LC, Kao WH, et al. The association of sudden cardiac death with inflammation and other traditional risk factors. Kidney International. 2008;**74**:1335-1342. DOI: 10.1038/ki.2008.449

[67] Allan CA, Strauss BJ, Burger HG, et al. Testosterone therapy prevents gain in visceral adipose tissue and loss of skeletal muscle in nonobese aging men. Journal of Clinical Endocrinology and Metabolism. 2008;**93**:139-146

[68] Paniagua R, Amato D, Vonesh E, Correa-Rotter R, Ramos A, Moran J, Mexican Nephrology Collaborative Study Group. Effects of increased peritoneal clearances on mortality rates in peritoneal dialysis: ADEMEX, a prospective, randomized, controlled trial. Journal of the American Society of Nephrology. 2002;**13**:1307-1320

[69] Mallamaci F, Tripepi G, Cutrupi S, Malatino LS, Zoccali C. Prognostic value of combined use of biomarkers of inflammation, endothelial dysfunction, and myocardiopathy in patients with ESRD. Kidney International. 2005;**67**:2330-2337

[70] Balakrishnan VS, Guo D, Rao M, Jaberm B, Tighiouart H, Freeman RL. Cytokine gene polymorphisms in hemodialysis patients: Association with comorbidity, functionality, and serum albumin. Kidney International. 2004;**65**:1449-1460

[71] Papaoikonomou S, Tentolouris N, Tousoulis D, Papadodiannis D, Miliou A, Papageorgiou N, Hatzis G, Stefanadis C. The association of the 174G>C polymorphism of interleukin 6 gene with diabetic nephropathy in patients with type 2 diabetes mellitus. Journal of Diabetes and its Complications. 2013;**27**(6):576-579. DOI: 10.1016/j.jdiacomp.2013.06.006

[72] Allison SJ. Anaemia: Targeting epigenetics in renal anaemia. Nature Reviews Nephrology. 2016;**12**(3):125. DOI: 10.1038/nrneph.2016.5

[73] Ronco C, Haapio M, House AA, Anavekar N, Bellomo R. Cardiorenal syndrome. Journal of the American College of Cardiology. 2008;**52**:1527-1539. DOI: 10.1016/j.jacc.2008.07.051

[74] McCullough PA, Kellum JA, Haase M, Müller C, Damman K, Murray PT, Cruz D, House AA, Schmidt-Ott KM, Vescovo G, Bagshaw SM, Hoste EA, Briguori C, Braam B, Chawla LS, Costanzo MR, Tumlin JA, Herzog CA, Mehta RL, Rabb H, Shaw AD, Singbartl K, Ronco C. Pathophysiology of the cardiorenal syndromes: Executive summary from the eleventh consensus conference of the Acute Dialysis Quality Initiative (ADQI). Contributions to Nephrology. 2013;**182**:82-98. DOI: 10.1159/000349966

[75] Cruz DN, Schmidt-Ott KM, Vescovo G, House AA, Kellum JA, Ronco C, McCullough PA. Pathophysiology of cardiorenal syndrome type 2 in stable chronic heart failure: Workgroup statements from the eleventh consensus conference of the Acute Dialysis Quality Initiative (ADQI). Contributions to Nephrology. 2013;**182**:117-136. DOI: 10.1159/000349968

[76] Granata A, Clementi A, Virzì GM, Brocca A, de Cal M, Scarfia VR, Zanoli L, Ronco C, Corrao S, Malatino L. Cardiorenal syndrome type 4: From chronic kidney disease to cardiovascular impairment. European Journal of Internal Medicine. 2016;**30**:1-6. DOI: 10.1016/j.ejim.2016.02.019

[77] Cruz DN, Bagshaw SM. Heart-kidney Interaction: Epidemiology of cardiorenal syndromes. International Journal of Nephrology. 2010;**2011**:35129111. DOI: 10.4061/2011/351291

[78] Cheung AK, Sarnak MJ, Yan G, Berkoben M, Heyka R, Kaufman A, Lewis J, Rocco M, Toto R, Windus D, Ornt D, Levey AS; HEMO Study Group. Cardiac diseases in maintenance hemodialysis patients: Results of the HEMO Study. Kidney International. 2004;**65**(6):2380-2389. DOI: 10.1111/j.1523-1755.2004.00657.x

[79] Burton JO, Jefferies HJ, Selby NM, McIntyre CW. Hemodialysis-induced repetitive myocardial injury results in global and segmental reduction in systolic cardiac function. Clinical Journal of the American Society of Nephrology. 2009;**4**(12):1925-1931. DOI: 10.2215/CJN.04470709

[80] Pinheiro da Silva AL, Vaz da Silva MJ. Type 4 cardiorenal syndrome. Revista Portuguesa de Cardiologia. 2016;**35**(11):601-616. DOI: 10.1016/j.repc.2016.06.007

[81] Clementi A, Virzì GM, Goh CY, Cruz DN, Granata A, Vescovo G, Ronco C. Cardiorenal syndrome type 4: A review. CardioRenal Medicine. 2013;**3**(1):63-70. DOI: 10.1159/000350397

[82] Vickery S, Webb MC, Price CP, John RI, Abbas NA, Lamb EJ. Prognostic value of cardiac biomarkers for death in a non-dialysis chronic kidney disease population. Nephrology, Dialysis, Transplantation. 2008;**23**(11):3546-3553. DOI: 10.1093/ndt/gfn341

[83] Sommerer C, Beimler J, Schwenger V, Heckele N, Katus HA, Giannitsis E, Zeier M. Cardiac biomarkers and survival in haemodialysis patients. European Journal of Clinical Investigation. 2007;**37**(5):350-356. DOI: 10.1111/j.1365-2362.2007.01785.x

[84] Wang AY, Lam CW, Yu CM, Wang M, Chan IH, Zhang Y, Lui SF, Sanderson JE. N-terminal pro-brain natriuretic peptide: An independent risk predictor of cardiovascular congestion, mortality, and adverse cardiovascular outcomes in chronic peritoneal dialysis patients. Journal of the American Society of Nephrology. 2007;**18**(1):321-330. DOI: 10.1681/ASN.2005121299

[85] Arikan H, Koc M, Tuglular S, Ozener C, Akoglu E. Elevated plasma levels of PAI-1 predict cardiovascular events and cardiovascular mortality in prevalent peritoneal dialysis patients. Renal Failure. 2009;**31(**6):438-445. DOI: 10.1080/08860220902963772

[86] D'Marco L, Bellasi A, Raggi P. Cardiovascular biomarkers in chronic kidney disease: State of current research and clinical applicability. Disease Markers. 2015;**2015**:586569. DOI: 10.1155/2015/586569

[87] Wasung ME, Chawla LS, Madero M. Biomarkers of renal function, which and when? Clinica Chimica Acta. 2015;**438**:350-357. DOI: 10.1016/j.cca.2014.08.039

[88] Ix JH, Shlipak MG, Chertow GM, Whooley MA. Association of cystatin C with mortality, cardiovascular events, and incident heart failure among persons with coronary heart disease: Data from the Heart and Soul Study. Circulation. 2007;**115**(2):173-179

[89] Patel PC, Ayers CR, Murphy SA, Peshock R, Khera A, de Lemos JA, Balko JA, Gupta S, Mammen PP, Drazner MH, Markham DW. Association of cystatin C with left ventricular structure and function: The Dallas Heart Study. Circulation. Heart Failure. 2009;**2**(2):98-104. DOI: 10.1161/CIRCHEARTFAILURE.108.807271

[90] Angelidis C, Deftereos S, Giannopoulos G, Anatoliotakis N, Bouras G, Hatzis G, Panagopoulou V, Pyrgakis V, Cleman MW. Cystatin C: An emerging biomarker in cardiovascular disease. Current Topics in Medicinal Chemistry. 2013;**13**(2):164-179

[91] Zachariah D, Olechowski B, Kalra PR. Clinical utility of biomarkers in chronic kidney disease and chronic heart failure. Journal of Renal Care. 2013;**39**(3):128-139. DOI: 10.1111/j.1755-6686.2013.12025.x

[92] Bolignano D, Lacquaniti A, Coppolino G, Donato V, Campo S, Fazio MR, Nicocia G, Buemi M. Neutrophil gelatinase-associated lipocalin (NGAL) and progression of chronic kidney disease. Clinical Journal of the American Society of Nephrology. 2009;**4**(2):337-344. doi: 10.2215/CJN.03530708

[93] Liu KD, Yang W, Anderson AH, Feldman HI, Demirjian S, Hamano T, He J, Lash J, Lustigova E, Rosas SE, Simonson MS, Tao K, Hsu CY; Chronic Renal Insufficiency Cohort (CRIC) study investigators. Urine neutrophil gelatinase-associated lipocalin levels do not improve risk prediction of progressive chronic kidney disease. Kidney International. 2013;**83**(5):909-914. DOI: 10.1038/ki.2012.458

[94] Furuya F, Shimura H, Yokomichi H, Takahashi K, Akiyama D, Asakawa C, Okamura A, Motosugi A, Haraguchi K, Yamagata Z, Kobayashi T. Neutrophil gelatinase-associated lipocalin levels associated with cardiovascular disease in chronic kidney disease patients. Clinical and Experimental Nephrology. 2014;**18**(5):778-783. DOI: 10.1007/s10157-013-0923-4

[95] Fassett RG, Venuthurupalli SK, Gobe GC, Coombes JS, Cooper MA, Hoy WE. Biomarkers in chronic kidney disease: A review. Kidney International. 2011;**80**(8):806-821. DOI: 10.1038/ki.2011.198

[96] Comnick M, Ishani A. Renal biomarkers of kidney injury in cardiorenal syndrome. Current Heart Failure Reports. 2011;**8**(2):99-105. DOI: 10.1007/s11897-011-0052-x

[97] Doi K, Katagiri D, Negishi K, Hasegawa S, Hamasaki Y, Fujita T, Matsubara T, Ishii T, Yahagi N, Sugaya T, Noiri E. Mild elevation of urinary biomarkers in prerenal acute kidney injury. Kidney International. 2012;**82**(10):1114-1120. DOI: 10.1038/ki.2012.266

[98] Vaidya VS, Niewczas MA, Ficociello LH, Johnson AC, Collings FB, Warram JH, Bonventre JV. Regression of microalbuminuria in type 1 diabetes is associated with lower levels of urinary tubular injury biomarkers, kidney injury molecule-1, and N-acetyl-β-D-glucosaminidase. Kidney International. 2011);**79**(4):464-470. DOI: 10.1038/ki.2010.404

[99] Damman K, Van Veldhuisen DJ, Navis G, Vaidya VS, Smilde TD, Westenbrink BD, Bonventre JV, Voors AA, Hillege HL. Tubular damage in chronic systolic heart failure is associated with reduced survival independent of glomerular filtration rate. Heart. 2010;**96**(16):1297-1302. DOI: 10.1136/hrt.2010.194878

[100] Hulthe J, McPheat W, Samnegård A, Tornvall P, Hamsten A, Eriksson P. Plasma interleukin (IL)-18 concentrations is elevated in patients with previous myocardial infarction and related to severity of coronary atherosclerosis independently of C-reactive protein and IL-6. Atherosclerosis. 2006;**188**(2):450-454. DOI: 10.1016/j.atherosclerosis.2005.11.013

[101] Formanowicz D, Wanic-Kossowska M, Pawliczak E, Radom M, Formanowicz P. Usefulness of serum interleukin-18 in predicting cardiovascular mortality in patients with chronic kidney disease—Systems and clinical approach. Scientific Reports. 2015;**5**:18332. DOI: 10.1038/srep18332

[102] Kovesdy CP, Quarles LD. The role of fibroblast growth factor-23 in cardiorenal syndrome. Nephron. Clinical Practice. 2013;**123**(3-4):194-201. DOI: 10.1159/000353593

[103] Pulido-Olmo H, García-Prieto CF, Álvarez-Llamas G, Barderas MG, Vivanco F, Aranguez I, Somoza B, Segura J, Kreutz R, Fernández-Alfonso MS, Ruilope LM, Ruiz-Hurtado G. Role of matrix metalloproteinase-9 in chronic kidney disease: A new biomarker of resistant albuminuria. Clinical Science (London). 2016;**130**:525-538. DOI: 10.1042/CS20150517

[104] Hsu TW, Kuo KL, Hung SC, Huang PH, Chen JW, Tarng DC. Progression of kidney disease in non-diabetic patients with coronary artery disease: Predictive role of circulating matrix metalloproteinase-2, -3, and -9. PLoS ONE. 2013;**8**(7):e70132. DOI: 10.1371/journal.pone.0070132

[105] Cozzolino M, Biondi ML, Galassi A, Turri O, Brancaccio D, Gallieni M. Matrix metalloproteinase-1 and matrix metalloproteinase-3 gene promoter polymorphisms are associated with mortality in haemodialysis patients. Nephrology, Dialysis, Transplantation. 2009;**24**(7):2207-2212. DOI: 10.1093/ndt/gfp061

[106] Pateinakis P, Papagianni A. Cardiorenal syndrome type 4-cardiovascular disease in patients with chronic kidney disease: Epidemiology, pathogenesis, and management. International Journal of Nephrology. 2011;**2011**:938651. DOI: 10.4061/2011/938651

[107] Clementi A, Virzì GM, Brocca A, de Cal M, Vescovo G, Granata A, Ronco C. Cardiorenal syndrome type 4: Management. Blood Purification. 2013;**36**(3-4):200-209. DOI: 10.1159/000356369

[108] Pfeffer MA, Burdmann EA, Chen CY, Cooper ME, de Zeeuw D, Eckardt KU, Feyzi JM, Ivanovich P, Kewalramani R, Levey AS, Lewis EF, McGill JB, McMurray JJ, Parfrey P, Parving HH, Remuzzi G, Singh AK, Solomon SD, Toto R; TREAT Investigators. A trial of darbepoetin alfa in type 2 diabetes and chronic kidney disease. New England Journal of Medicine. 2009;**361**(21):2019-2032. DOI: 10.1056/NEJMoa0907845

[109] Palmer SC, Navaneethan SD, Craig JC, Johnson DW, Tonelli M, Garg AX, Pellegrini F, Ravani P, Jardine M, Perkovic V, Graziano G, McGee R, Nicolucci A, Tognoni G,

Strippoli GF. Meta-analysis: Erythropoiesis-stimulating agents in patients with chronic kidney disease. Annals of Internal Medicine. 2010;**153**(1):23-33. DOI: 10.7326/0003-4819-153-1-201007060-00252

[110] Wrone EM, Hornberger JM, Zehnder JL, McCann LM, Coplon NS, Fortmann SP. Randomized trial of folic acid for prevention of cardiovascular events in end-stage renal disease. Journal of the American Society of Nephrology. 2004;**15**(2):420-426

[111] House AA. Cardio-renal syndrome type 4: Epidemiology, pathophysiology and treatment. Seminars in Nephrology. 2012;**32**(1):40-48. DOI: 10.1016/j.semnephrol.2011.11.006

[112] Macleod AM, Campbell M, Cody JD, Daly C, Donaldson C, Grant A, Khan I, Rabindranath KS, Vale L, Wallace S. Cellulose, modified cellulose and synthetic membranes in the haemodialysis of patients with endstage renal disease. Cochrane Database of Systematic Reviews. 2005;(3):CD003234

[113] House AA, Wells GA, Donnelly JG, Nadler SP, Hébert PC. Randomized trial of high-flux vs low-flux haemodialysis: Effects on homocysteine and lipids. Nephrology, Dialysis, Transplantation. 2000;**15**(7):1029-1034

[114] Chauveau P, Nguyen H, Combe C, Chêne G, Azar R, Cano N, Canaud B, Fouque D, Laville M, Leverve X, Roth H, Aparicio M; French Study Group for Nutrition in Dialysis. Dialyzer membrane permeability and survival in hemodialysis patients. American Journal of Kidney Disease. 2005;**45**(3):565-571. DOI: 10.1053/j.ajkd.2004.11.014

[115] Honda H, Suzuki H, Hosaka N, Hirai Y, Sanada D, Nakamura M, Nagai H, Ashikaga E, Matsumoto K, Mukai M, Watanabe M, Akizawa T. Ultrapure dialysate influences serum myeloperoxidase levels and lipid metabolism. Blood Purification. 2009;**28**(1):29-39. DOI: 10.1159/000210035

[116] Fassett RG, Driver R, Healy H, Coombes JS. Cardiovascular disease in peritoneal dialysis patients. Panminerva Medica. 2009;**51**(3):151-161

[117] Gajjala PR, Fliser D, Speer T, Jankowski V, Jankowski J. Emerging role of post-translational modifications in chronic kidney disease and cardiovascular disease. Nephrology, Dialysis, Transplantation. 2015;**30**(11):1814-1824. DOI: 10.1093/ndt/gfv048

[118] Gillery P, Jaisson S, Gorisse L, Pietrement C. Role of protein carbamylation in chronic kidney disease complications. Néphrologie & Thérapeutique. 2015;**11**(3):129-134. DOI: 10.1016/j.nephro.2014.12.004

[119] Hegab Z, Gibbons S, Neyses L, Mamas MA. Role of advanced glycation end products in cardiovascular disease. World Journal of Cardiology. 2012;**4**(4):90-102. DOI: 10.4330/wjc.v4.i4.90

[120] Busch M, Franke S, Rüster C, Wolf G. Advanced glycation end-products and the kidney. European Journal of Clinical Investigation. 2010;**40**(8):742-755. DOI: 10.1111/j.1365-2362.2010.02317.x

[121] Stephen EA, Venkatasubramaniam A, Good TA, Topoleski LD. The effect of oxidation on the mechanical response and microstructure of porcine aortas. Journal of Biomedical Materials Research. Part A. 2014;**102**(9):3255-3262. DOI: 10.1002/jbm.a.34998

[122] Hsu SP, Chiang CK, Yang SY, Chien CT. N-acetylcysteine for the management of anemia and oxidative stress in hemodialysis patients. Nephron. Clinical Practice. 2010;**116**(3):c207-c216. DOI: 10.1159/000317201

[123] Aluganti Narasimhulu C, Selvarajan K, Brown M, Parthasarathy S. Cationic peptides neutralize Ox-LDL, prevent its uptake by macrophages, and attenuate inflammatory response. Atherosclerosis. 2014;**236**(1):133-141. DOI: 10.1016/j.atherosclerosis.2014.06.020

Chapter 2

Disorders in the System of Mineral and Bone Metabolism Regulators—FGF-23, Klotho and Sclerostin—in Chronic Kidney Disease: Clinical Significance and Possibilities for Correction

Ludmila Y. Milovanova, Victor V. Fomin,
Lidia V. Lysenko (Kozlovskaya), Nikolay A. Mukhin,
Svetlana Y. Milovanova, Marina V. Taranova,
Yuriy S. Milovanov, Vasiliy V. Kozlov and
Aigul Zh. Usubalieva

Additional information is available at the end of the chapter

http://dx.doi.org/10.5772/intechopen.69298

Abstract

The chapter discusses the current understanding of the system of mineral and bone metabolism regulators—FGF-23, Klotho and sclerostin—disturbances in chronic kidney disease (CKD). In the chapter we presented the date, including our own results, which allow to suggest the change in the ratio of FGF-23-Klotho-sclerostin in CKD as an early biomarker not only for the chronic kidney damage but also for high cardiovascular (CV) risk. Results of studies show that disorders in FGF-23-Klotho-sclerostin ratio correlate with the frequency and severity of hypertension, vascular calcification, cardiac remodelling, anaemia, malnutrition, inflammation and strong aggravate CV risk in CKD. It was found independent from blood pressure (BP) action of increased serum FGF-23 on the myocardium as well as the correlation of serum high-sensitive troponin I with increased serum FGF-23 and low Klotho levels in CKD patients. At the same time, it was shown that renoprotective therapy, including renin-angiotensin blockers, low-protein diet with amino/keto acid supplementation and phosphate binders, erythropoiesis stimulators, vitamin D metabolites used to get the target levels of BP, serum phosphorus, haemoglobin, parathyroid hormone and nutritional status disorders correction can reduce the risk of CV events, as the major cause of death in CKD patients.

Keywords: chronic kidney disease, FGF-23, Klotho, sclerostin, vascular calcification, cardiac remodelling

1. Introduction

Chronic kidney disease (CKD) is a global problem that has not only medical but also great social and economic importance, due to a significant prevalence in the population (10–15%), high mortality rate from cardiovascular complications (CVC), as well as the need for high-cost treatment for the end CKD stage (dialysis, transplantation). As compared with general population, mortality rate due to CVC in patients with chronic renal failure is 10 times higher, and in young people, this risk is higher by 100 or more time. Many patients with CKD die from CVC on pre-dialysis stages, not reaching the end stage of CKD [1, 2].

Among cardiovascular damage in CKD, the progressive both cardiac remodelling and vascular calcification have leading contribution, which together lead to an urgently high cardiovascular mortality in patients with CKD [3, 4]. Understanding of the early mechanisms of arterial calcification as well as left ventricular hypertrophy (LVH) is important for the development of new therapeutic strategies aimed for cardiovascular morbidity reducing, pre-dialysis period prolonging and overall survival of CKD patients improving.

Clarification of CKD progression mechanisms and possible early markers of CVC has led to interest in studying of the identified in recent years factors such as morphogenetic proteins—fibroblast growth factor-23 (FGF-23), Klotho protein and sclerostin glycoprotein—which were estimated initially only as bone-mineral metabolism regulators in CKD [5].

Nowadays, the broader functional role of FGF-23, Klotho and sclerostin in organism has become understandable, including them significance as humoral factors involved in the processes of remodelling and calcification of the heart and vessels in CKD [6, 7]. Furthermore, the accumulated recently data allow to consider these factors as a possible therapeutic option for reducing mortality in CKD patients, but new randomized trials are still needed to clarify the individual mechanisms of their influence on remodelling and calcification of the heart and blood vessels as well as the optimal therapeutic modalities for correction of these disturbances.

The aim of the review was to systematize accumulated information and to establish the significance of the changes in serum levels of morphogenetic proteins (FGF-23, Klotho) and sclerostin glycoprotein, based on available literature data, including the results of our own studies, to assess renal and cardiac prognosis and possibilities for improving of cardio-renoprotective strategy in CKD.

2. FGF-23, Klotho and sclerostin in mineral bone disorders (MBD) in CKD

Disorders of phosphorus-calcium metabolism begin to be detected already on the 3A stage of CKD, when serum phosphorus starts to increase in serum due to glomerular filtration rate (GFR) decreasing [8]. PTH and vitamin D (calcitriol) were considered as main phosphor-regulating hormones for a long time. However, in recent years, it has been established, including our data, that FGF-23 begins to increase in serum in response to phosphorus retention, earlier than PTH [8, 9], that allows to reconsider the traditional concept of secondary hyperparathyroidism (SGPT) pathogenesis.

FGF-23, produced by osteocytes, is a phosphaturic hormone that maintains a normal serum phosphorus concentration by increasing excretion of phosphorus in the urine and reducing its absorption from the gastrointestinal tract by inhibiting synthesis of 1,25-dihydroxyvitamin D in kidneys. Physiological stimuli for FGF-23 secretion are both a diet with an excess of phosphorus content and an increase in $1,25(OH)_2D_3$ levels in circulation [5, 8]. In the kidneys, FGF-23 suppresses $1,25(OH)_2D_3$ formation by inhibiting 1α-hydroxylase enzyme activity, which converts $25(OH)D_3$ transition to $1,25(OH)_2D_3$, as well as FGF-23 stimulates the formation of 24-hydroxylase, which converts $1,25(OH)_2D_3$ into its inactive metabolites. At the same time, FGF-23 suppresses the expression of the sodium-phosphorus co-transporters of both types (IIa and IIc) located on the apical surface of the epithelial cells of the proximal renal tubules; as a result, renal excretion of phosphorus increases [5, 8, 10].

At the same time, a date on the direct blocking effect of FGF-23 on PTH secretion was obtained [11]. It was found that FGF-23 stimulates mitogen-activated protein kinase (PKA) pathway, and so it inhibits the expression of PTH mRNA and PTH secretion both in vivo in rats and in vitro in parathyroid cell culture [11]. Since PTH is the inducer of $1,25(OH)_2D_3$ gene expression, the suppression of PTH, caused by FGF-23, reduces the serum level of $1,25(OH)_2D_3$, thereby closing the negative feedback of vitamin D homeostasis.

As the renal 1α-hydroxylase is inhibited and secretion of $1,25(OH)_2D_3$ is decreased, hypocalcaemia occurs, which stimulates PTH overproduction [12]. Thus, normal levels of calcium and phosphorus in serum are maintained that is successful at the early CKD stages.

Initially, at the early CKD, the increase in FGF-23 is a compensatory response aimed at normalizing phosphorus serum levels while decreasing the functioning nephron number [8, 12]. The serum FGF-23 level increases in parallel with the progressive decrease in kidney function, and the serum phosphorus does not increase significantly until GFR falls <30 mL/min/1.73 m^2 [5, 8]. When this stage of CKD is reached, the above compensation mechanism becomes ineffective, and constant hyperphosphatemia occurs that stimulates the increasing secretion of FGF-23 and PTH [8]. By the time when patients reach the end stage of CKD, FGF-23 level exceeds its normal range by 100 or more times [8].

To realize its effects in the kidneys, FGF-23 needs a co-receptor which is a transmembrane form of Klotho protein [5, 10]. Klotho was originally identified as an "ageing suppressor" [13]. The Klotho gene encodes a transmembrane protein, which is expressed predominantly in the epithelial cells of distal tubules in the kidneys, in parathyroid glands (PTG) and in the cerebral vascular plexus. Two forms of Klotho protein were found: transmembrane and secreted forms, each of which has different functions. The membrane Klotho form acts as an obligate co-receptor for FGF-23, inducing the excretion of phosphate in the urine. Secreted Klotho form (sKlotho) is detected in human serum and cerebrospinal fluid. It was found that it is formed as a result of Klotho protein cleavage from the cell membrane of the distal tubules of the kidneys [5, 10]. The decrease of Klotho protein expression in the kidneys due to CKD advancement allows to consider it as an early diagnostic marker of kidney damage [5, 14].

Unlike the membrane form, the secreted form of Klotho has systemic effects: it regulates endothelial production of NO [15], maintains the integrity and permeability of the endothelium [16] and calcium homeostasis in the kidneys [17] and suppresses intracellular signals of insulin and insulin-like growth factor-1 as mechanisms evolutionarily associated with life expectancy [18]. The low serum level of sKlotho is associated with an increase of CVC [6] and all causes mortality [19].

In recent years, there is increasing evidence that sKlotho decreasing, as CKD advancement, occurs early (2–3A stage of CKD) and may be also an important reason for the inducing of FGF-23 serum increase. Koh et al. [20], based on the analysis of the kidney biopsy that results in ten patients with a histological nephrosclerosis, found a significant decrease in the expression of Klotho mRNA as well as in sKlotho level and also the role of Klotho deficiency as nephrosclerosis advances, in the development of numerous complications of CKD, including uncontrolled FGF-23 serum increase.

The reduced expression of Klotho transmembrane form on the surface of parathyroid glands (PTGs) cell membranes (Klotho is also a co-receptor for FGF-23 in PTGs) at advanced stages of CKD is attributed to the resistance of PTG receptors to FGF-23, even in FGF-23 maximum concentrations [10, 12, 21].

In recent years, data on the important role of sclerostin glycoprotein in CKD are accumulating [22, 23]. Sclerostin, synthesized by osteocytes, blocks Wnt signalling pathway that leads to suppression of bone formation, as a result of decreased osteoblast differentiation and proliferation and osteocyte apoptosis [24]. The level of sclerostin increases as CKD advances [22, 25].

To date, sclerostin is an established regulator of bone mineralization, while its role in the pathophysiology of vessels in CKD is actively explored [22, 26]. It is important to determine the clinical significance of changes in sclerostin metabolism in CKD, because the relationship between adynamic bone disease (ABD) and calcification of the heart and blood vessels in patients with CKD is considered proven [27]. At the same time, available-to-date publications on the role of sclerostin in ectopic calcification still remain contradictory [22, 23, 25, 26].

It has been shown in experimental studies that in the case of hyperphosphatemia, the function of the skeleton as a phosphorus reservoir is blocked, although the need of bone in phosphorus, on the contrary, is increased, which stimulates a rising of its level in the blood, and soft tissues and vessels become a new reservoir for phosphate deposition [27].

Thus, in patients with end CKD stages, hyperphosphatemia, Klotho's and $1{,}25(OH)_2D_3$ deficiency and increased PTH and sclerostin occur, despite a very high level of FGF-23. At the same time, the frequency of ABD associated with a relatively low PTH and high sclerostin serum levels increases [12, 24, 27]. These changes, together with a decreased calcium excretion, may be responsible for the development of such complications of CKD as renal osteodystrophy, cardiovascular calcification following CVC and adverse outcomes in CKD [6, 7, 26].

It is suggested that an increase in sclerostin serum levels leads to a slowdown in osteogenesis in CKD. At the same time, there are reasons to believe that this mechanism is blocked in CKD and an increase in sclerostin is directed mainly to the inhibition of the extraosteal calcification [22, 25]. In addition it is believed that an increase in sclerostin expression by osteocytes in CKD causes bone resistance to PTH [24].

According to the results of recent studies, a disorder of the FGF-23-Klotho-sclerostin ratio in CKD is an early biomarker of the degree of chronic renal damage, preceded to the changes in other established markers of CKD advancement such as hyperphosphatemia, hyperparathyroidism and hypovitaminosis D, considering early as emerging cardiovascular risk factors in CKD patients [5, 26]. In addition, in interventional trials, intake of phosphate binders, cinacalcet or active vitamin D did not exert a consistently beneficial effect to reduce in cardiovascular event rate [28].

2.1. The relation of FGF-23, Klotho and sclerostin with cardiovascular remodelling and calcification in CKD

Mineral bone disorders (MBD) in CKD are the main contributor in CVC risk and in general prognosis of this patient cohort (**Figure 1**).

If the increase in FGF-23 serum levels at early CKD stages is adaptive, then the rapid FGF-23 rising from 3B CKD stage acquires a pathological significance. It was shown that an increase in serum FGF-23 level in CKD 3B-5 stages is associated with an endothelium dysfunction, Left ventricular hypertrophy (LVH) and an increase in cardiovascular mortality [7, 29–31].

It is also believed that a markedly increased FGF-23 level in CKD leads to a non-selective binding of it to FGF receptors in the heart, which are usually activated by local growth factors, such as FGF-2 [32]. Thus, an elevated FGF-23 level was directly associated with an increased risk of LVH development, which was detected with prolonged exposure with FGF-2 in experiment. In addition, it was found that an increase in left ventricular mass index (LVMI) accompanied with increased serum FGF-23 was independent from serum phosphorus level [7, 9].

FGF-23 is an earlier, than phosphorus, marker of CVC in patients with CKD, even when a phosphorus serum level is within the normal range [8, 9]. The pathogenetic relationship

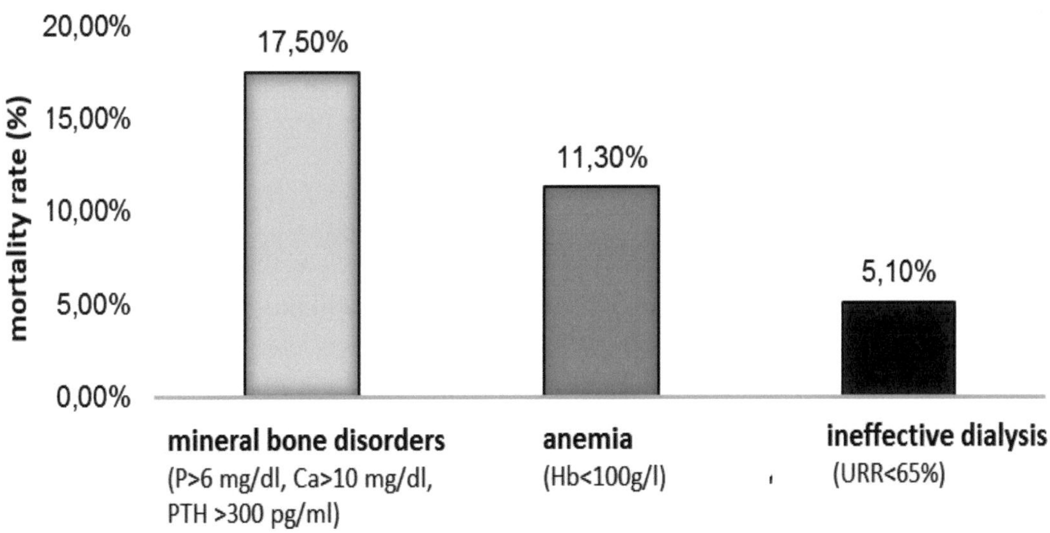

Figure 1. The position of MBD among the main causes of mortality in CKD haemodialysis patients (according to Block GA et al. J. Am. Soc. Nephrol. 2004).

between FGF-23 serum level and LVH was fully confirmed in the fundamental clinical work of Faul and Ansel [7] which showed that an increase in serum FGF-23 levels can directly lead to LVH development in CKD patients. The study consists of several stages; at the first stage, more than 3000 patients with renal insufficiency were examined for serum FGF-23 and echocardiography (EchoCG) at baseline and 1 year later. Each increase in serum FGF-23 on 1 logarithmic unit was associated with an increase in LVMI on 1.5 g/m^2. After 2.9 ± 0.5 years, the researchers re-examined 411 patients who had normal EchoCG parameters at the beginning of the study. In 84 (20%) patients with normal blood pressure (BP) levels, LVH was firstly detected. At the same time, each increase in FGF23 on 1 logarithmic unit led to an increase in the frequency of LVH de novo detection by 4.4 times; and significantly high levels of FGF-23 caused a sevenfold increase in the frequency of LVH detection, independently of the arterial hypertension (AH).

In order to confirm the hypothesis of the direct influence of FGF-23 on cardiomyocytes, Kardami [32] conducted the experimental study in which an effect of exogenous FGF-23 on the cardiomyocytes of newborn rats was evaluated using immunohistochemical and morphometric analysis. As a result, the hypertrophy of cardiomyocytes was revealed, as well as the increase in them, a level of alpha-actinin protein that indicates an increase of sequentially connected sacrometer units in the cardiomyocytes, and an increase in expression of heavy embryonic beta-myosin chains and depression of mature alpha-myosin chains. This switching of heavy chains from mature to embryonic isoforms indicates on the reactivation of embryonic gene programme, which is associated with hypertrophic transformation.

In the work of Di Marco et al. [33], prohypertrophic effect of FGF-23 and FGF-2 on cardiomyocytes was noted, which disappeared after the use of FGF-23 receptor inhibitor, PD173074, that authors consider as evidence of direct FGF-23 action, independently of Klotho protein. It is important to note that the use of PD173074 prevented the development of LVH in rats, despite the presence of hypertension in them.

According to our data [34], an increase in serum FGF-23 levels was associated with a moderately elevated level of troponin I. At the same time, in the patients with increased central BP (>120/80 mm Hg) as well as with normal central BP (90–120/60–79 mm Hg), mean levels of FGF-23 were about the same [629 ± 118 and 489 ± 85, respectively], indicating, an independent from the BP, FGF-23 action on the myocardium. The association of troponins with ischaemic heart disease and their role as predictors of an unfavourable cardiovascular outcome is known that also allows to suggest FGF-23 as an important prognostic cardiomarker in CKD.

In addition, it was established [35] that an increase in serum FGF-23 levels accelerated the development of vascular arteriosclerosis almost by sixfold, with the direct correlation with vascular calcification. However, in multivariate analysis, this relationship was statistically weak, which may indicate a possible indirect effect of FGF-23 on vascular calcification. Further obtained data indicate the effect of FGF-23 on fetuin A level, which is known to be synthesized by osteoblasts and is an inhibitor of vascular smooth muscle cell (VSMS) calcification [35, 36].

In the prospective cohort ArMORR study [37] involving 10,044 patients, it was shown that a high FGF-23 serum level of patients, starting treatment with programmed HD, is an independent predictor of annual mortality and the patients with high levels of FGF-23 from a higher quartile had a sixfold increase in the risk of mortality compared to similar patients from the lower quartile according to multidimensional corrected model.

In another prospective the mild to moderate kidney disease (MMKD) study [38] involving 227 patients with nondiabetic CKD 1–4 stages, the patients were followed up for 53 months to assess the progression of the nephropathy. Based on the results, an independent direct relationship between increased serum FGF-23 level and CKD progression rate was established. FGF-23 was recognized as an important independent predictor of adverse renal and cardiovascular prognosis, and in addition, in the regression Cox analysis, phosphorus levels lost prognostic value after adjustment to serum FGF-23 level.

Accumulating recent data allow to consider FGF-23 as an earlier and important predictor of mortality than serum phosphorus and PTH levels in patients with CKD. Elevated serum FGF-23 level is currently considered as an independent trigger factor in the pathogenesis of uremic cardiomyopathy and vascular calcification that served as the basis for suggesting FGF-23 *as a new uremic toxin*, earlier than PTH [39].

At the same time, part of the pathological effects of FGF-23 may be due to Klotho deficiency in CKD advancement. It has been shown that kidneys are the main producers of Klotho forms in organism [5, 10, 14], so CKD is a state of Klotho deficiency. Deficit of Klotho causes development of multiple systemic manifestations (i.e. premature ageing syndrome), an integral part of which is severe cardiovascular impairments [6, 13, 15]. According to recent update, it has been proved now that Klotho downregulation is not merely an early biomarker for kidney damage but also plays a pathogenic independent role in the advancing of CKD as well as in principal complications of CKD, important part of which is vascular calcification [6, 9]. As it was recently summarized, Klotho's anti-calcification effect is possibly via at least three mechanisms: a phosphaturic hormone, the preservation of GFR and a direct effect on soft tissues including the vascular smooth muscle [6, 21]. In experiment Klotho overexpression slowed down CKD advancement, improves phosphate metabolism and protects the vasculature from calcification [5, 6, 10].

The role of soluble Klotho form in phosphate homeostasis was recognized as soon as Klotho was discovered, because Klotho-deficient mouse demonstrates severe hyperphosphatemia [10, 13, 18]. This was further confirmed by the fact that there was low serum phosphate in Klotho-overexpressing mice [18]. A patient with homozygous missense mutation (H193R) in Klotho gene had severe calcinosis, dural and carotid artery calcifications, severe hyperphosphatemia, hypercalcemia and high-serum 1,25$(OH)_2$ vitamin D and FGF-23. This mutation conceivably destabilizes KL1 domain of Klotho, thereby attenuating production of membrane-bound and sKlotho protein [40]. Therefore, Klotho is now considerable as a novel candidate gene for genetic hyperphosphatemia and calcinosis.

It was established that a decrease in Klotho level is also possible due to the inhibition of its extrarenal production. In this connection, the results of Takeshita et al. [41] study, indicating the presence of Klotho gene expression in sinoatrial node and a high rate of sudden cardiac death due to arrhythmias caused by dysfunction of sinoatrial node in mice with blocked Klotho gene, are interesting.

One of the most important effects of Klotho and sclerostin is its ability to inhibit Wnt signal pathway and through it to slow down vascular calcification [42]. Reduction of serum Klotho levels impairs this protective effect. Besides this, it has been demonstrated that Klotho mitigates the increased cell senescence and apoptosis triggered by oxidative stress in endothelial cells [43] and Klotho also suppresses TNF-β-induced expression of intracellular adhesion molecule-1 and vascular cell adhesion molecule-1, attenuates NF-kappaB activation and reverses the inhibition of eNOS phosphorylation by TNF-α. Thus Klotho protein also protects the vascular endothelium by inhibition of endothelial inflammation [44].

The most definitive study to date of the direct effects of Klotho on the endothelium was conducted by Kusaba et al. [16]. Klotho-deficient mice have increased VEGF-mediated calcium influx, downregulation of vascular endothelial cadherin, increased apoptosis and excessive permeability of vessels. The KL2 domain of Klotho protein binds directly to VEGF receptor 2 and endothelial transient-receptor potential Ca^{2+} channel 1 on the extracellular side and promotes their co-internalization, thereby reducing the Ca^{2+}-activated and caspase-mediated destruction of catenin and vascular endothelial cadherin on the cell surface. Thus, it may be one more effect of soluble Klotho's protein cardioprotection.

In vitro studies have shown that along with the increase in phosphaturia, stabilization of GFR and regulation of vascular endothelial permeability, Klotho suppresses Na-dependent capture of phosphorus by the endothelium and vascular smooth muscle cell (VSMC) and prevents differentiation of VSMC and mineralization induced by hyperphosphatemia [5, 14].

In our study, an association of increased serum FGF-23 and low Klotho levels with the presence of inflammation (as C-reactive protein level increasing) as well as with protein-energy deficiency, and proteinuria, was found [45]. These data are in agreement with the results of other authors [44, 46] who consider CKD as a state of chronic inflammation, based on the consideration of elevated C-reactive protein level as a nonspecific marker of inflammation and endothelial dysfunction in CKD patients. Frequent coexistence triad—malnutrition, inflammation and atherosclerosis (MIA) syndrome—contributes to the risk of CVC in CKD [2, 3, 47]. The obtained data clearly indicate that circulating form of Klotho protein functions as a humoral factor that protects the cardiovascular system from the development of inflammatory endothelial changes and prevents the progression of atherosclerosis and pathological calcification [5, 14–16].

Less understood is the role of sclerostin in CV calcification processes in CKD. Our data go in agreement with the results of authors, who demonstrated a protective effect of sclerostin in calcification in CKD [22, 48, 49]. Its inhibitory effect on osteogenesis and negative association of sclerostin with level of parathyroid hormone as uremic toxin can attest in favour of this date [48, 49].

Viaene et al. [50] showed that in patients on haemodialysis, the serum concentration of sclerostin is higher than in general population. In the future, these data will be repeatedly confirmed by the results of other studies devoted to identify the role of sclerostin in patients on regular haemodialysis [23, 49].

Emerging evidence indicates that Wnt plays a role in vascular biology including vascular calcification, angiogenesis and atherosclerosis [42]. Wnt signalling occurs when the Wnt ligand binds to co-receptors, Frizzled and low-density lipoprotein receptor-related protein (LRP), which induces β-catenin translocation to the nucleus to regulate the transcription of Wnt target genes. The Wnt pathway is involved in many aspects of biology including cell survival, stem cell development and cell differentiation, including bone and vascular lineages [24, 42].

Register et al. [25] found that high sclerostin was associated with less calcified carotid plaque in diabetic African American men and was not associated with aortic or coronary calcification. Authors' hypothesis to explain this situation is that increased overproduction of sclerostin may be a physiological adaptation to increased calcification.

Sclerostin slows the canonical Wnt signalling pathway and inhibits osteoblast activity and bone formation by sequestering LRP5 and LRP6 [24, 42]. Retarding the Wnt signalling pathway by using a dominant-negative LRP has been depicted to significantly reduce VSMC proliferation. In addition to VSMC proliferation, animal models of intimal thickening have revealed increased β-catenin levels, which suggest the involvement of the Wnt-β-catenin pathway also in VSMC migration. Moreover, Wnt proteins are also known to promote the migration of various cell types, including monocytes and endothelial cells. Furthermore, the Wnt pathway has been described to play an important role in the regulation of endothelial inflammation, vascular calcification and mesenchymal stem cell differentiation. As a result, considering the fact that atherosclerosis and calcification are both an actively regulated and progressive process, we might speculate that high sclerostin levels might be indicative of a sort of defensive mechanism that may attenuate the upregulation of the canonical Wnt pathway and lead to the restoration of quiescent Wnt signalling observed under healthy conditions [24, 49].

Sclerostin has been demonstrated to be upregulated in VSMC, which previously transformed into osteocytic phenotype under calcifying circumstances [22, 24]. Recently, it has been suggested that increased circulating sclerostin levels might protect dialysis patients from cardiovascular calcification and that low bone-specific alkaline phosphatase activity may be the causal pathway [23, 49]. Sclerostin is a potent inhibitor of alkaline phosphatase activity, which inactivates the potent calcification inhibitor, the inorganic pyrophosphate. Accumulating data suggest that Wnt signalling pathway inhibitor overexpression in calcifying vasculature (advanced carotid plaques and calcified aortas) might be vasculoprotective and anti-calcific [25, 49].

PTH increases FGF-23 expression via Wnt and protein kinase (PKA) signalling pathways by blocking the inhibitory effect of sclerostin (**Figure 2**).

According to several authors, the overexpression of sclerostin by osteocytes in patients on haemodialysis is associated with a decrease in overall cause's mortality, including CVC, in dialysis patients [49].

In the same time, more research for confirmation of sclerostin role in FGF-23-Klotho-sclerostin system as a protector of pathogenic transformation of VSMC, triggered by phosphate and FGF-23, is seen as a priority. It is likely that sclerostin confronts effects of low Klotho levels and high levels of FGF-23, allowing for some time to maintain a certain compensatory balance in the system of FGF-23-Klotho-sclerostin. Increasing levels of sclerostin in CKD are likely directed at suppression of processes of calcification, but cannot fully inhibit them, because

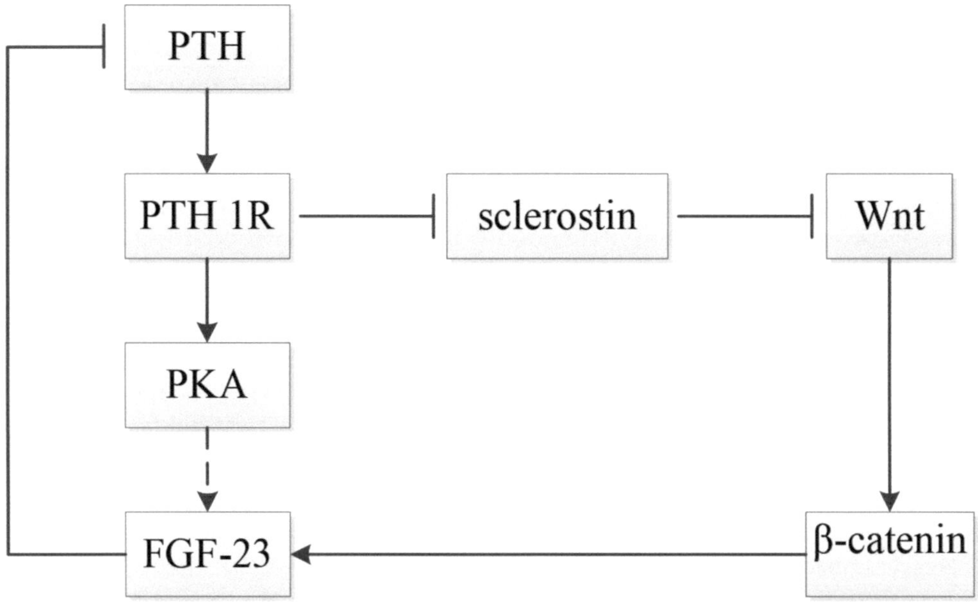

Figure 2. The relationship between PTH, FGF-23 and sclerostin (materials of ISN Nexus Symposium «Bone and the Kidney» September 2012, Copenhagen, Denmark).

reduction of Klotho may be much more potent stimulus for progression of calcification, and increased PTH suppresses sclerostin. Because levels of sclerostin increase as CKD progresses and as levels of Klotho at the same time reduce, some authors may mistakenly interpret the role of sclerostin as a factor, which potentiates calcification. In reality (the results of the multivariate analysis), it is likely that dramatic fall of Klotho levels in the course of CKD outbalances and levels down protective effects of sclerostin.

To sum up, we can consider all three factors (FGF-23, Klotho, sclerostin) as a discrete system of factors influencing cardiovascular risk. Apparently, such high CV risk is determined by joint effect of all of these three factors that appear along with early CKD stages and connect not only between themselves but also with traditional factors, which snowballed quickly following added, potentiate one another as CKD advanced and thereby strongly increase the risk of CV mortality. Influence of each group of these factors may have different impacts depending on the stage of CKD. Importantly, date indeed suggests that the FGF-23-Klotho-sclerostin axis may be a potential novel target in cardio-renal medicine.

3. Possibilities for correction of FGF-23, soluble Klotho and sclerostin serum disorders in CKD by traditional renoprotective therapy

The appearance preliminary results of few clinical trials indicate the possibility of influencing traditional renoprotective therapy such as early correction of arterial hypertension, anaemia, hyperphosphatasemia and nutritional status disorders on the maintenance of Klotho protein synthesis and FGF-23 overproduction suppression [51–53].

Since the serum FGF-23 level (as more earlier marker of MBD than PTH in CKD) rises before serum phosphorus increases as CKD advances, a preventive decrease in phosphorus diet content in CKD patients with elevated serum FGF-23 levels and the use of phosphate-binding drugs (for the control of serum phosphorus levels below 6.5 mg/dL) in CKD advancing are becoming an important therapeutic task in CKD patients. It can contribute not only in the prevention of SGPT but of CVC in CKD.

In our study [51], in the group of CKD 5D, patients who managed to reach and maintain the target level of serum phosphorus (0.9–1.45 mmol/L), compared to the matched group of patients with uncorrected hyperphosphatemia (>1.45 mmol/L), lower FGF-23 and PTH ($p < 0.01$ and $p < 0.05$ respectively) in serum were noted, mainly among those patients who used phosphate-binding drugs that did not contain calcium (sevelamer hydrochloride) for correction of hyperphosphatasemia.

Among 17 patients who received low-protein diet (LPD) in combination with phosphate binders for at least 12 months before starting HD and who achieved the target level of serum phosphorus during the first year of treatment with regular HD, the formation of SGPT was noted significantly less ($\chi^2 = 8, 2$; $p < 0.05$) than among those patients who has begun correction of elevated serum phosphorus simultaneously starting with haemodialysis treatment. In these patients, CVC such as worsening of the functional class of angina pectoris, acute coronary syndrome and acute myocardial infarction [51] were also reliably less noted.

In experimental studies, increased Klotho expression was accompanied by a decrease in proteinuria and a significant decrease in angiotensin II in the hypertensive chronic glomerulonephritis mice [54, 55].

Data on the role of the asymmetric dimethylarginine complex 17/transforming growth factor-α/endothelial growth factor (ADAM17/TGF-α/EGFR) induced both due to renin-angiotensin system (RAS) activation and calcitriol deficiency, in the restructuring of the PTGs and in the decrease of Klotho expression in kidneys, allows to suggest the importance of the effective blockade of RAS by renin angiotensin blockers as well as D-hormone deficiency correction for the prevention and treatment of SGPT [55]. Our preliminary results [53, 56] confirm the experimental studies on the ability of AT II blockers to maintain the renal production of sKlotho protein.

It has been reported that angiotensin II and aldosterone, through the initiation of oxidative stress, have the ability to low Klotho expression in rat kidneys, even in minimal concentrations, while exogenous sKlotho infusion contributed to the inversion of renal damage caused by angiotensin II [55].

In our study in patients with CKD stages 1–5D [56] when comparing the patients with hypertension who were receiving antihypertensive monotherapy, the highest serum levels of Klotho protein were observed in those of them whose target BP level was achieved primarily through angiotensin II receptor blockers, compared to those who were administered with another drug group or have not reached the target blood pressure level ($p = 0.008$ and $p = 0.067$ respectively).

On experimental model of mice with CKD and arterial hypertension (AH), it was established that one of the mechanisms of sKlotho cardioprotection is also its ability to block the calcium channels in cardiomyocytes (TRPC6) that contributes to more adequate correction of AH and slower remodelling of the left ventricular myocardium [57].

A number of studies have shown that hypoxia due to anaemia is an independent factor of sKlotho protein production reduction as CKD advances [5, 6, 14]. According to our data, in patients with CKD with anaemia who managed to reach the target haemoglobin with the help of epoetin and iron and maintain it in this range and, as a result, eliminating the hypoxia of vital organs, including the kidneys, the preservation of decreasing of sKlotho protein was noted [58].

According to the results of our study [52], the use of Low Protein Diet (LPD) in combination with keto/amino acids, during not less than 12 months, in patients with 3B–4 stages of CKD, can prevent the development of nutritional status disorders, as well as stimulate sKlotho expression and suppress FGF-23 production. In addition, in these group patients, impairment of vascular damping function (according to the assessment of pulse wave velocity and augmentation indices by «SphygmoCor» device) as well as cardiac (by EchoCG, semiquantitative scale) and aorta calcification (by Kauppila method), and the formation of LVH, was less common.

In addition, according to our data, in patients with CKD 3B–4 stages using of LPD (0.6 g protein per kg body weight/day) supplemented with calcium salts of keto acids, it was possible to achieve and maintain the target level of serum phosphorus and calcium by using lower doses of phosphate-binding drugs, compared with the patients who used LPD, but did not take keto/amino acids [51, 52].

Maintenance of the phosphorus and calcium target serum levels can be a factor that inhibits FGF-23 overproduction and reduces the risk of ectopic mineralization and FGF-23-dependent LVH in CKD 3B–4 stages [51].

It is known that sKlotho paracrine functions include the activation of calcium channel receptors (TRPVs), especially TRPV5 and TRPV6 [14, 59]. TRPV5 are located mainly in the distal renal tubules and participate in the reabsorption of calcium in the kidneys [14]. TRPV6 is expressed in intestinal epithelial cells, where it is involved in the intestinal calcium absorption [14, 59]. In mice with a defect in Klotho gene expression, an increase in the serum level of phosphorus and calcium was revealed [5, 14]. Taking into account the participation of sKlotho in providing the constancy of serum calcium concentration by changing its reabsorption in the kidneys and intestines, it can be assumed that as a result of the intake of calcium salts of keto acids, it is possible to stimulate sKlotho production with its effect on the prevention of transient hypercalcaemia episodes in CKD advancement.

4. Conclusion

Understanding of the role of Klotho, FGF-23 and sclerostin in CKD is important, because it is known that mortality from cardiovascular complications in 20-year-old patients with terminal kidney disease is comparable with such of 80-year-old subjects in total population

[2]. And this very high mortality risk cannot be explained solely by influence of traditional CVD risk factors, which are highly prevalent in patients with CKD as well as by traditional CKD factors such as phosphorus and PTH, correction of which did not result to enough beneficial effects on cardiovascular survival.

Initial disturbances of mineral bone metabolism begin early, already with 3A stage of CKD, with an increase in serum FGF-23 and sclerostin and decrease of Klotho levels. The manifestation of these early changes may be as an increase in phosphorus excretion. From this moment, cardiovascular risk begins to be pawned, although the levels of phosphorus and PTH in serum are usually normal yet.

The accumulated data allow to consider the disturbances in FGF-23-Klotho-sclerostin ratio as one of the early markers of CKD advancement, disorders of mineral metabolism developing and cardiovascular prognosis. Alteration of the FGF-23/sKlotho/sclerostin ratio in serum as CKD advancement is accompanied by the development of vascular calcification, formation of cardiac remodelling and increasing risk of death from cardiovascular events, independently of the serum phosphorus and PTH levels. Changing the ratio of FGF-23, sKlotho and sclerostin can be regarded as independent early marker of cardiovascular and overall prognosis of patients with CKD.

In the reduction of Klotho expression in the kidneys, the role of ischemia, oxidative stress, intracellular elevation of angiotensin II and inflammation was established. These changes require careful correction to maintain Klotho's production as a potent strong cardio-renoprotective factor.

The preliminary results obtained on the positive effects of hypertension and anaemia correction on sKlotho protein maintenance, as well as the possibility of the FGF-23 overproduction suppression by correcting hyperphosphatemia, demonstrate the need for a personalized approach to the choice of cardio-renoprotective therapy from the early stages of CKD based on the degree of morphogenetic proteins and sclerostin system dysfunction as well as open prospects for studying of cardio-nephroprotective strategy in the new aspect.

Acknowledgements

This work was supported by Russian Science Foundation (grant №.14-15-00947 2014).

Author details

Ludmila Y. Milovanova*, Victor V. Fomin, Lidia V. Lysenko (Kozlovskaya), Nikolay A. Mukhin, Svetlana Y. Milovanova, Marina V. Taranova, Yuriy S. Milovanov, Vasiliy V. Kozlov and Aigul Zh. Usubalieva

*Address all correspondence to: ludm.milovanova@gmail.com

I.M. Sechenov First Moscow State Medical University, Moscow, Russian Federation

References

[1] Couser WG, Remuzzi G, Mendis S, et al. The contribution of chronic kidney disease to the global burden of major noncommunicable diseases. Kidney International. 2011;**80**(12):1258-1270. DOI: 10.1038/ki.2011.368

[2] Go AS, Chertow GM, Fan D, et al. Chronic kidney disease and the risks of death, cardiovascular events, and hospitalization. New England Journal of Medicine. 2004;**351**:1296-1305. DOI: 10.1056/NEJMoa041031

[3] Garland JS, Holden RM, Groome PA, et al. Prevalence and associations of coronary artery calcification in patients with stages 3 to 5 CKD without cardiovascular disease. American Journal of Kidney Disease. 2008;**52**(5):849-858. DOI: 10.1053/j.ajkd.2008.04.012

[4] Middleton RJ, Parfrey PS, Foley RN. Left ventricular hypertrophy in the renal patient. Journal of the American Society of Nephrology. 2001;**12**:1079-1084.

[5] Hu MC, Shiizaki K, Kuro-o M, et al. Fibroblast growth factor 23 and Klotho: Physiology and pathophysiology of an endocrine network of mineral metabolism. Annual Review of Physiology. 2013;**75**:503-533. DOI: 10.1146/annurev-physiol-030212-183727

[6] Semba RD, Cappola AR, Sun K, et al. Plasma klotho and cardiovascular disease in adults. Journal of American Geriatrics Society. 2011;**59**:1596-1601. DOI: 10.1111/j.1532-5415.2011.03558.x

[7] Faul C, Ansel P. FGF-23 induces left ventricular hypertrophy. Journal of Clinical Investigation. 2011;**121**(11):4393-4408. DOI: 10.1172/JCI46122

[8] Isakova T, Wahl P, Vargas GS, et al. Fibroblast growth factor 23 is elevated before parathyroid hormone and phosphate in chronic kidney disease. Kidney International 2011;**79**:1370-1378. DOI: 10.1038/ki.2011.47

[9] Milovanova LY, Kozlovscaya LV, Markina MM. Morphogenetic proteins—Fibroblast growth factor-23 (FGF-23) and Klotho in the serum of patients with chronic kidney disease. Clinical Medicine. 2015;**93**(12):32-38. DOI: 616.61-036.12-06:616.1]-07

[10] Razzaque MS, Lanske B. The emerging role of the fibroblast growth factor-23-klotho axis in renal regulation of phosphate homeostasis. Journal of Endocrinology. 2007;**194**(1):1-10. DOI: 10.1677/JOE-07-0095

[11] Ben-Dov IZ, Galitzer H, Lavi-Moshayoff V, et al. The parathyroid is a target organ for FGF-23 in rats. Journal of Clinical Investigation. 2007;**117**:4003-4008. DOI: 10.1172/JCI32409

[12] Bergwitz C, Jüppner H. Regulation of phosphate homeostasis by PTH, vitamin D, and FGF23. Annual Review of Medicine. 2010;**61**:91-104. DOI: 10.1146/annurev.med.051308.111339

[13] Kuro-o M, Matsumura Y, Aizawa H, et al. Mutation of the mouse klotho gene leads to a syndrome resembling ageing. Nature 1997;**390**:45-51. DOI: 10.1038/36285

[14] Kuro-o M. Klotho and chronic kidney disease – Whats new? Nephrology, Dialysis, Transplantation. 2009;**24**(6):1705-1708. DOI: 10.1093/ndt/gfp069

[15] Nagai R, Saito Y, Ohyama Y, et al. Endothelial dysfunction in the klotho mouse and downregulation of klotho gene expression in various animal models of vascular and metabolic diseases. Cellular and Molecular Life Sciences. 2000;**57**:738-746. DOI: 10.1007/s000180050038

[16] Kusaba T, Okigaki M, Matui A, et al. Klotho is associated with VEGF receptor-2 and the transient receptor potential canonical-1 Ca^{2+} channel to maintain endothelial integrity. Proceedings of the National Academy of Sciences of the United States of America. 2010;**107**:19308-19313. DOI: 10.1073/pnas.1008544107

[17] Imura A, Tsuji Y, Murata M, et al. Alpha-Klotho as a regulator of calcium homeostasis. Science. 2007;**316**:1615-1618. DOI: 10.1126/science.1135901

[18] Kurosu H, Yamamoto M, Clark JD, et al. Suppression of aging in mice by the hormone Klotho. Science. 2005;**309**:1829-1833. DOI: 10.1126/science.1112766

[19] Semba RD, Cappola AR, Sun K, et al. Plasma klotho and mortality risk in older community-dwelling adults. Journals of Gerontology. Series A, Biological Sciences and Medical Sciences. 2011;**66**:794-800. DOI: 10.1093/gerona/glr058

[20] Koh N, Fujimori T, Nishiguchi S, et al. Severely reduced production of klotho in human chronic renal failure kidney. Biochemical and Biophysical Research Communications. 2001;**280**(4):1015-1020. DOI: 10.1006/bbrc.2000.4226

[21] Vervloet M, Larsson T. Fibroblast growth factor-23 and Klotho in chronic kidney disease. Kidney International Supplements. 2011;**1**:130-135. http://dx.doi.org/10.1038/kisup.2011.29

[22] Claes KJ, Viaene L, Heye S, et al. Sclerostin: Another vascular calcification inhibitor? Journal of Clinical Endocrinology and Metabolism. 2013;**98**(8):3221-3228. DOI: 10.1210/jc.2013-1521

[23] Brandenburg VM, et al. Relationship between sclerostin and cardiovascular calcification in hemodialysis patients: A cross-sectional study. BMC Nephrology. 2013;**14**:219. DOI: 10.1186/1471-2369-14-219

[24] Moester MJ, Papapoulos SE, Löwik CW, et al. Sclerostin: Current knowledge and future perspectives. Calcified Tissue International. 2010;**87**(2):99-1077. DOI: 10.1007/s00223-010-9372-1

[25] Register TC, Hruska KA, Divers J, et al. Sclerostin is positively associated with bone mineral density in men and women and negatively associated with carotid calcified atherosclerotic plaque in men from the african american-diabetes heart study. Journal of Clinical Endocrinology and Metabolism. 2014;**99**(1):315-321. DOI: 10.1210/jc.2013-3168

[26] Hsu B-G, Liou H-H, Lee C-J, et al. Serum sclerostin as an independent marker of peripheral arterial stiffness in renal transplantation recipients a cross-sectional study. Medicine (Baltimore). 2016;**95**(15):e3300. DOI: 10.1097/MD.0000000000003300

[27] Brandenburg VM, Floege J. Adynamic bone disease—bone and beyond. NDT Plus. 2008;**3**:135-147. DOI: 10.1093/ndtplus/sfn040

[28] Seiler S. Associations of FGF-23 and Klotho with cardiovascular outcomes among patients with CKD stage 2-4. Clinical Journal of the American Society of Nephrology. 2014;**9**(6):1049-1058. DOI: 10.2215/CJN.07870713

[29] Gutiérrez OM, Januzzi JL, Isakova T, et al. Fibroblast growth factor-23 and left ventricular hypertrophy in chronic kidney disease Circulation 2009;**119**(19):2545-2552. DOI: 10.1161/CIRCULATIONAHA.108.844506

[30] Yilmaz MI, Sonmez A, Saglam M, et al. FGF-23 and vascular dysfunction in patients with stage 3 and 4 chronic kidney disease. Kidney International. 2010;**78**:679-685. DOI: 10.1038/ki.2010.194

[31] Gutierrez O, Mannstadt M, Isakova T, et al. Fibroblast growth factor 23 and mortality among hemodialysis patients. New England Journal of Medicine. 2008;**359**:584-592. DOI: 10.1056/NEJMoa0706130

[32] Kardami E. Fibroblast growth factor 2 isoforms and cardiac hypertrophy. Cardiovascular Research. 2004;**63**(3):458-466. DOI: https://doi.org/10.1016/j.cardiores.2004.04.024

[33] Di Marco GS, Reuter S, Kentrup D, et al. Treatment of established left ventricular hypertrophy with fibroblast growth factor receptor blockade in an animal model of CKD. Nephrology, Dialysis, Transplantation. 2014;**10**:1-8. DOI: 10.1093/ndt/gfu190

[34] Milovanova LY, Kozlovskaya LV, Milovanova SY, et al. Associations of fibroblast growth factor 23, soluble Klotho, troponin I in CKD patients. International Research Journal. 2016;**9**(51):65-69. DOI: 10.18454/IRJ.2016.51.074

[35] Majd A, Mirza I, Hansen T, et al. Relationship between circulating FGF23 and total body atherosclerosis in the community. Nephrol. Dial. Transplant. 2009;**24**(10):3125-3131. DOI: https://doi.org/10.1093/ndt/gfp205

[36] Coen G, Ballanti P, Silvestrini G, et al. Immunohistochemical localization and mRNA expression of matrix Gla-protein and fetuin-A in bone biopsies of hemodialysis patients. Virchows Archiv. 2009;**454**:263-271. DOI: 10.1007/s00428-008-0724-4

[37] Gutiérrez OM, Mannstadt M, Isakova T, et al. Fibroblast growth factor 23 and mortality among patients undergoing hemodialysis. New England Journal of Medicine. 2008;**359**(6):584-592. DOI: 10.1056/NEJMoa0706130.

[38] Fliser D, Kollerits B, Neyer U, et al. Fibroblast growth factor 23 (FGF-23) predicts progression of chronic kidney disease. The Mild to Moderate Kidney Disease (MMKD) study. Journal of the American Society of Nephrology. 2007;**18**(9):2601-2608. DOI: 10.1681/ASN.2006080936

[39] Kuczera P, Adamczak M, Wiecek A. Fibroblast growth factor-23—A potential uremic toxin. Toxins (Basel). 2016;**8**(12):369. DOI: 10.3390/toxins8120369

[40] Ichikawa S, Imel EA, Kreiter ML, et al. A homozygous missense mutation in human KLOTHO causes severe tumoral calcinosis. Journal of Clinical Investigation 2007; **117**:2684-2691. DOI: 10.1172/JCI31330

[41] Takeshita K, Fujimori T, Kurotaki Y, et al. Sinoatrial node dysfunction and early unexpected death of mice with a defect of klotho gene expression. Circulation. 2004;**109**(14):1776-1782. DOI: 10.1161/01.CIR.0000124224.48962

[42] Monroe DG, McGee-Lawrence ME, Oursler MJ, et al. Update on Wnt signaling in bone cell biology and bone disease. Gene. 2012;**492**(1):1-18. DOI: S0378-1119(11)00650-0 [pii]

[43] Yamamoto M, Clark JD, Pastor JV, et al. Regulation of oxidative stress by the anti-aging hormone klotho. Journal of Biological Chemistry. 2005;**280**:38029-38034.

[44] Maekawa Y, Ishikawa K, Yasuda O, et al. Klotho suppresses TNF-alpha-induced expression of adhesion molecules in the endothelium and attenuates NF-kappaB activation. Endocrine. 2009;**35**:341-346. DOI: 10.1007/s12020-009-9181-3

[45] Milovanova LIu, Milovanov IuS, Kozlovskaia LV et al. New markers of cardio-renal links in chronic kidney disease. Terapevticheskii Arkhiv. 2013;**85**(6):17-24. DOI: https://www.ncbi.nlm.nih.gov/pubmed/23866594

[46] Yeun JY. C-Reactive protein predicts all-cause and cardiovascular mortality in hemodialysis patients. American Journal of Kidney Diseases. 2000;**35**:469-476. DOI: http://dx.doi.org/10.1016/S0272-6386(00)70200-9

[47] KDIGO 2012 clinical practice guideline for the evaluation and management of chronic kidney disease. Kidney Int. 2013;3 (Suppl.1) KDIGO-CKD-MBD 2009Work Group. KDIGO clinical practice guideline for the diagnosis, evolution, prevention, and treatment of chronic kidney disease-mineral and bone disorder (CKD-MBD). Kidney International. 2009;**76**(Suppl. 113):1-130

[48] Milovanova LYu, Milovanov YuS, Kudryavtseva DV, et al. Role of the morphogenetic proteins FGF-23 and Klotho and the glycoprotein sclerostin in the assessment of the risk of cardiovascular diseases and the prognosis of chronic kidney disease. Terapevticheskii Arkhiv. 2015;**87**(6):10-16. DOI: https://www.ncbi.nlm.nih.gov/pubmed/26281189

[49] Drechsler C, Evenepoel P, Vervloet MG. High levels of circulating sclerostin are associated with better cardiovascular survival in incident dialysis patients: Results from the NECOSAD study. Nephrology, Dialysis, Transplantation. 2015;**30**(2):288-293. DOI: 10.1093/ndt/gfu301

[50] Viaene L, Behets G, Claes K, et al. Sclerostin: Another bone-related protein related to all-cause mortality in hemodialysis? Nephrology, Dialysis, Transplantation. 2013;**28**(12):3024-3030. DOI: 10.1186/1471-2369-15-190

[51] Mukhin NA, Milovanov YS, Kozlovskaya LV, et al. The serum level of the morphogenetic protein fibroblast growth factor 23 (FGF-23) as a marker for the efficiency of hyperphosphatemia therapy with phosphate-binding agents in chronic kidney disease. Terapevticheskii Arkhiv. 2016;**88**(4):41-45. DOI: https://www.ncbi.nlm.nih.gov/pubmed/27070162

[52] Milovanova LY, Dobrosmislov IA, Milovanov YS. Influence of essential amino acids ketoanalogs and protein restriction to phosphoric-calcium metabolism regulators production—morphogenetic proteins (FGF-23 and Klotho) in CKD patients 3B-4 stages. Nephrology. 2016;**20**(2):15-20. DOI: http://nefr.elpub.ru/jour/article/view/170/171

[53] Milovanova LY, Kozlovscaya LV, Milovanova SY, et al. Influence of traditional cardio-nephroprotective therapy on cardiovascular risk markers (FGF-23, Klotho) in patients with chronic kidney disease. International Research Journal. 2016;**7**(38 part 5):39-41. DOI: 10.18454/IRJ.2227-6017

[54] Maltese G, Karalliedde J. The putative role of the antiageing protein klotho in cardiovascular and renal disease. International Journal of Hypertension. 2012;**12**:5. DOI: 10.1155/2012/757469

[55] Yoon HE, Ghee JY, Piao S, et al. Angiotensin II blockage upregulates the expression of Klotho, the anti-ageing gene, in an experimental model of chronic cyclosporine nephropathy. Nephrology, Dialysis, Transplantation. 2011;**26**:800-813. DOI: https://doi.org/10.1093/ndt/gfq537

[56] Milovanova LY, Mukhin NA, Kozlovskaya LV, et al. Decreased serum levels of Klotho protein in CKD patients: Clinical importance. Annals of the Russian Academy of Medical Science. 2016;**71**(4):288-296. DOI: 10.15690/vramn581

[57] Xie J, Cha S-K, An S-W, et al. Cardioprotection by Klotho through downregulation of TRPC6 channels in the mouse heart. Nature Communications. 2012;**3**:1238-1242. DOI: 10.1038/ncomms2240

[58] Milovanov YS, Mukhin NA, Kozlovskaya LV, et al. Impact of anemia correction on the production of the circulating morphogenetic protein α-Klotho in patients with Stages 3B—4 chronic kidney disease: A new direction of cardionephroprotection. Terapevticheskii Arkhiv. 2016;**88**(6):21-25. DOI: 10.17116/terarkh201688621-25

[59] Cha SK, Ortega B, Kurosu H, et al. Removal of sialic acid involving Klotho causes cell-surface retention of TRPV5 channel via binding to galectin-1. Proceedings of the National Academy of Science of the United States of America. 2008;**105**:9805-9810. DOI: 10.1073/pnas.0803223105

Chapter 3

Mechanisms and Clinical Implications of Vascular Calcifications in Chronic Kidney Disease

Cristina Capusa and Daria Popescu

Additional information is available at the end of the chapter

http://dx.doi.org/10.5772/intechopen.72717

Abstract

Chronic kidney disease (CKD), a major public health problem that affects up to 10–13% of the general population worldwide, imposes considerable socio-economic burden due to both the need for renal replacement therapy and, even more important, the negative influence on the overall patients' health status. Cardiovascular (CV) diseases are the main cause of death in CKD patients and are triggered not only by the traditional CV risk factors but also by specific, uremia-related, factors. Among these, calcium-phosphate and bone metabolism disorders play a central role. Abnormalities of mineral metabolism occur early, evolve silently as the kidney function deteriorates, and are associated with CV morbidity and mortality, mainly by the development of valvular and vascular calcifications. This chapter aims to summarize the recent knowledge on the types and mechanisms of arterial calcifications, as well as their clinical implications, in the setting of CKD. The issue is significant for both nephrologists and cardiologists and could be an example of the requirement for interdisciplinary collaboration in the medical practice.

Keywords: atherosclerosis and arteriosclerosis, arterial stiffness, calcifications, cardiovascular morbidity, chronic kidney disease

1. Introduction

The prevalence of chronic kidney disease (CKD) is constantly growing [1] largely due to the shift in age distribution of the population toward individuals older than 60 years, in which CKD is more common, accounted for by the combined effect of physiologic decline in glomerular filtration rate (GFR) and systemic atherosclerosis, and also due to increasing prevalence of arterial hypertension, diabetes mellitus, and obesity, all risk factors for CKD. Notably, the mortality of CKD patients is higher than their non-CKD counterparts, predominantly with respect to cardiovascular mortality. Abnormalities of arterial and left ventricular functions, such as arterial stiffness, atherosclerosis and arteriosclerosis, left ventricular hypertrophy, and systolic and end-diastolic stiffness, which are common in CKD patients, were incriminated [2]. The pathophysiology of cardiovascular disease (CVD) in CKD is complex, with both traditional and uremia-related risk factors being involved. Among the latter, calcium-phosphate metabolism anomalies are more and more debated, and the concept of chronic kidney disease-mineral and bone disorder (CKD-MBD) has been adopted. It is a broad term that refers to a systemic disorder of mineral metabolism due to the kidneys' failure to maintain homeostasis of calcium (Ca), phosphate (PO_4), and active vitamin D, which leads to maladaptive alterations in related hormones, namely fibroblast growth factor-23 (FGF23) and parathyroid hormone (PTH), and results in defective bone architecture and extraskeletal calcifications [3, 4]. CKD-MBD occurs early in the course of CKD, progresses as kidney function declines, and it is manifested by three separate, but interrelated, components that are not necessarily present concurrently in all patients, any combination of these component being possible [4]:

1. Changes in biochemistry profile (Ca, PO_4, vitamin D, PTH, FGF23, and alkaline phosphatase—ALP), which reflect mineral and hormonal abnormalities;
2. Bone abnormalities regarding turnover, mineralization, volume, linear growth, or strength; and
3. Soft tissue (vascular, valvular, and periarticular) calcifications.

The vascular calcifications at least partially account for increased cardiovascular (CV) risk in CKD patients, so it is worth to draw attention on the mechanisms involved in their development.

2. Types and characteristics of vascular calcification in chronic kidney disease

Even at early ages, CKD patients develop vascular calcifications at all the levels (large vessel arteries such as the aorta, medium arteries like the coronary arteries, as well as small-caliber arteries of the skin), in a much greater proportion than the general population, and the prevalence and severity of arterial and valvular calcifications increase as kidney function decreases [5].

The main types of arterial calcifications, both commonly seen in CKD, are distinguished by their location in the structure of the arterial wall (**Figure 1**) and their association with atherosclerotic plaque formation:

1. *Atherosclerosis* consists in the calcification of the intimal layer in association with cellular necrosis, inflammation, atherosclerotic plaques, and lipid deposition [6]. This type of calcification is related to traditional risk factors such as arterial hypertension and dyslipidemia (**Table 1**). The vessel lumen is eccentrically reduced and deformed due to patchy calcification of the atherosclerotic plaques [7]. It produces arterial stenosis which accounts for tissular ischemia and infarction and may predispose to plaque rupture generating life-threatening thrombi.
2. *Arteriosclerosis*, which represents the calcification of the medial layer, occurs in the elastic lamina of large-caliber and medium- to small-size arteries. It seems to be independent of atherosclerosis, although both can coexist [6, 7]. Medial calcification was known initially as

Mönckeberg's sclerosis, and it has radiographically been described as "railroad tracks" on the peripheral arteries of upper and lower limbs [6, 8]. This type of calcification is related to non-traditional risk factors such as hyperphosphatemia, excess PTH, and cytokines of chronic inflammation (**Table 1**), and it is more prevalent in patients with CKD and diabetes [6]. The vessel lumen is reduced concentrically due to amorphous mineral that forms circumferentially along or within one or more elastic lamellae of the media [7]. It induces arterial stiffness, which contributes to increased pulse pressure and, consequently, to left ventricular hypertrophy and altered coronary perfusion [9, 10].

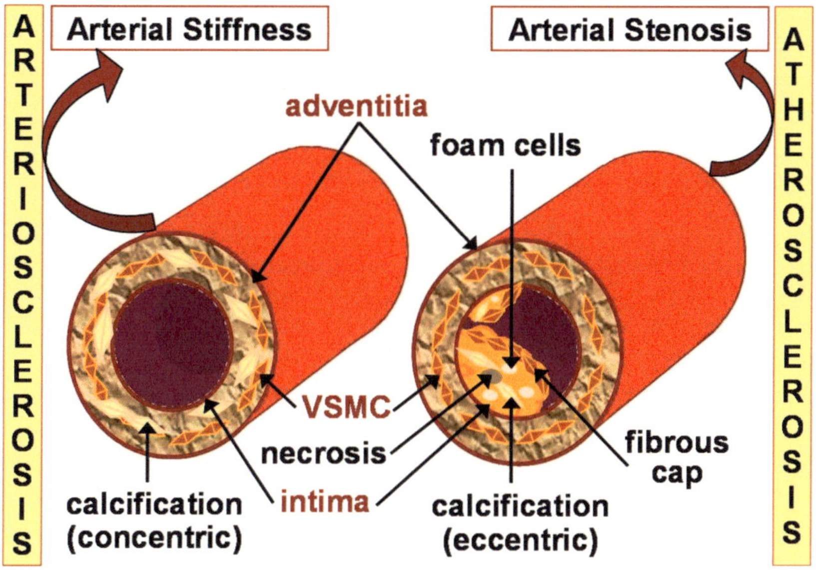

Figure 1. Main types of arterial calcifications and their consequences. VSMCs, vascular smooth muscle cells.

Traditional risk factors	Non-traditional (CKD-related) risk factors
Arterial hypertension	Hyperphosphatemia, high calcium-phosphate product
Dyslipidemia	Hyper- or hypoparathyroidism
Diabetes mellitus	High dosage of vitamin D metabolites
Smoking	Chronic inflammation
Old age	Oxidative stress
Family history of premature coronary heart disease	Metabolic abnormalities: hypoalbuminemia, hyperhomocysteinemia
	Decrease of calcification inhibitors (Fetuin-A)
	Anemia

CKD: chronic kidney disease.

Table 1. Risk factors for vascular calcification in chronic kidney disease patients (modified from Román-García et al. [5]).

These two types of calcifications encountered in CKD also vary based on their localization on the arterial tree. Intimal calcifications are found more proximally, while medial ones have a predilection for distal sites [10].

Etiologically, vascular calcifications may be categorized as metastatic calcifications, those which arise from systemically high calcium and phosphate product, or dystrophic calcifications, which take place under pathologic conditions of cell death or apoptosis [9]. *Metastatic calcifications* occur when the calcium-phosphate product exceeds its solubility in serum resulting in its deposition in healthy, extraskeletal tissue such as the arterial wall, the viscera, the conjunctiva, articulations, or tumors [8]. In contrast, *dystrophic calcifications* result from the de novo deposition of calcium and phosphate in diseased or damaged tissue. This occurs when cells die as a result of direct injury or apoptosis and release their intracellular calcium contents which can serve as a foundation for further calcium deposition [8].

3. Pathogenesis of vascular calcifications in chronic kidney disease

3.1. Overview on the molecular basis of mineralization and vascular calcifications

Although not yet entirely elucidated, the process of vascular calcification was extensively studied and the bulk of its steps were unveiled. The common feature to almost all physiologic mineralization mechanisms, either inside the bone or in extra-osseous tissues, involves matrix vesicles, which form the nidus for hydroxyapatite crystals nucleation [11]. These matrix vesicles are membrane-bound particles of 20–200 nm where mineral crystals are arranged by interaction with specific regulators, like membrane transporters and enzymes, with crucial roles in the influx of calcium and phosphate ions into the vesicles [9]. For example, tissue nonspecific alkaline phosphatase hydrolyzes pyrophosphate and generates inorganic phosphate, which is further transported through the vesicle membrane by the sodium-phosphate cotransporter type III [12]. On the other hand, annexins function as ion channels and provide a way for calcium to enter inside the matrix vesicle, where the accumulation of both divalent ions induces crystalline nucleation [9, 12].

In the bone, matrix vesicles bud off from the plasma membrane of chondrocytes or osteoblasts, at the epiphyseal plate of growing bone and are released into the premineralized organic matrix where they serve as a vehicle for the interaction of calcium and phosphate ions to form hydroxyapatite and initiate mineralization of the organic substance [11]. Hydroxyapatite crystals that are released from vesicles serve as templates for subsequent crystal formation, creating the lattice of the bone [9, 13]. Therefore, matrix vesicles have an osteogenic role.

Growing body of evidence supports significant resemblance between bone and vascular calcifications, leading to the belief that ectopic calcifications and normal osteogenesis are driven alike. Indeed, many cellular and molecular signaling processes are identical in vascular calcification and osteogenesis. Among these, matrix vesicle release and expression of mineralization-regulating proteins by vascular smooth muscle cells (VSMCs) are seen in the vessel wall [14]. Consequently, vascular calcification is also considered a regulated biomineralization process.

The balance among promoters and inhibitors of calcification plays the key role during mineralization (**Figure 2**).

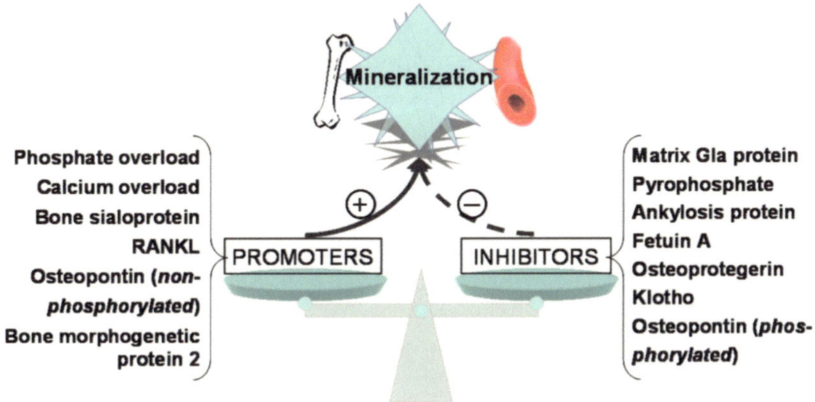

Figure 2. Regulating molecules of the mineralization/calcification processes. RANKL, receptor activator of nuclear factor-kB ligand; (+), stimulation; (−), inhibition.

The main known inhibitor molecules involved in both bone and extra-osseous sites calcification, are:

1. *Matrix GLA protein* (MGP, matrix γ-carboxyglutamate protein), an extracellular protein has roles in normal bone formation as well as inhibition of vascular calcification [15, 16]. The inactive MGP (desphospho-uncarboxylated MGP, dp-ucMGP) needs two subsequent modifications (serine phosphorylation and glutamate carboxylation) in order to exert its function [17]. Circulating levels of dp-uc MGP are considered a biomarker associated with cardiovascular risk and mortality, severity of the vascular damage, and all-cause mortality [17]. MGP is able to bind calcium and hydroxyapatite, thanks to its vitamin K-dependent γ-carboxylation, inhibiting their precipitation and mineralization [16]. MGP synthesis has been detected in cartilage, lung, heart, kidney, arteries, and calcified atherosclerotic plaques attesting to MGP's role in inhibition of soft tissue calcifications [18]. In addition, recent works suggested a link between MGP and renal microvasculature, and argued in favor of a possible renoprotective action of activated MGP and, consequently, emphasized the importance of having adequate vitamin K stores [17].

2. *Osteoprotegerin* (OPG) is a soluble cytokine and tumor necrosis factor (TNF) receptor-like molecule that acts as an inhibitor of osteoclast differentiation by binding the receptor activator of nuclear factor κB-ligand (RANKL), thus blocking RANKL-mediated activation of osteoclasts [11, 19]. OPG is present in many human tissues: bone (osteoblasts), vessels (endothelial and vascular smooth muscle cells), lung, heart, liver, kidney, hypothalamus, lymphoid organs and B-cells, bone marrow, articular chondrocytes, and breasts [19, 20]. Its expression in bone is regulated by osteoblasts through the same pathway that regulates bone formation, indicating RANKL/OPG ratio is a major determinant of bone mass and OPG has an osteoprotective role [21]. However, its functions in the vascular system are still a matter of debate. While experimental studies sustain an anti-calcification role (due to

inhibition of apoptotic passive calcification and the alkaline phosphatase-mediated osteogenic differentiation of vascular cells), elevated serum levels of OPG were found in various cardiovascular diseases and were hypothesized as a promoter of atherosclerosis progression [19]. Osteoprotegerin expression was significantly lower and RANKL was identified in calcified valves of human aortic stenosis, indicating that in the absence of inhibition by OPG, RANKL may promote matrix calcification and induce the expression of osteoblast-associated genes (bone alkaline phosphatase and osteocalcin) [22].

3. *Extracellular pyrophosphate* (PPi) is a small molecule made of two phosphate ions linked by an ester bond, which regulates cell differentiation and serves as an essential physiologic inhibitor of calcification by negatively interfering with hydroxyapatite formation and crystal growth [11]. PPi is produced from the hydrolyses of extracellular adenosine-5′-triphosphate by the enzyme ectonucleotide pyrophosphatase/phosphodiesterase [23]. On the other hand, alkaline phosphatase (ALP) catalyzes the hydrolysis of phospho-monoesters (including PPi) with release of inorganic phosphate (P_i) in order to avoid accumulation of this mineralization inhibitor, thus ensuring normal bone mineralization [11, 24]. However, through this action, ALP also acts as a powerful inducer of vascular calcification partially as a result of increased PPi degradation [23].

4. *Fetuin-A*, a circulating glycoprotein from the cystatin superfamily of proteins, produced by the liver, functions as a potent inhibitor of de novo hydroxyapatite formation from supersaturated mineral solutions, and it also acts as a negative acute phase reactant, thus being downregulated in acute and chronic systemic inflammation [25–27]. In experimental and clinical studies, it was shown that serum containing fetuin-A inhibited precipitation of calcium salts in a dose-dependent manner, and its serum concentrations were inversely correlated to C-reactive protein, calcifications, and cardiovascular and all-cause mortality, even when the serum calcium-phosphate product was close to the normal range [26, 28]. Hence, it was assumed that a major link between low fetuin-A levels and mortality consists of promoting accelerated cardiovascular calcification [26].

Other main factors with essential contribution to the processes of mineralization and calcification are those involved in the signaling pathways, like:

1. *Bone morphogenetic proteins* (BMPs) are cytokines with multiple functions, which modulate gene expression through phosphorylation of regulatory Smad transcription factors [16, 27]. Smad6 and Smad7 proteins act as negative regulators and thus are crucial to limit the osteogenic vascular response induced by BMPs [27]. For example, BMP 2—a protein that belongs to the transforming growth factor-β (TGF-β) superfamily of cell regulatory proteins—is involved in both osteogenic and chondrogenic differentiation of multipotent mesenchymal progenitors and drives the formation of cartilage and bone [29]. It also participates in vascular calcification probably through inducing osteoblastic differentiation of VSMCs. Conversely, BMP 7, primarily expressed in the kidney where it is required for the normal development of the organ, was found to restore the bone anabolic balance, reduce serum phosphate levels, and reduce vascular calcification [27].

2. *Core-binding factor alpha 1* (Cbfa1), also known as runt-related transcription factor 2 (Runx2), is a nuclear protein essential for osteoblastic development and skeletal morphogenesis, and it is believed to be the switch that turns a mesenchymal cell into an osteoblast [11, 13, 30]. It acts

as a scaffold for the interaction of nucleic acids and regulatory factors that are involved in the expression of a number of downstream proteins essential for osteoblastic differentiation, such as type I collagen, osteocalcin, and osteopontin [13].

3. *Type I collagen* makes up over 90% of the organic component of bone where it forms the framework necessary for mineralization [13, 31]. It was shown that ex vivo cells grown on type I collagen were found to mineralize three times faster and incorporate two times more calcium than cells grown in plastic media. Moreover, rapidly mineralizing cells generate a matrix that contains three times the amount of collagen type I and fibronectin but 70% less collagen type IV than their non-mineralizing counterparts. These findings indicate a regulatory role of the matrix composition on arterial calcification development [31].

4. *Osteocalcin* is a protein secreted by active osteoblasts into the extracellular matrix where it binds hydroxyapatite via 3 γ-carboxylated glutamic acid residues during bone mineralization. For this reason, it is often used as a marker for bone formation [32].

5. *Osteopontin*, also known as secreted phosphoprotein 1 or bone sialoprotein 1, is an extracellular structural component of bone (of the non-collagenous organic bone matrix) and an important modulator of bone mineralization, which can either promote or inhibit hydroxyapatite formation, depending on its post-translational modifications [11, 15]. Non-phosphorylated osteopontin shows a stimulatory effect on calcification, while phosphorylation of osteopontin converts it into a potent inhibitor of ectopic calcifications, proportional to the number of phosphorylated sites [33]. Overexpression of osteopontin was found in human atherosclerotic plaques, in calcified smooth muscle cells, in medial layers of arteries of diabetic patient, and calcified heart valves, suggesting it intervenes in the development of ectopic calcifications [34].

In conclusion, mineralization and calcification processes are tightly regulated through the complex interactions of various tissular and circulating molecules, many of which suffer profound changes in chronic kidney disease.

3.2. How does chronic kidney disease favor vascular calcifications?

3.2.1. *Imbalance between pro- and counter-calcification factors*

Vascular calcifications in CKD patients are thought to arise due to disruptions in the balance between promoters and inhibitors of calcification, leading to osteoblastic transformation of vascular smooth muscle cells (VSMCs) [5, 35]. Because VSMCs and osteoblasts derive from a similar mesenchymal cell precursor, VSMCs can be induced to differentiate along osteoblastic lines. The process involves an increase in calcification promoters, decrease in calcification inhibitors, and formation of calcification vesicles culminating with the induction of a cellular phenotypic change from VSMCs to osteoblast-like cells [5].

Concerning *promoters of calcification*, it is recognized that the osteoblastic differentiation, which is the initial step in vascular calcification, is revealed by the expression of pro-calcification factors such as Cbfa1 and BMP on vascular cells [13, 15]. In vitro experiments showed that changes in serum composition like those that occurred in the course of CKD may upregulate expression of Cbfa1, while in vivo studies found higher expression of Cbfa1 in both the media and intima of calcified arteries compared to non-calcified arteries of the same patients, thus emphasizing the important role of Cbfa1 in vascular calcifications [5, 36]. In addition, since positive immunostaining for bone matrix proteins (like osteonectin, osteopontin, bone sialoprotein, alkaline phosphatase, and type I collagen) were more common than overt calcifications but were proportional with their extent, it appears that the deposition of these proteins precedes calcification [36]. Another modulator of calcification—osteocalcin—has been detected in VSMCs where it may potentially regulate their glucose utilization, promoting a phenotypic change in these cells [32]. Furthermore, an inverse correlation between osteopontin plasma levels and glomerular filtration rate (GFR) was reported, suggesting that reduced renal excretion due to impaired kidney function may lead to increased circulating levels [37]. Increased osteopontin and other promoters of calcification in CKD can be accounted for by different mechanisms also. For example, in experimental settings, high concentrations of phosphorus, uremic serum, oxidized lipids, cytokines, and high glucose (abnormalities commonly seen in CKD patients as well) were able to stimulate the VSMCs and vascular pericytes to produce bone-forming transcription factors and proteins [36]. Taken together, these findings suggest that biochemical changes that occur during the progression of CKD (hyperphosphatemia, hypercalcemia, accumulating uremic toxins, cytokines, oxidized lipoproteins, and advanced glycation end products) tip the balance in favor of promoters of vascular calcification.

On the other hand, abnormalities of *calcification inhibitors* can also contribute to the pathogenesis of vascular calcifications in CKD. For example, lower levels of matrix Gla protein were associated with decreased kidney function, probably because metabolic abnormalities due to CKD, such as vitamin D deficiency, may suppress MGP production. Alternatively, MGP may be lost from circulation as it binds to hydroxyapatite crystals in vascular calcifications. Regardless of the mechanism, reduced plasma MGP has been suggested as a marker for the presence and severity of vascular calcifications in patients with CKD [38]. Also, lower levels of circulating fetuin-A were described in CKD and were associated with coronary artery calcification, valvular calcifications, and increased mortality in dialysis patients [36].

These changes in the levels of both promoters and inhibitors of vascular calcification, that occur in CKD patients, ultimately culminate in the *transdifferentiation of VSMCs to an osteoblast phenotype* through an active, cell-mediated, osteogenic process, with the release of calcium matrix vesicles that can nucleate hydroxyapatite and form the first nidus for calcification [11, 30]. The process is driven by upregulation of bone-forming transcription factors and proteins on VSMCs, such as Cbfa1 and bone morphogenetic protein 2, which control the expression of osteogenic proteins (osteocalcin, osteonectin, alkaline phosphatase, collagen type I, and bone sialoprotein). Exposure to high levels of calcium, phosphate, cytokines, and so on, along with the deficit of calcification inhibitors (such as fetuin-A, matrix Gla protein, pyrophosphate) are required for the cells' phenotypic switch [39]. The transformed cells deposit collagen and non-collagenous proteins in the arterial wall and incorporate calcium and phosphorus into matrix vesicles to initiate mineralization and crystal growth. The overall positive calcium and phosphorus balance from CKD patients supports both the cellular transformation and the generation of matrix vesicles [36].

3.2.2. Mineral metabolism abnormalities and vascular calcifications

Elevated calcium levels have long been implicated in the vascular calcifications observed in CKD patients. Early on, these patients are usually hypocalcemic as a result of calcitriol deficiency, but treatment with calcium salts and vitamin D derivatives can induce a positive calcium balance or even overt hypercalcemia [30]. In this context, it is possible that in patients with advanced kidney disease, calcium that is absorbed from the gastrointestinal tract cannot be excreted by the failing kidneys nor can it be deposited in bones with altered turnover (either high or low turnover is detrimental) and is therefore deposited at extra-osseous sites, such as the vascular bed [5, 6]. Calcium changes in the external milieu have a direct effect on the nearby cells. Normally, VSMCs recognize these changes via the membrane such as calcium sensing receptor (CaR) and a G-protein-coupled receptor, which was shown to be downregulated in calcified arteries from CKD patients, suggesting that calcium sensing is disrupted in these patients [6, 40]. In response to elevated extracellular calcium, VSMCs release calcium-laden vesicles, as an attempt to prevent intracellular calcium overload. When the vesicles do not contain enough calcification inhibitors (as in CKD), this adaptive response in fact promotes extracellular matrix calcification by serving as a site of origin for propagated calcification [35].

Besides calcium, *hyperphosphatemia* that is so common in advanced CKD, has emerged as a major culprit of vascular calcifications [41]. Increased serum levels of phosphate induce osteoblastic transformation of VSMCs, while the decrease of phosphatemia reduces the expression of proteins responsible for active bone mineral deposition in vascular cells [15, 35]. As suggested by in vitro studies, phenotypic transformation of VSMCs in response to hyperphosphatemia is mediated by Pit-1 (a type III sodium-phosphate cotransporter), which allow the influx of phosphate into VSMCs and predisposes the cells to undergo mineralization. It was observed that the first step of vascular calcification requires an increased uptake of calcium and phosphate by the VSMCs [42].

In addition to sodium-phosphate cotransport, alkaline phosphatase is necessary for the uptake of phosphorus into the cell and the subsequent induction of osteopontin. Moreover, VSMCs treated with pooled uremic sera from CKD patients also increased expression of osteopontin and mineral deposition, suggesting that uremic serum plays a role in vascular calcifications [43].

Clinical data also support the link between elevated phosphate and vascular calcifications. For example, in a population-based cohort without CKD, serum phosphate levels at the upper end of normal range were associated with aortic valve sclerosis and mitral annular calcification, independent of PTH or calcium values [44]. Moreover, each 1 mg/dL increase in serum phosphate appears to predict higher risk for de novo coronary artery calcification (CAC) over time, with an impact similar to traditional cardiovascular risk factors, in relatively healthy subjects [45]. As in general population, phosphate serum concentration correlated with a greater risk of ectopic calcification in patients with moderate CKD (stage 3), as each 1 mg/dL increase in phosphatemia, even within normal laboratory ranges, was associated with a 21, 33, 25, and 62% higher prevalence of coronary and thoracic arteries, aortic and mitral valves calcifications, respectively [46].

Furthermore, in the presence of increased phosphate, even modest increases in calcium can substantially exacerbate calcification, by inducing nucleation of basic calcium-phosphate and, consequently, the growth of nascent vesicles that are released from both viable and apoptotic VSMCs [47]. The dominant role of phosphate is further supported by experimental studies which showed that dietary phosphate restriction in FGF23-null mice (an animal model characterized by hyperphosphatemia, markedly elevated circulating calcitriol levels, extensive vascular calcifications, and early mortality) yielded complete resolution of ectopic calcifications, a result which was not obtained with the vitamin D-deficient diet [48].

The relationship between *vitamin D* and vascular calcification appears to follow a biphasic dose-response curve, with adverse effects associated with very high and very low calcidiol levels [49]. At certain levels, vitamin D promotes bone formation by increasing the expression of critical matrix proteins in osteoblasts, leading to the incorporation of calcium into bone, thus taking it away from the vasculature. In addition, vitamin D may also prevent vascular calcifications through modulation of inflammatory responses [50]. Indeed, in dialysis patients, serum levels of calcidiol were inversely correlated with the extent of coronary calcifications [51], and clinical observations revealed that vitamin D receptor agonists were associated with decreased deposition of calcium, improved therapeutic outcomes, and survival benefits, independent of baseline levels of calcium, phosphate, parathyroid hormone, measured comorbidities, and kidney function [6, 15, 52].

However, vitamin D excess was associated with medial calcification and arterial stiffness [49]. Indeed, high doses of vitamin D may actually increase the risk of vascular calcification in CKD owing to its effects on increasing intestinal calcium and phosphate absorption, as well as the mobilization of these minerals from bone, leading to hypercalcemia and hyperphosphatemia, especially in patients already taking calcium-based phosphate binders [13, 50, 52]. Besides its indirect effects due to interactions with the other major factors involved in osteoblastic transformation of VSMCs, vitamin D appears to directly induce the phenotypic switch through the vitamin D receptors on VSMCs resulting in upregulation of proteins involved in calcium transport and mineralization such as osteopontin and osteocalcin [35, 53].

Taken together, these data suggest that excess calcitriol can promote vascular calcifications through several interrelated mechanisms, while moderate physiological or pharmacological doses are beneficial (by suppressing the expression of osteoblastic genes in VSMCs). Debate also exists concerning the potential differential effects and benefits of native vitamin D as compared to active vitamin D receptor agonists, with an assumption that early administration of nutritional supplementation in CKD patients may prevent vascular calcification [54]. However, this remains to be proven by future research.

Secondary hyperparathyroidism may also be involved, indirectly, in the osteoblastic transformation of VSMCs since its excessive action on bone resorption results in hypercalcemia and hyperphosphatemia [55]. Also, arterial hypertension which may result from persistently increased parathyroid hormone (PTH), through the stimulation of renin-angiotensin-aldosterone and sympathetic nervous systems, is another indirect pathway to endothelial dysfunction and arterial calcification [56]. Despite these pathogenetic links, the exact contribution of PTH on vascular calcification is not known yet. In various clinical trials, therapies directed to decrease PTH (parathyroidectomy and calcimimetics) provided discordant results on prevention or regression of vascular calcifications [57–59]. Moreover, both hyperparathyroidism (which induce high bone turnover and activation of osteoclasts with calcium and phosphorus release into the circulation) and suppressed PTH (which induce adynamic bone disease with low bone turnover and reduce uptake of calcium and phosphate into the bone) were associated with extensive arterial calcifications [60]. Consequently, it was hypothesized that parathyroid hormone does not exert a direct intervention in the pathogenesis of vascular calcification in CKD, so its exact role on this matter remains to be elucidated.

The relationships of *Fibroblast growth factor 23* (FGF23) and its receptor—*Klotho*—with calcifications were also investigated, but conflicting results were reported. Some authors found an association of increased FGF23 with carotid artery calcification in stages 3 and 4 CKD patients [61], and with abdominal aortic calcifications in hemodialysis patients [62], while others observed contrary findings [63]. To date, it is not clear whether FGF23 can directly act on vascular cells to promote or inhibit matrix calcification. It is possible that the involvement of FGF23 in vascular calcification would be only indirect, through the related calcium-phosphate metabolism disturbances [64]. Alternatively, since FGF23 needs Klotho as mandatory co-receptor and Klotho (which controls the dedifferentiation of VSMCs by blocking the expression sodium-phosphate cotransporters) decreases from the early stages of CKD, the ability of FGF23 to interact with vascular cells is consequently altered [64, 65]. Despite the fact that experimental data are congruent to suggest that the effect of Klotho is protective against vascular calcifications, it still remains unknown whether or not Klotho is expressed in the vessel wall [64]. Thus, no definitive conclusions regarding the direct effects of FGF23 or Klotho on VSMCs functions can be drawn based on the current state of knowledge.

4. Clinical consequences of vascular calcifications in chronic kidney disease

Observational studies point to cardiovascular disease (CVD) as the leading cause of morbidity and mortality in CKD patients. The annual 2014 report of the United States Renal Data System estimates that, in patients with CKD, the prevalence of CVD is 69.8% compared to 34.8% in patients without renal disease, and these numbers increase with decline in kidney function [66]. In fact, the risk of any cardiovascular (CV) event seems to increase as estimated glomerular filtration rate (eGFR) decreases, ranging from a 43% increase in risk with an estimated GFR of 45–59 mL/min/1.73 m^2 to a 600% increase in cardiovascular (CV) risk at an estimated GFR of less than 15 mL/min/1.73 m^2 [67].

The burden of CVD in patients with CKD is, at least in part, accounted for by the presence of non-traditional risk factors, which are much more prevalent in this group. Among these, mineral metabolism abnormalities and vascular calcifications are commonly seen. For example, Russo et al. reported that 40% of patients with stage 3 CKD had coronary artery calcification compared with only 13% of the control subjects with no renal impairment [68]. Similar data were found in our own experience: a cross-sectional, unicentric study that enrolled 110 stable CKD patients not on renal replacement therapy, and 34 age- and gender-matched patients without CKD showed higher prevalence of coronary artery disease (defined as past myocardial infarction, angor pectoris associated with electrocardiographic or ultrasound indices, coronary angioplasty or bypass) in CKD (49% vs. 19%, $p = 0.001$). In addition, more CKD patients than Controls had valvular (38% vs. 17%, $p = 0.02$), and vascular calcification (carotid plaques 60% vs. 29%, $p = 0.02$ and abdominal aorta calcifications 54% vs. 26%, $p = 0.003$), irrespective of the CKD stage [69].

4.1. Arterial stiffness

Clinical consequences of vascular calcifications in CKD include loss of arterial elasticity with resultant rise in arterial stiffness due to reduced compliance of large arteries, lower delivery of oxygen to the tissues, and endothelial dysfunction. Arterial stiffness represents the functional disturbance of vascular calcification and predominantly results from greater medial calcification. The main consequence of arterial stiffness is increased pulse pressure, which contributes to left ventricular hypertrophy and impaired coronary perfusion by increasing ventricular afterload and reducing coronary blood flow during diastole [70]. In response to higher pressure or flow, the arterial wall undergoes a remodeling process, which consists of either reorganization of cellular and noncellular elements (eutrophic remodeling) or increased muscle mass (hypertrophic remodeling), both with significant impact on altered arterial function, that is, the reduced ability to buffer pressure, and pulsatile flow oscillations [71].

Aortic pulse wave velocity, an accurate and reproducible parameter of arterial stiffness and a marker of cardiovascular dysfunction, is linked to several other CV risk factors such as microalbuminuria and proteinuria, vascular calcifications, and left ventricular hypertrophy [72]. Wang and coworkers, in a study on 102 non-dialysis CKD patients, found an inverse relation between pulse wave velocity and estimated glomerular filtration rate, with a significant stepwise increase in pulse wave corresponding to the advance in CKD from stage 1 to 5 [73], suggesting that arterial stiffness increases with decreased kidney function. Contrary to this result, but in line with others which did not detect independent associations between eGFR and aortic stiffness [74, 75], in a cross-sectional, single-center study on 135 stable patients (79% with CKD), we found increased cardio-ankle vascular index (CAVI, a stiffness marker less influenced by blood pressure than pulse wave velocity) in 73% subjects, irrespective of chronic kidney disease presence and severity [76].

It is largely accepted that arterial stiffness is a powerful independent predictor of mortality and CVD in advanced CKD, as well as in general population [70].

More debatable is the influence of arterial stiffness on kidney function. In theory, besides the effects on myocardium, the decreased compliance of the large arteries would be followed by the transmission of cyclic blood flow from the aorta to peripheral microcirculations in various organs (including the kidneys) because its transformation in the physiological continuous capillary flow fails. Consequently, the protective autoregulatory mechanisms of the glomerular microcirculation are overpassed, and renal tissue becomes more vulnerable to the high blood pressure–related damage, favoring the decline in glomerular filtration [71]. Despite these pathogenetic explanations, clinical studies yielded conflicting results, as mentioned earlier. The majority of large population-based studies (adult or elderly cohorts) seem to support an independent association of aortic stiffness (measured by carotid-femoral pulse wave velocity) with the risk of incident CKD, but not with the risk of CKD progression (even if, the latter is not a unanimously reported result) [71].

The presence of arterial stiffness in CKD patients is important also from the therapeutic point of view, since numerous trials investigating the efficacy of anti-hypertensive drugs in cardiologic cohorts showed significant differences among various therapeutic regimens with regard to central hemodynamic parameters. Thus, it was found that calcium channel blockers but not beta-blockers, lower the central pulse pressure [77], so the presence of arterial stiffness could impact the choice of blood-pressure-lowering medication in CKD patients.

4.2. Atherosclerotic cardiovascular disease

Atherosclerotic lesions, which refer to intimal deposition of material with consecutive occlusive consequences, are highly prevalent in CKD patients mainly due to traditional CV risk factors. Specific features of atherosclerosis in chronic kidney disease comprise a higher proportion of calcified plaques among atherosclerotic plaques and a greater intervention of inflammatory stimuli than in general population [71]. Atherosclerosis represents one link between serum calcium and CVD with the content of coronary artery calcium emerging as a predictor of coronary heart disease [78]. Indeed, Budoff et al. showed a graded relationship between decreased kidney function in CKD patients and higher coronary artery calcification scores [79], connecting calcium and kidney function with the development of cardiovascular disease, in particular ischemic heart disease.

Even in the general population, lower level of kidney function was associated with increased 5-year probability of atherosclerotic cardiovascular disease [80]. Many studies found an inverse association between the glomerular filtration rate and the risk of occurrence or progression of atherosclerosis. For example, a cross-sectional retrospective study on almost 450 subjects with moderate to severe CKD (eGFR below 60 mL/min) and acute coronary syndrome suggested that estimated kidney function is an independent risk factor for atherosclerotic multivessel cardiovascular disease, as the decreased eGFR independently predicted a three-vessel coronary stenosis, with a magnitude dependent on the severity of renal impairment. The risk was seven times higher in patients with CKD stages 4–5 than in those with stage 1 CKD [81].

However, it should be mentioned that a significant proportion of cardiovascular death among CKD patients is not strictly related to atherosclerosis (i.e., it is not due to myocardial infarction, stroke, and heart failure), as the main event is sudden cardiac death which has a multifactorial causation [82].

Atherosclerotic lesions are usually accompanied by impairment of the endothelium. Endothelial function is often abnormal in CKD patients, who have diminished endothelium-dependent dilatation compared with controls and increased von Willebrand factor, regardless of the stage of renal disease and coexisting risk factors, suggesting that atherosclerosis may develop early in the progression of chronic kidney disease [83]. Besides common factors like age, hypertension, diabetes, smoking, dyslipidemia, and atherosclerosis, endothelial dysfunction is also accounted for by retention of uremic toxins, fluid overload, anemia, phosphate load, increased FGF23, increased homocysteine, enhanced oxidative stress, impaired nitric oxide metabolism (accumulation of asymmetrical dimethyl L-arginine), accumulation of advanced glycation end products, proinflammatory cytokines, and impaired angiogenesis [84].

Vascular calcifications of the large arteries, like abdominal aorta (assessed by the lumbar aortic calcification score—ACS) is not only a predictor of the cardiovascular morbidity and mortality, but it could also provide an indirect estimation of the intrarenal vascular status, as we found in a cross-sectional study that enrolled 77 stages 2–5 non-dialysis CKD patients, older than 50 years, and with known atherosclerotic disease. This study described increased aortic calcification as eGFR declines and found that higher lumbar aortic calcification score was independently associated with lower ankle-brachial index and higher intima-media thickness, suggesting a relationship of abdominal calcifications with the extension of atherosclerosis in other territories [85]. In addition, the novel finding of the study was the ability of an aortic calcification score >5 to predict with 65% sensitivity and 68% specificity a pathologic (<0.7) renal resistive index (marker of intrarenal atherosclerotic lesions on Doppler ultrasound) [85].

4.3. Calcific uremic arteriolopathy

Previously referred to as *calciphylaxis*, this is another form of vascular calcification almost exclusive to chronic kidney disease patients with kidney failure, although some cases were scarcely reported in non-CKD patients. Female gender, hyperphosphatemia, high alkaline phosphatase, and low serum albumin are among the risk factors of calcific uremic arteriolopathy [86]. It is typically found in end-stage kidney disease, obese, diabetic females, often associated with secondary hyperparathyroidism, hypercalcemia, hyperphosphatemia, malnutrition, chronic warfarin therapy, or hypercoagulability [87].

Calcific uremic arteriolopathy involves diffuse medial calcification of small- to medium-sized subcutaneous arteries and arterioles of up to 50-μm diameter, with intimal fibroproliferative occlusions that lead to necrosis. Histological abnormalities include intimal hyperplasia, inflammation, obliterative endovascular fibrosis, arteriolar medial calcification, and thrombotic cutaneous ischemia. The result is dermal, subdermal, and adipose tissue necrosis with subsequent skin ulceration. Calciphylaxis occurs independent of osteogenic activity, when the physiological calcium phosphate solubility threshold exceeds 60 mg^2/dL^2 [13, 86].

Overt clinical signs include livedo reticularis advancing to patches of ischemic necrosis and painful skin ulcers, especially on the legs, thighs, abdomen, or breasts. Often, the initial presenting complaint is a dull deep dermal pain with periods of neuritic-type dysesthesia associated with palpable subcutaneous nodules or dermal plaques, which evolve to livedo reticularis and then nonhealing ulcerations [7, 88]. These lesions predispose the patients to life-threatening skin necrosis or acral gangrene susceptible to supra-infectious complications. Dermal fat, lung, and mesentery are most commonly affected [7, 86].

Sepsis, which is also the main cause of death due to calcific uremic arteriolopathy, and amputation are among the severe morbidities associated with this obliterative disease.

5. Conclusions

In chronic kidney disease, even in non-dialysis stages, the prevalence of atherosclerotic lesions, vascular calcifications, and arterial stiffness are significantly higher as compared to patients of same-age without kidney damage. Because the interplay of multiple factors is responsible for the arterial disorders in CKD, the exact mechanism involved is still a matter of debate. Therefore, the best therapeutic approach to minimize the adverse impact of CKD-related mineral and bone disorder on the patients' outcome is not yet known and controversies exist especially regarding the influence of intestinal phosphate binders and vitamin D receptor activators on arterial calcifications.

Author details

Cristina Capusa[1,2]* and Daria Popescu[1]

*Address all correspondence to: ccalexandr@yahoo.com

1 "Carol Davila" University of Medicine and Pharmacy, Bucharest, Romania

2 "Dr. Carol Davila" Teaching Hospital of Nephrology, Bucharest, Romania

References

[1] Hill NR, Fatoba ST, Oke JL, Hirst JA, O'Callaghan CA, Lasserson DS, Hobbs FDR. Global prevalence of chronic kidney disease: A systematic review and meta-analysis. PLoS One. 2016;**11**(7):e0158765. DOI: 10.1371/journal.pone.0158765

[2] Matsushita K, van der Velde M, Astor BC, Woodward M, Levey AS, de Jong PE, Coresh J, Gansevoort RT. For the Chronic Kidney Disease Prognosis Consortium. Association of estimated glomerular filtration rate and albuminuria with all-cause and cardiovascular mortality in general population cohorts: A collaborative meta-analysis. Lancet. 2010;**375**: 2073-2081. DOI: 10.1016/S0140-6736(10)60674-5

[3] Kidney Disease: Improving Global Outcomes (KDIGO) CKD Work Group. KDIGO 2012 clinical practice guideline for the evaluation and management of chronic kidney disease. Kidney International. 2013;(Suppl. 3):S1-S150. DOI: 10.1038/kisup.2012.73

[4] Kidney Disease Improving Global Outcomes (KDIGO) CKD-MBD Work Group. KDIGO clinical practice guideline for the diagnosis, evaluation, prevention, and treatment of chronic kidney disease-mineral and bone disorder (CKD-MBD). Kidney International. 2009;(Suppl. 113):S1-S130. DOI: 10.1038/ki.2009.188

[5] Román-García P, Rodríguez-García M, Cabezas-Rodríguez I, López-Ongil S, Díaz-López B, Cannata-Andía JB. Vascular calcification in patients with chronic kidney disease: Types, clinical impact and pathogenesis. Medical Principles and Practice. 2011;**20**:203-211. DOI: 10.1159/000323434

[6] Mizobuchi M, Towler D, Slatopolsky E. Vascular calcification: The killer of patients with chronic kidney disease. Journal of the American Society of Nephrology. 2009;**20**(7):1453-1464. DOI: 10.1681/ASN.2008070692

[7] Thompson B, Towler DA. Arterial calcification and bone physiology: Role of the bone-vascular axis. Nature Reviews. Endocrinology. 2012;**8**:529-543. DOI: 10.1038/nrendo.2012.36

[8] Alfrey AC. The role of abnormal phosphorus metabolism in the progression of chronic kidney disease and metastatic calcification. Kidney International. 2004;**66**:S13-S17. DOI: 10.1111/j.1523-1755.2004.09003.x

[9] Demer LL, Tintut Y. Vascular calcification pathobiology of a multifaceted disease. Circulation. 2008;**116**:2938-2948. DOI: 10.1161/CIRCULATIONAHA.107.743161

[10] Amann K. Media calcification and intima calcification are distinct entities in chronic kidney disease. Clinical Journal of the American Society of Nephrology. 2008;**3**(6):1599-1605. DOI: 10.2215/CJN.02120508

[11] Ronchetti I, Boraldi F, Annovi G, Cianciulli P, Quaglino D. Fibroblast involvement in soft connective tissue calcification. Frontiers in Genetics. 2013;**4**(22):1-16. DOI: 10.3389/fgene.2013.00022 eCollection 2013

[12] Hasegawa T, Yamamoto T, Tsuchiya E, Hongo H, Tsuboi K, Kudo A, Abe M, Yoshida T, Nagai T, Khadiza N, Yokoyama A, Oda K, Ozawa H, de Freitas PHL, Li M, Amizuka N. Ultrastructural and biochemical aspects of matrix vesicle-mediated mineralization. Japanese Dental Science Review. 2017;**53**(2):34-45. DOI: 10.1016/j.jdsr.2016.09.002

[13] Johnson RC, Leopold JA, Loscalzo J. Vascular calcification pathobiological mechanisms and clinical implications. Circulation Research. 2006;**99**:1044-1059. DOI: 10.1161/01.RES.0000249379.55535.21

[14] Duer MJ, Friscić T, Proudfoot D, Reid DG, Schoppet M, Shanahan CM, Skepper JN, Wise ER. Mineral surface in calcified plaque is like that of bone. Further evidence for regulated mineralization. Arteriosclerosis, Thrombosis, and Vascular Biology. 2008;**28**: 2030-2034. DOI: 10.1161/ATVBAHA.108.172387

[15] Cozzolino M, Brancaccio D, Gallieni M, Slatopolsky E. Pathogenesis of vascular calcification in chronic kidney disease. Kidney International. 2005;**68**:429-436. DOI: 10.1111/j.1523-1755.2005.00421.x

[16] Hruska KA, Mathew S, Lund RJ, Memon I, Saab G. The pathogenesis of vascular calcification in the chronic kidney disease mineral bone disorder (CKD-MBD): The links between bone and the vasculature. Seminars in Nephrology. 2009;**29**(2):156-165. DOI: 10.1016/j.semnephrol.2009.01.008

[17] Epstein M. Matrix Gla-Protein (MGP) not only inhibits calcification in large arteries but also may be renoprotective: Connecting the dots. eBioMedicine. 2016;**4**:16-17. DOI: 10.1016/j.ebiom.2016.01.026

[18] Schurgers LJ, Cranenburg EC, Vermeer C. Matrix Gla-protein: The calcification inhibitor in need of vitamin K. Thrombosis and Haemostasis. 2008;**100**(4):593-603. DOI: 10.1160/TH08-02-0087

[19] Van Campenhout A, Golledge J. Osteoprotegerin, vascular calcification and atherosclerosis. Atherosclerosis. 2009;**204**(2):321-329. DOI: 10.1016/j.atherosclerosis.2008.09.033

[20] Liu W, Zhang X. Receptor activator of nuclear factor-κB ligand (RANKL)/RANK/osteoprotegerin system in bone and other tissues. Molecular Medicine Reports. 2015;**11**:3212-3218. DOI: 10.3892/mmr.2015.3152

[21] Boyce BF, Xing L. Biology of RANK, RANKL, and osteoprotegerin. Arthritis Research & Therapy. 2007;**9**(1):S1-S7. DOI: 10.1186/ar2165

[22] Kaden JJ, Bickelhaupt S, Grobholz R, Haase KK, Sarikoç A, Kiliç R, Brueckmann M, Lang S, Zahn I, Vahl C, Hagl S, Dempfle CE, Borggrefe M. Receptor activator of nuclear factor κB ligand and osteoprotegerin regulate aortic valve calcification. Journal of Molecular Cell Biology. 2003;**36**(1):57-66. DOI: 10.1016/j.yjmcc.2003.09.015

[23] Villa-Bellosta R, Egido J. Phosphate, pyrophosphate, and vascular calcification: A question of balance. European Heart Journal. 2017;**38**:1801-1804. DOI: 10.1093/eurheartj/ehv605

[24] Narisawa S, Harmey D, Yadav MC, O'Neill CW, Hoylaerts MF, Millán JL. Novel inhibitors of alkaline phosphatase suppress vascular smooth muscle cell calcification. Journal of Bone and Mineral Research. 2007;**22**(11):1700-1710. DOI: 10.1359/jbmr.070714

[25] Jahnen-Dechent W, Heiss A, Schäfer C, Ketteler M. Fetuin-A regulation of calcified matrix metabolism. Circulation Research. 2011;**108**:1494-1509. DOI: 10.1161/CIRCRE SAHA.110.234260

[26] Hermans MM, Brandenburg V, Ketteler M, Kooman JP, van der Sande FM, Boeschoten EW, Leunissen KM, Krediet RT, Dekker FW. For the Netherlands cooperative study on the adequacy of dialysis (NECOSAD). Association of serum fetuin-A levels with mortality in dialysis patients. Kidney International. 2007;**72**(2):202-207. DOI: 10.1038/sj.ki.5002178

[27] Schoppet M, Shroff RC, Hofbauer LC, Shanahan CM. Exploring the biology of vascular calcification in chronic kidney disease: What's circulating? Kidney International. 2008;**73**(4):384-390. DOI: 10.1038/sj.ki.5002696

[28] Westenfeld R, Schafer C, Smeets R, Brandenburg VM, Floege J, Ketteler M, Jahnen-Dechent W. Fetuin-A (AHSG) prevents extraosseous calcification induced by uraemia and phosphate challenge in mice. Nephrology, Dialysis, Transplantation. 2007;**22**:1537-1546. DOI: 10.1093/ndt/gfm094

[29] Shea CM, Edgar CM, Einhorn TA, Gerstenfeld LC. BMP treatment of C3H10T1/2 mesenchymal stem cells induces both chondrogenesis and osteogenesis. Journal of Cellular Biochemistry. 2003;**90**:1112-1127. DOI: 10.1002/jcb.10734

[30] Shanahan CM, Crouthamel MH, Kapustin A, Giachelli CM. Arterial calcification in chronic kidney disease: Key roles for calcium and phosphate. Journal of the American Heart Association. 2011;**109**:697-711. DOI: 10.1161/CIRCRESAHA.110.234914

[31] Watson KE, Parhami F, Shin V, Demer LL. Fibronectin and collagen I matrixes promote calcification of vascular cells in vitro, whereas collagen IV matrix is inhibitory. Arteriosclerosis, Thrombosis, and Vascular Biology. 1998;**18**:1964-1971. DOI: 10.1161/01.ATV.18.12.1964

[32] Kapustin AN, Shanahan CM. Osteocalcin: A novel vascular metabolic and osteoinductive factor? Arteriosclerosis, Thrombosis, and Vascular Biology. 2011;**31**:2169-2171. DOI: 10.1161/ATVBAHA.111.233601

[33] Jono S, Peinado C, Giachelli CM. Phosphorylation of osteopontin is required for inhibition of vascular smooth muscle cell calcification. The Journal of Biological Chemistry. 2000;**275**(26):20197-20203. DOI: 10.1074/jbc.M909174199

[34] Kahles F, Findeisen HM, Bruemmer D. Osteopontin: A novel regulator at the cross roads of inflammation, obesity and diabetes. Molecular Metabolism 2014;**3**(4):384-393. DOI: 10.1016/j.molmet.2014.03.004

[35] Shroff RC, McNair R, Skepper JN, Figg N, Schurgers LJ, Deanfield J, Rees L, Shanahan CM. Chronic mineral dysregulation promotes vascular smooth muscle cell adaptation and extracellular matrix calcification. Journal of the American Society of Nephrology. 2010;**21**(1): 1103-1112. DOI: 10.1681/ASN.2009060640

[36] Moe SM, Chen NX. Mechanisms of vascular calcification in chronic kidney disease. Journal of the American Society of Nephrology. 2008;**19**(2):213-216. DOI: 10.1681/ASN.2007080854

[37] Lorenzen J, Krämer R, Kliem V, Bode-Boeger SM, Veldink H, Haller H, Fliser D, Kielstein JT. Circulating levels of osteopontin are closely related to glomerular filtration rate and cardiovascular risk markers in patients with chronic kidney disease. European Journal of Clinical Investigation. 2010;**40**:294-300. DOI: 10.1111/j.1365-2362.2010.02271.x

[38] Parker BD, Ix JH, Cranenburg ECM, Vermeer C, Whooley MA, Schurgers LJ. Association of kidney function and uncarboxylated matrix Gla protein: Data from the Heart and Soul Study. Nephrology, Dialysis, Transplantation. 2009;**24**(7):2095-2101. DOI: 10.1093/ndt/gfp024

[39] Montezano AC, Zimmerman D, Yusuf H, Burger D, Chignalia AZ, Wadhera V, van Leeuwen FN, Touyz RM. Vascular smooth muscle cell differentiation to an osteogenic phenotype involves TRPM7 modulation by magnesium. Hypertension. 2010;**56**:453-462. DOI: 10.1161/HYPERTENSIONAHA.110.152058

[40] Molostvov G, James S, Fletcher S, Bennett J, Lehnert H, Bland R, Zehnder D. Extracellular calcium-sensing receptor is functionally expressed in human artery. American Journal of Physiology. Renal Physiology. 2007;**293**(3):F946-F955. DOI: 10.1152/ajprenal.00474.2006

[41] Giachelli CM. The emerging role of phosphate in vascular calcification. Kidney International. 2009;**75**(9):890-897. DOI: 10.1038/ki.2008.644

[42] Shroff R, Long DA, Shanahan CM. Mechanistic insights into vascular calcification in CKD. Journal of the American Society of Nephrology. 2013;**24**(2):179-189. DOI: 10.1681/ASN.2011121191

[43] Chen NX, O'Neill KD, Duan D, Moe SM. Phosphorus and uremic serum up-regulate osteopontin expression in vascular smooth muscle cells. Kidney International. 2002;**62**:1724-1731. DOI: 10.1046/j.1523-1755.2002.00625.x

[44] Linefsky JP, O'Brien KD, Katz R, de Boer IH, Barasch E, Jenny NS, Siscovick DS, Kestenbaum B. Association of serum phosphate levels with aortic valve sclerosis and annular calcification. Journal of the American College of Cardiology. 2011;**58**(3):291-297. DOI: 10.1016/j.jacc.2010.11.073

[45] Tuttle KR, Short RA. Longitudinal relationships among coronary artery calcification, serum phosphorus, and kidney function. Clinical Journal of the American Society of Nephrology. 2009;**4**(12):1968-1973. DOI: 10.2215/CJN.01250209

[46] Adeney KL, Siscovick DS, Ix JH, Seliger SL, Shlipak MG, Jenny NS, Kestenbaum BR. Association of serum phosphate with vascular and valvular calcification in moderate CKD. Journal of the American Society of Nephrology. 2009;**20**:381-387. DOI: 10.1681/ASN.2008040349

[47] Reynolds JL, Joannides AJ, Skepper JN, McNair R, Schurgers LJ, Proudfoot D, Jahnen-Dechent W, Weissberg PL, Shanahan CM. Human vascular smooth muscle cells undergo vesicle-mediated calcification in response to changes in extracellular calcium and phosphate concentrations: A potential mechanism for accelerated vascular calcification in ESRD. Journal of the American Society of Nephrology. 2004;**15**(11):2857-2867. DOI: 10.1097/01.ASN.0000141960.01035.28

[48] Stubbs JR, Liu S, Tang W, Zhou J, Wang Y, Yao X, Quarles LD. Role of hyperphosphatemia and 1,25-dihydroxyvitamin D in vascular calcification and mortality in fibroblastic growth factor 23 null mice. Journal of the American Society of Nephrology. 2007;**18**:2116-2124. DOI: 10.1681/ASN.2006121385

[49] Tilman BD, Massy ZA. Role of vitamin D in vascular calcification: Bad guy or good guy? Nephrology, Dialysis, Transplantation. 2012;**27**:704-1707. DOI: 10.1093/ndt/gfs046

[50] Rodriguez M, Martinez-Moreno JM, Rodríguez-Ortiz ME, Muñoz-Castañeda JR, Almaden Y. Vitamin D and vascular calcification in chronic kidney disease. Kidney & Blood Pressure Research. 2011;**34**:261-268. DOI: 10.1159/000326903

[51] London GM, Guérin AP, Verbeke FH, Pannier B, Boutouyrie P, Marchais SJ, Mëtivier F. Mineral metabolism and arterial functions in end-stage renal disease: Potential role of 25-hydroxyvitamin D deficiency. Journal of the American Society of Nephrology. 2007;**18**(2):613-620. DOI: 10.1681/ASN.2006060573

[52] Cozzolino M, Ketteler M, Zehnder D. The vitamin D system: A crosstalk between the heart and kidney. European Journal of Heart Failure. 2010;**12**:1031-1041. DOI: 10.1093/eurjhf/hfq112

[53] Hsu JJ, Tintut Y, Demer LL. Vitamin D and osteogenic differentiation in the artery wall. Clinical Journal of the American Society of Nephrology. 2008;**3**(5):1542-1547. DOI: 10.2215/CJN.01220308

[54] Hou YC, Liu WC, Zheng CM, Zheng JQ, Yen TH, Role LKC. of vitamin D in uremic vascular calcification. BioMed Research International. 2017;**2017**:2803579. DOI: 10.1155/2017/2803579

[55] Cunningham J, Locatelli F, Rodriguez M. Secondary hyperparathyroidism: Pathogenesis, disease progression, and therapeutic options. Clinical Journal of the American Society of Nephrology. 2011;**6**:913-921. DOI: 10.2215/CJN.06040710

[56] Palit S, Kendrick J. Vascular calcification in chronic kidney disease: Role of disordered mineral metabolism. Current Pharmaceutical Design. 2014;**20**(37):5829-5833. DOI: 10.2174/1381612820666140212194926

[57] Bleyer AJ, Burkart J, Piazza M, Russell G, Rohr M, Carr JJ. Changes in cardiovascular calcification after parathyroidectomy in patients with ESRD. American Journal of Kidney Diseases. 2005;**46**:464-469. DOI: 10.1053/j.ajkd.2005.04.035

[58] Raggi P, Chertow GM, Torres PU, Csiky B, Naso A, Nossuli K, Moustafa M, Goodman WG, Lopez N, Downey G, Dehmel B, Floege J. The ADVANCE study: A randomized study to evaluate the effects of cinacalcet plus low-dose vitamin D on vascular calcification in patients on hemodialysis. Nephrology, Dialysis, Transplantation. 2011;**26**:1327-1339. DOI: 10.1093/ndt/gfq725

[59] Chertow GM, Block GA, Correa-Rotter R, et al. For EVOLVE trial investigators. Effect of cinacalcet on cardiovascular disease in patients undergoing dialysis. The New England Journal of Medicine. 2012;**367**:2482-2494. DOI: 10.1056/NEJMoa1205624

[60] Schlieper G, Schurgers L, Brandenburg V, Reutelingsperger C, Floege J. Vascular calcification in chronic kidney disease: An update. Nephrology, Dialysis, Transplantation. 2016;**31**(1):31-39. DOI: 10.1093/ndt/gfv111

[61] Nakayama M, Kaizu Y, Nagata M, Ura Y, Ikeda H, Shimamoto S, Kuma K. Fibroblast growth factor 23 is associated with carotid artery calcification in chronic kidney disease patients not undergoing dialysis: A cross-sectional study. BMC Nephrology. 2013;**14**:22. DOI: 10.1186/1471-2369-14-22

[62] Lee YT, Ng HY, Chiu TTY, Li LC, Pei SN, Kuo WH, Lee CT. Association of bone-derived biomarkers with vascular calcification in chronic hemodialysis patients. Clinica Chimica Acta. 2016;**452**:38-43. DOI: 10.1016/j.cca.2015.10.031

[63] Scialla JJ, Lau WL, Reilly MP, Isakova T, Yang HY, Crouthamel MH, Chavkin NW, Rahman M, Wahl P, Amaral AP, Hamano T, Master SR, Nessel L, Chai B, Xie D, Kallem RR, Chen J, Lash JP, Kusek JW, Budoff MJ, Giachelli CM, Wolf M, for Chronic Renal Insufficiency Cohort Study Investigators. Fibroblast growth factor 23 is not associated with and does not induce arterial calcification. Kidney International. 2013;**83**(6):1159-1168. DOI: 10.1038/ki.2013.3

[64] Yamada S, Giachelli CM. Vascular calcification in CKD-MBD: Roles for phosphate, FGF23, and Klotho. Bone. 2017;**100**:87-93. DOI: 10.1016/j.bone.2016.11.012

[65] MC H, Shi M, Zhang J, Quiñones H, Griffith C, Kuro-o M, Moe OW. Klotho deficiency causes vascular calcification in chronic kidney disease. Journal of the American Society of Nephrology. 2011;**22**(1):124-136. DOI: 10.1681/ASN.2009121311

[66] United States Renal Data System. 2014 USRDS annual data report: Epidemiology of kidney disease in the United States. Bethesda, MD: National Institutes of Health, National Institute of Diabetes and Digestive and Kidney Diseases; 2014. Available from https://www.usrds.org/2014/download/V1_Ch_04_Cardiovascular-Disease_14.pdf [Accessed 2017.10.08]

[67] Go AS, Chertow GM, Fan D, McCulloch CE, Hsu C. Chronic kidney disease and the risks of death, cardiovascular events, and hospitalization. The New England Journal of Medicine. 2004;**351**:1296-1305. DOI: 10.1056/NEJMoa041031

[68] Russo D, Palmiero G, De Blasio AP, Balletta MM, Andreucci VE. Coronary artery calcification in patients with CRF not undergoing dialysis. American Journal of Kidney Diseases. 2004;**44**(6):1024-1030. DOI: 10.1053/j.ajkd.2004.07.022

[69] Badulescu M, Capusa C, Stancu S, Blaga V, Ilyes A, Anghel C, Mircescu G. Cardiovascular abnormalities prevalence in non-dialysis chronic kidney disease patients. In: Abstracts to the XLVIIIth ERA-EDTA Congress, Praga, 23-26 June 2011. NDT Plus. 2011;**4**(suppl 2): 4.s2.48. DOI: 10.1093/ndtplus/4.s2.48

[70] Toussaint ND, Kerr PG. Vascular calcification and arterial stiffness in chronic kidney disease: Implications and management. Nephrology (Carlton). 2007;**12**(5):500-509. DOI: 10.1111/j.1440-1797.2007.00823.x

[71] Garnier AS, Briet M. Arterial stiffness and chronic kidney disease. Pulse. 2015;**3**:229-241. DOI: 10.1159/000443616

[72] Bellasi A, Ferramosca E, Ratti C. Arterial stiffness in chronic kidney disease: The usefulness of a marker of vascular damage. International Journal of Nephrology. 2011;**2011**:734832. DOI: 10.4061/2011/734832

[73] Wang MC, Tsai WC, Chen JY, Huang JJ. Stepwise increase in arterial stiffness corresponding with the stages of chronic kidney disease. American Journal of Kidney Diseases. 2005;**45**(3):2044-2053. DOI: 10.1053/j.ajkd.2004.11.011

[74] Briet M, Bozec E, Laurent S, Fassot C, London GM, Jacquot C, Froissart M, Houillier P, Boutouyrie P. Arterial stiffness and enlargement in mild-to-moderate chronic kidney disease. Kidney International. 2006;**69**:350-357. DOI: 10.1038/sj.ki.5000047

[75] Hermans MM, Henry R, Dekker JM, Kooman JP, Kostense PJ, Nijpels G, Heine RJ, Stehouwer CD. Estimated glomerular filtration rate and urinary albumin excretion are independently associated with greater arterial stiffness: The Hoorn Study. Journal of the American Society of Nephrology. 2007;**18**:1942-1952. DOI: 10.1681/ASN.2006111217

[76] Capusa C, Boitan B, Stefan G, Barsan L, Blaga V, Mircescu G. Age and malnutrition markers are predictors of arterial stiffness in adults with and without chronic kidney disease. In: Abstracts to the LIIth ERA-EDTA Congress, London, 28-31 May 2015. Nephrology Dialysis Transplantation. 2015;**30**(suppl 3):iii491. DOI: 10.3252/pso.eu.52era.2015

[77] Dudenbostel T, Glasser SP. Effects of antihypertensive drugs on arterial stiffness. Cardiology in Review. 2012;**20**(5):259-263. DOI: 10.1097/CRD.0b013e31825d0a44

[78] Detrano R, Guerci AD, Carr JJ, Bild DE, Burke G, Folsom AR, Liu K, Shea S, Szklo M, Bluemke DA, O'Leary DH, Tracy R, Watson K, Wong ND, Kronmal RA. Coronary calcium as a predictor of coronary events in four racial or ethnic groups. The New England Journal of Medicine. 2008;**358**(13):1336-1345. DOI: 10.1056/NEJMoa072100

[79] Budoff MJ, Rader DJ, Reilly MP, Mohler ER 3rd, Lash J, Yang W, Rosen L, Glenn M, Teal V, Feldman HI, for CRIC Study Investigators. Relationship of estimated GFR and coronary artery calcification in the CRIC (Chronic Renal Insufficiency Cohort) study. American Journal of Kidney Diseases. 2011;**58**(4):519-526. DOI: 10.1053/j.ajkd.2011.04.024

[80] Manjunath G, Tighiouart H, Ibrahim H, MacLeod B, Salem DN, Griffith JL, Coresh J, Levey AS, Sarnak MJ. Level of kidney function as a risk factor for atherosclerotic cardiovascular outcomes in the community. Journal of the American College of Cardiology. 2003;**41**(1):47-55. DOI: 10.1016/S0735-1097(02)02663-3

[81] Olechnowicz-Tietz S, Gluba A, Paradowska A, Banach M, Rysz J. The risk of atherosclerosis in patients with chronic kidney disease. International Urology and Nephrology. 2013;**45**(6):1605-1612. DOI: 10.1007/s11255-013-0407-1

[82] Whitman IR, Feldman HI, Deo R. CKD and sudden cardiac death: Epidemiology, mechanisms, and therapeutic approaches. Journal of the American Society of Nephrology. 2012;**23**(12):1929-1939. DOI: 10.1681/ASN.2012010037

[83] Thambyrajaha J, Landraya MJ, McGlynnb FJ, Jonesa HJ, Wheelerb DC, Townenda JN. Abnormalities of endothelial function in patients with predialysis renal failure. Heart. 2000;**83**:205-209. DOI: 10.1136/heart.83.2.205

[84] Goligorsky MS. Pathogenesis of endothelial cell dysfunction in chronic kidney disease: A retrospective and what the future may hold. Kidney Research and Clinical Practice. 2015; **34**(2):76-82. DOI: 10.1016/j.krcp.2015.05.003

[85] Stefan G, Capusa C, Stancu S, Petrescu L, Nedelcu ED, Andreiana I, Mircescu G. Abdominal aortic calcification and renal resistive index in patients with chronic kidney disease: Is there a connection? Journal of Nephrology. 2014;**27**(2):173-179. DOI: 10.1007/s40620-013-0021-4

[86] Disthabanchong S. Vascular calcification in chronic kidney disease: Pathogenesis and clinical implication. World Journal of Nephrology. 2012;**1**(2):43-53. DOI: 10.5527/wjn.v1.i2.43

[87] Schiffrin EL, Lipman M, Mann JFE. Chronic kidney disease: Effects on the cardiovascular system. Circulation. 2007;**116**(1):85-97. DOI: 10.1161/CIRCULATIONAHA.106.678342

[88] Sowers KM, Hayden MR. Calcific uremic arteriolopathy: Pathophysiology, reactive oxygen species and therapeutic approaches. Oxidative Medicine and Cellular Longevity. 2010;**3**(2):109-121. DOI: 10.4161/oxim.3.2.5

Chapter 4

Cardiovascular Risk Factors: The Old Ones and a Closer Look to the Mineral Metabolism

Ana Paula Silva, Anabela Malho Guedes and
Pedro Leão Neves

Additional information is available at the end of the chapter

http://dx.doi.org/10.5772/intechopen.69323

Abstract

Patients with chronic kidney disease (CKD) are particularly susceptible to cardiovascular complications, and cardiovascular disease (CVD) accounts for more than 50% of all deaths in this population. Cardiac diseases are independently associated with a deterioration of renal function and worsening of existing kidney disease. On the other hand, chronic kidney disease is an independent risk factor for increased cardiovascular morbidity and mortality. It has a complex pathogenesis, and traditional risk factors are not able to fully explain its high incidence and prevalence. Several substances have been identified, and they seem to play important roles in different physiological functions. This chapter will review traditional risk factors such as hypertension, diabetes, dyslipidemia, and left ventricular hypertrophy. The most relevant bibliography will be referred, and also interventional studies will be discussed. Other new emerging factors associated with the osteomineral metabolism have been described, mainly in advanced stages of CKD, and frequently are associated with higher cardiovascular risk, which in turn will contribute to the unfavorable prognosis of this population.

Keywords: cardiovascular risk factors, chronic kidney disease, mineral metabolism

1. Introduction

The burden of chronic kidney disease (CKD) throughout the world is steadily increasing. Patients with CKD face a particularly high risk of cardiovascular disease (CVD). Cardiovascular events, regardless of the stage of kidney disease, are the leading cause of premature death in patients with CKD, with the rate of CVD progression being twice as common compared with the general population [1–3]. Over the last 30 years, it has become clear that the risk of CVD increases early in the course of progressive kidney disease and that the epidemiology, pathophysiology, prevention, and treatment of CVD and CKD are closely related and interdependent [4].

In this chapter, we initially describe the epidemiology of CKD and cardiovascular risk in CKD. We then discuss the common risk factors for CVD (traditional and nontraditional) and key aspects of its pathophysiology.

1.1. CKD epidemiology

Patients with CKD represent an important segment of the population (7–10%) [5], which is projected to grow worldwide at a rate of 8% annually, with the fastest growth expected in developing nations [4, 6]. The National Health and Nutrition Examination Surveys (NHANES III and IV) stated that a moderate degree of renal impairment (glomerular filtration rate (GFR) 15–59ml/min/1.73m^2, as estimated by the Modification of Diet in Renal Disease (MDRD) formula) had 4.2 and 3.7% prevalence, respectively [5, 7]. In the AusDiab study, the prevalence of moderate renal failure (GFR<60, >30 ml/min/m^2) as assessed by the Cockcroft-Gault method was even more alarming, reaching 11% [5, 8]. The PREVEND study showed an incidence rate of moderate renal insufficiency of 4.2% in 4 years [9].

In a retrospective cohort study by the Kaiser Permanente Center, only a minority of patients (about 1%) with mild-to-moderate renal insufficiency developed ESRD over a 5-year follow-up [10]. However, as many as 19 and 24% of patients with mild and moderate renal insufficiency, respectively, died, mostly because of atherosclerotic complications, during the same 5 years. Thus, the true risk of renal insufficiency is cardiovascular rather renal [5, 10].

1.2. Cardiovascular risk in CKD

The prevalence of CVD, including stroke, peripheral vascular disease, sudden death, coronary artery disease (CAD), and congestive heart failure, is about twice of that observed in general population and is increased over the entire span of CKD [4]. Coronary artery disease (CAD) is a leading cause of death among people with advanced CKD [4]. In addition, the onset of CVD frequently is premature when compared to general population [11]. In the last decade, the high frequency of renal impairment as an epiphenomenon of cardiovascular damage and/or cardiac dysfunction has been fully recognized [5]. The Cardiovascular Health Study analysis demonstrated that in every 10 mL/min per 1.73 m^2 decrease in glomerular filtration rate (GFR), the risk of CVD and all-cause mortality increased by 5 and 6%, respectively [11]. It can be estimated that the (fully adjusted) risk associated with moderate renal insufficiency is about 40% higher than normal [10]. The risk increases linearly as renal function deteriorates until the GFR <15ml/min. Cardiovascular risk in patients who reach the end-stage phase of renal disease is staggering, being 5 times higher than normal in 85- to 95-year-old ESRD patients and 65 and 500 times higher than normal in those 45–54 years old and 25–35 years old, respectively [12].

On the other hand, in US Medicare patients admitted to the hospital with myocardial infarction and heart failure, the prevalence of moderate renal failure (creatinine clearance <60 ml/min/1.73 m^2) was very high, 60 and 52%, respectively, and these patients had a high risk of renal disease progression [13].

Traditional risk factors for development of CVD include hypertension, diabetes, dyslipidemia, smoking, increased body mass index, older age, male gender, physical inactivity, stress, and positive family history [11]. The same traditional risk factors can incite renal dysfunction. As renal function deteriorates, nontraditional risk factors play an increasing role both in glomerular filtration rate (GFR) loss and in cardiovascular damage [5]. The higher mortality from CVD persists even after adjusting for most of the traditional risk factors, suggesting the possible contributions of uremia-related, nontraditional risk factors. It seems that CVD and CKD can initiate, enhance, and perpetuate each other, eventually leading to vicious circle and premature death [11]. This has led to the current understanding that the pathophysiology of CVD in CKD involves a complex interplay of both the traditional and nontraditional, uremia-related risk factors [2], sequentially considering traditional risk factors as dominant for triggering initial renal damage and cardiovascular events in the general population, but with nontraditional risk factors becoming increasingly important as renal function worsens [5].

Mineral metabolism disorders are a part of those uremia-related risk factors mentioned, but for their complexity and multiplicity of interplay mechanisms, as for their hidden precocious action on cardiovascular balance makes it obligatory to explore more deeply.

2. Traditional risk factors

2.1. Hypertension

Hypertension is simultaneously a cause and a consequence of chronic kidney disease (CKD), and this strong relationship has been recognized since the nineteenth century. As the renal function declines, the prevalence of hypertension increases, and for that reason, more than 80% of the patients beginning renal replacement therapy have high blood pressure [14]. The physiopathology of hypertension associated with CKD is complex and multifactorial, mainly in the late stages of CKD. In addition to the well-known factors such as increased intravascular volume and excessive activity of the RAS, there are new recognized players such as increased activity of the sympathetic nervous system, endothelial dysfunction, and alterations of several neural and humoral factors that increase the blood pressure [15]. Although hypertension is clearly a risk factor of cardiovascular disease in the general population, when we look to the renal population, this association is less evident due to the reverse epidemiology phenomenon [15, 16]. In CKD patients, hypertension is associated with ischemic heart disease, heart failure, and left ventricular hypertrophy [17–20]. Secondary analysis from randomized controlled trials such as the HOPE, IDNT, and ADVANCE studies demonstrated that hypertension treatment in CKD patients can reduce the risk of cardiovascular events [21–23]. Recently, the SPRINT study [24] showed that treatment of systolic blood pressure to a lower target (120 vs. 140 mmHg) reduced 25% of the composite CV outcome. However, in this study, less than 30% of the patients had CKD, and diabetic patients were excluded. There is a bulk of evidence that treating patients to lower blood pressure levels increases morbidity and mortality, mainly in elderly patients [17, 18, 24, 25]. The real challenge is how far we should go when we treat renal patients. The KDIGO guidelines recommend that the blood pressure should be less than 140/90 mmHg in CKD nondiabetic patients and less than 130/80 mmHg in CKD diabetic patients and nondiabetic proteinuric patients [26]. Kovesdy et al. proved that the optimal blood pressure in patients with CKD seems to be 130 to 159/70 to 89 mm Hg [18], and Agarwal [17] pointed out that higher levels of systolic and lower levels of diastolic blood pressure are associated with poorer cardiovascular outcomes. We should treat carefully our renal patients, lowering their systolic values but paying attention to the diastolic values. This concern is especially important in the elderly patients [27]. Regarding dialysis patients, there is a suggestion that treating hypertension decreases cardiovascular morbidity and mortality [28, 29], but there are no randomized controlled studies addressing the target of the blood pressure.

2.2. Diabetes

Diabetes mellitus is a major cause of CKD, and in most Western countries, the proportion of incident dialysis patients are between 22 and 44% [30].

Diabetes mellitus is a well-known risk factor of cardiovascular disease since the Framingham and other population-based studies. Once the renal population is under an increased risk of cardiovascular disease, not unexpectedly in patients with diabetic nephropathy, this risk increases exponentially. In fact, the NHANES III showed that the standardized mortality of patients with diabetes and CKD was 31.1% compared with a standardized mortality of 11.5% in patients with diabetes and of 7.7% in patients without diabetes or CKD [31]. The mechanisms of how diabetes increases atherogenesis are multiple, associated to hyperglycemia itself (*via* the polyol pathway, protein kinase C, AGEs, hexosamine pathway) and associated to other circumstances such as dyslipidemia, obesity, insulin resistance, and prothrombotic and proinflammatory states [32]. In the early stages of diabetic nephropathy, the presence of microalbuminuria is a harbinger of an increased cardiovascular risk [33], and this risk increases as the nephropathy progresses [34]. Diabetes continues to raise the risk of morbidity and mortality throughout the spectrum of kidney disease. Diabetic patients on dialysis maintain a poorer prognosis when compared with nondiabetic patients [35–37].

The treatment strategy includes the reduction of the progression of diabetic nephropathy with antagonists of the renin-angiotensin system [38, 39], the control of glycemia, and all the complex conditions associated.

2.3. Dyslipidemia

The presence of alterations of the lipid profile is frequent in the early stages of renal disease. Renal patients have, in general, lower levels of HDL, LDL, and total cholesterol and higher levels of triglycerides. There is a clustering of low HDL and elevated Lp(a) and TG-rich apolipoprotein B (ApoB) containing VLDL and LDL [40]. The increased concentration of triglyceride-rich lipoproteins in renal patients is due to delayed catabolism and to the increased hepatic production [41]. The severity of hypercholesterolemia is also associated with the level of proteinuria in CKD predialysis patients. In HD patients, the serum lipid profile is similar of predialysis patients, but PD patients have higher total and LDL cholesterol values and increased concentrations of small-dense LDL and apolipoprotein B [41]. Although dyslipidemia is clearly a risk factor of cardiovascular disease in the general population in kidney patients, this relationship is not straightforward. Chronic kidney disease is characterized by increased oxidative stress and inflammation, and these are the two major players responsible for the increased atherosclerosis in this group of patients [42–44]. This fact can explain, in part, why there is a solid association between inflammation and cardiovascular disease, and patients with low cholesterol may have poorer outcomes [45–47]. This phenomenon is called reverse epidemiology [45]. However, Koch et al. also found a positive association between cholesterol values and the risk for cardiovascular events in CKD individuals [48].

Regarding therapy, statins improve the lipid profile and exert several pleiotropic effects. Nevertheless, concerning the cardiovascular outcomes, the timing of the initiation of the therapy is critical. The Prospective Pravastatin Pooling Project that included three studies has shown that pravastatin reduced significantly the CV composite outcome only in patients with moderate renal insufficiency [49]. We also found in an observational study that statins plus vitamin D reduced cardiovascular mortality in predialysis patients [50]. The SHARP trial also demonstrated the benefit of simvastatin plus ezetimibe in predialysis but not in patients already on dialysis [51]. This data according with the AURORA and 4D studies had not shown greater survival in patients on dialysis treated with statins when compared with placebo [52, 53]. The lack of benefit of using statins in dialysis patients can have several reasons: high mortality of dialysis patients due to sudden death and cardiomyopathy, existence of other pathways contributing to cardiovascular disease, or just because it is too late to interfere with the natural history of atherosclerosis [54]. Regarding prevention of cardiovascular disease in renal patients, there is a strong evidence of benefit in using statins only in predialysis patients, but their use is not recommended in dialysis patients [55]. The utilization of fibrates is not recommended in patients with advanced renal failure, and other approaches such as niacin, ezetimibe, or Ω-3 polyunsaturated fatty acids need randomized controlled studies to validate their effectiveness.

2.4. Left ventricular hypertrophy

Left ventricular hypertrophy (LVH) is an established risk factor of cardiovascular morbidity and mortality in the general and also in the renal population. Its prevalence increases as the renal function deteriorates. It is estimated to be around 25% in the early stages of CKD and rises to 75 to 90% at the initiation of renal replacement therapy [56]. There are several factors associated to LVH in CKD. As it happens in the general population [57], age, hypertension, and existence of previous heart disease increase the risk of LVH in renal patients [58]. In these patients, other specific factors related to their condition also influence the left ventricular mass, such as anemia, disturbances of the mineral metabolism, inflammation, and oxidative stress [59, 60]. Concerning the mineral metabolism, recent studies revealed associations between vitamin D, FGF23, and Klotho with LVH [56, 59, 61]. In dialysis patients, the volume status, the presence of arteriovenous fistula, and the time on renal replacement therapy are also relevant aspects [56, 58, 62]. LVH contributes to a greater prevalence of ventricular arrhythmias and ischemic heart disease [63], as was demonstrated in the 4D study [52].

Therefore, it is vital to reduce the left ventricular mass, to control as far as possible the modifiable risk factors, such as the anemia, the mineral metabolism, the blood pressure, and the hypervolemia as was shown in quite a few studies [64, 65]. This reduction of the LVH is associated with diminution of the cardiac events and death [66].

3. Chronic kidney disease: mineral metabolism and cardiovascular risk

3.1. Phosphorus

In recent years, numerous epidemiological studies have shown a link between high phosphorus (P*i*) levels and cardiovascular outcomes, in both the chronic renal failure population and the population as a whole.

The link between P*i* and morbidity and mortality was demonstrated some years ago, initially in the CKD population on dialysis in the classic study conducted by Block et al. [67], and was later confirmed by several other cohort studies both in individuals with CKD and in individuals with normal renal function [68–71]. Analysis of the Dialysis Outcomes and Practice Patterns Study (DOPPS) showed that serum P*i* levels higher than 6.1 mg/dl at the start of the study were associated with an increased risk of death from any cause and from cardiovascular disease compared to P*i* levels within the normal reference range [68]. Very low P*i* levels were also associated with increased mortality, perhaps reflecting the poor nutritional status of these patients [68]. It is also known that high concentrations of P*i* are associated with the presence of vascular, valvular, and soft tissue calcifications in this population [72] even at earlier stages of CKD [73]. These observations were later extended to the general population, and, surprisingly, even P*i* levels at the upper limits of normal were found to be associated with greater cardiovascular disease (CARE post hoc analysis) [69]. This analysis showed that, after 5 years of follow-up, there was a positive, gradual association between baseline serum P*i* levels and mortality due to any cause, conferring a 27% increase in the risk of death for each 1 mg/dL increase in serum P*i*. The Framingham Heart Study cohort [74] and the Atherosclerosis Risk in Communities Study (ARIC) also showed an increased cardiovascular mortality in patients with higher levels of P*i* [71]. These last two studies draw attention to the fact that the serum P*i* levels were still within the normal range. At least two studies showed a correlation between P*i* and the severity of coronary lesions on angiography [75, 76]. This information emphasizes the possibly important role of P*i* in the processes of calcification and atherogenesis [76]. It is interesting to observe that the authors also demonstrated that P*i* was a predictor for atherosclerosis in other sites, such as the carotid arteries, [77, 78] as well as the left ventricular hypertrophy (LVH) in the general population [79]. The mechanisms by which P*i* increases mortality and the incidence of cardiovascular events have not yet been established, but it seems likely that it contributes directly, as a result of its participation in the pathogenesis of vascular calcification and in the atherosclerosis process, [80] and indirectly, by raising FGF23 levels [81]. Hyperphosphatemia, by raising parathyroid hormone (PTH) levels, can also have, indirectly, a harmful effect on cardiomyocytes [82, 83] and interfere with the mechanisms that regulate vascular calcification [84]. This mechanism would also explain the relationship between vascular calcification and serum *Pi* in the presence of hyperphosphatemia, as seen in the CKD population. Vascular calcification is one of the mechanisms proposed for *Pi*-related cardiovascular risk. In vitro studies show that *Pi* participates actively in the vascular calcification process. Smooth muscle cells grown in a *Pi*-rich medium transdifferentiate into osteoblast-like cells. *Pi* is able to enter the smooth muscle cell via the type III sodium-phosphate cotransporter (PiT-1), activate a nuclear transcription factor called Cbfa-1/RUNX-2, and stimulate cell transdifferentiation [85, 86]. The smooth muscle cells acquire phenotypical characteristics similar to osteoblasts and begin to express osteopontin, osteocalcin, alkaline phosphatase, and type I collagen, promoting an authentic "ossification" of the vascular tissue [87]. *Pi* overload is also associated with increased production of reactive oxygen species [88], changes in angiogenesis, epithelial migration, and survival of endothelial cells [89].

One of the biggest difficulties in interpreting the harmful effects of *Pi* in vivo is to determine if they are the result of their direct action or indirect mechanisms, e.g., via an increase in FGF23 and PTH. However, there is quite a few data demonstrating that the reduction of *Pi* levels was associated with improvement in endothelial dysfunction, aortic stiffness, and left ventricular hypertrophy [90] and slowing of the progression of vascular calcification [91]. Furthermore, it was also shown that controlling *Pi* through dietary restriction or with the use of sevelamer was effective in reducing mortality in uremic mice with established vascular calcification [92].

Although experimental studies suggest that a better control of *Pi* levels is associated with a beneficial effect on the cardiovascular system, including mortality, interpretation of these findings is still controversial. Nevertheless, such findings are considered a strong evidence implicating *Pi* as a cardiovascular disease-promoting agent and, as such, an important therapeutic target.

3.2. Vitamin D and PTH

The role played by vitamin D and PTH in cardiovascular function appears to be much more important than was originally thought. The discovery of a protein that binds to calcium, which is calcitriol-dependent and which is present in the myocardium, the vascular smooth muscle, and the endothelium, offered a clearer view on this subject [93–98].

In an experimental context of vitamin D deficiency, it was observed that calcitriol normalizes the contractility of disorganized myocardial areas, promoting regulation of myocyte proliferation and hypertrophy [94]. It also stimulates the production of prostacyclin in the vascular smooth muscle tissue, which prevents thrombus formation, cell adhesion, and proliferation of smooth muscle tissue [97]. Calcitriol is also known to suppress the synthesis and secretion of atrial natriuretic peptide and increase production of the matrix protein carboxyglutamic acid, which has a protective effect against arterial calcification [98, 99].

The recent discovery of the 25(OH)D-1 hydroxylase enzyme—whose activity is regulated by the action of PTH and by estrogenic compounds—in the vascular smooth muscle cell has also contributed to the growing importance of vitamin D in vascular function [93, 96]. Cardiac tissue cells have receptors for both PTH and PTH-related peptides, which affect the physiology of the cardiovascular cell in a different way from the action they exert on classic bone tissue

[100]. PTH-related peptide is produced by the vascular smooth muscle cells, which regulate the arterial smooth muscle tissue proliferation rate, producing positive chronotropic and inotropic effects, not attributable to PTH, in isolated cardiomyocytes [96]. PTH is responsible for the expression of fetal proteins in the cardiomyocytes and, if present in excess, may be related to hypertrophic growth of the myocytes [100]. In animal studies, a relation between PTH levels and a permissive role in fibroblast activation and cardiac fibrosis has been observed, possibly via transformation of growth factor 1, a promoter of cardiac fibrosis [82, 101, 102].

Zittermann et al. [100] proposed various mechanisms to explain the relation between vitamin D deficiency and cardiovascular disease. One of these suggests that the matrix Gla protein—synthesized by the chondrocytes and the vascular smooth muscle and stimulated by calcitriol—is an important inhibitor of vascular calcification. They also mention the important role that inflammatory processes play in the development of adverse cardiovascular effects and the fact that interleukin 6 and tumor necrosis factor (TNF), which are stimulators of C-reactive protein, are suppressed by calcitriol, unlike interleukin 10, whose production is stimulated. The renin-angiotensin-aldosterone system, which is responsible for regulating blood pressure, electrolytes, and volemic status, is regulated by calcitriol via reduction of plasma renin activity and the angiotensin II concentration [99, 103].

In addition to these mechanisms, PTH and vitamin D are significantly involved in the osteoprotegerin/RANKL/RANK pathway, a fact that could make it the connecting link between bone tissue and cardiovascular diseases [104, 105]. Calcitriol, on the other hand, reduces expression of osteoprotegerin [106, 107].

A link between vitamin D deficiency and cardiovascular disease can be found in a number of studies, which demonstrated a 30–50% higher cardiovascular morbidity and mortality associated with reduced sun exposure caused by changes in season or latitude [108–110]. One fact that supports this thesis is that cardiovascular mortality rates are lower in the European countries with greater sun exposure and higher during the winter months [110].

Despite the negative association between vitamin D deficiency and cardiovascular disease described in multiple studies [111–114], clinical trials have failed to convincingly demonstrate a benefit of vitamin D supplements on cardiovascular (CV) health. One such study was the PRIMO trial, which showed no improvement in ventricular mass index or any other remodeling parameters by administering paricalcitol, a selective activator of vitamin D receptors, to patients with chronic renal failure [115]. However, experiments performed in vitro and in several animal models of LV pressure overload show that vitamin D supplements attenuate LV hypertrophy, reduce cardiac fibrosis, and decrease the expression of collagen, fibronectin, and transforming growth factor-β, along with an improvement of the systolic and diastolic function [116, 117].

3.3. FGF23

Fibroblast growth factor 23 (FGF23) is a phosphaturic protein and an inhibitor of 1α-hydroxylase, the enzyme responsible for calcitriol synthesis. Its discovery has enabled a better understanding of chronic kidney disease-related mineral and bone disorders (CKD-MBD) [118, 119].

Recent experimental and clinical studies have confirmed the role of FGF23 in the physiology of MBD and CV disease [120]. FGF23 is produced by osteocytes and osteoblasts, and it acts on the kidneys in the proximal tubular cells, increasing renal excretion of phosphorus and decreasing 1,25-dihydroxivitamin D [1,25(OH)D] [118, 121, 122].

Elevated FGF23 is observed after dietary ingestion due to a resulting increase in intestinal absorption of phosphorus after administration of PTH in experimental work with CKD [123, 124]. The rise in FGF23 associated with the resulting decrease in intestinal absorption of phosphorus, mediated by the decrease in calcitriol, contributes to maintaining adequate blood phosphate levels in the initial stages of kidney disease [125]. In CKD, there are concomitant increases in the levels of phosphorus, PTH, and FGF23, which reflects an increased production and decreased degradation, leading to their accumulation to levels much higher than those in the general population [126].

The action of FGF23 is obtained only when it is bound to the FGFR1c receptor associated with the Klotho cofactor. The Klotho protein is specifically expressed in the distal tubule of the normal kidney, but it is produced in many other tissues and organs [118, 127, 128]. The main targets of FGF23 are defined by the expression of the FGFR1c-Klotho complex. However, important actions of FGF23 on cardiomyocytes occur even in the absence of Klotho, via intracellular mechanisms that are not yet fully understood [129]. Elevated FGF23 levels imply an increase in the mortality rate adjusted for classic CV-KD factors and other traditional CKD markers [71–73].

This link between elevated serum levels of FGF23 and the occurrence of relevant clinical events was initially established in patients with kidney disease who were on hemodialysis [130, 131]. Faul et al. in a cohort study of 3000 patients demonstrated that, in the early stages of kidney disease, FGF23 is an independent risk factor for LVH [132]. The cardiac hypertrophic effects of FGF23 are mediated by FGFR-dependent activation of the calcineurin nuclear factor of the activated T-cell (NFAT) signaling cascade, but do not require Klotho as a co-receptor [133].

The available studies that evaluated FGF23 and cardiovascular changes or events in the general population have a limitation, because their samples included individuals with CKD. Keeping this fact in mind, links were found between FGF23 and LVH, endothelial dysfunction, and total body atherosclerosis as assessed by magnetic resonance imaging in the community [134]. Recently, an analysis of the cohort participating in the Heart and Soul Study, which included 833 patients with coronary artery disease, established FGF23 as a predictor of events in this population [135]. This study included patients with CKD, but the results remained the same after adjusting for this variable.

FGF23 is also being linked to severe aortic and coronary artery calcifications and is considered a marker of CV disease in patients with CKD [136, 137]. One of the mechanisms may be related to a decrease in fetuin-A. Fetuin-A is synthesized by the hepatocytes, is secreted into the blood, and accumulates in the skeleton during bone mineralization due to its high affinity for hydroxyapatite. It is considered an inhibitor of CV disease and represents the most important inhibitor of the formation of circulating hydroxyapatite [138, 139]. Another mechanism that would explain the vascular calcifications associated with FGF23 would be through hyperphosphatemia.

Scialla et al. studied the link between FGF23, P, and coronary calcification as measured by CT scan of the aorta in 1501 subjects with CKD. They concluded that FGF23 was not directly associated with calcification of the aorta and coronary arteries, but rather with phosphorus levels. This group found a link between the severity of the calcification and FGF23 and concluded that FGF23 may be a marker of surveillance and not of the genesis of vascular calcification [140].

3.4. Klotho

The Klotho protein is a potential marker for vascular events. Suppression of the Klotho gene in animal models causes extensive aging-like phenotypes, including atherosclerosis, ectopic calcification, infertility, skin atrophy, and severe hypoglycemia [141], while its overexpression increases life span by 20–30%, in animal models [142]. The Klotho protein is present mainly in the distal tubules of the kidney and in the cerebral choroid plexus, but it can be posttranslationally processed and released into the bloodstream, with the free extracellular domain functioning as a hormone [143, 144]. Its presence in vascular tissue is still a topic of debate [145].

An important physiological property attributed to circulating Klotho is the start of a pathway that inhibits insulin and IGF1 signaling, which contributes to the integrity of the microcirculation and of a healthy endothelium [146, 147].

In chronic kidney disease, serum levels of Klotho are decreased, contributing to increased cardiovascular risk in this population. Tests have been carried out in wild-type and transgenic mice, where it was observed that KL-/- mice with chronic kidney disease (CKD) showed early calcification of the soft tissues compared to wild-type mice (KL+/+) that also had CKD. Mice with CKD that overexpress Klotho (preserved levels of Klotho) showed greater phosphaturia and, consequently, better renal function and less calcification of tissues compared to wild-type mice with CKD [148].

The role of Klotho in uremic myocardiopathy is not yet fully understood. However, in animal models, we know that ventricular hypertrophy is associated with increased expression of transient receptor potential canonical (TRPC6) channels, whose expression is regulated by different mechanisms. Recently, Xie et al. demonstrated that Klotho can inhibit the cardiac TRPC6 channels, thereby protecting the myocardium against excessive/pathological remodeling [149, 150].

The cardioprotective mechanisms of Klotho and the role of FGF23 in the cardiac fibrosis of CKD are not yet fully explained. However, some studies have demonstrated that there are several factors responsible for this complex process: (1) cardiac fibrosis and hypertrophy are associated with primary genetic Klotho deficiency or secondary deficiency associated with aging and CKD; (2) cardiac hypertrophy precedes cardiac fibrosis and is associated with left ventricular dysfunction; (3) high levels of phosphate and low serum levels of Klotho correlate with more cardiac hypertrophy and fibrosis in all the studied models; (4) even in the absence of Klotho, important actions of FGF23 on the cardiomyocytes occur by an intracellular route that is not clarified, promoting cardiac hypertrophy [151, 152].

The role of emerging factors like FGF23 and Klotho in cardiovascular risk in both the early and late stages of chronic kidney disease is not entirely perceptible. The entire process involves direct and indirect mechanisms that contribute to this high cardiovascular risk.

4. Conclusions

Chronic kidney disease is an independent risk factor for increased cardiovascular morbidity and mortality. It has a complex pathogenesis, and traditional risk factors are not able to fully explain its high incidence and prevalence. Several substances have been identified, and they seem to play important roles in different physiological functions.

The CKD mineral disease is another player in this complex puzzle and is one of the factors responsible for this high cardiovascular risk of this population in the early or late stages of the CKD.

Author details

Ana Paula Silva*, Anabela Malho Guedes and Pedro Leão Neves

*Address all correspondence to: anapassionara@gmail.com

Nephrology Department, Centro Hospitalar do Algarve, Algarve Biomedical Center, Faro, Portugal

References

[1] Zoccali C, Mallamaci F, Tripepi G. Traditional and emerging cardiovascular risk factors in end-stage renal disease. Kidney Int. 2003;**63**:105-110

[2] Yerram P, Karuparthi PR, Hesemann L, Horst J, Whaley-Connell A. Chronic kidney disease and cardiovascular risk. Journal of the American Society of Hypertension. 2007 May-Jun;**1**(3):178-184

[3] Kidney Disease Outcome Quality Initiative. K/DOQI clinical practice guidelines for chronic kidney disease: Evaluation, classification, and stratification. American Journal of Kidney Diseases. 2002;**39**(Suppl 2):S1-S246

[4] Tonelli M, Karumanchi A, Thadhani R. Epidemiology and mechanisms of uremia-related cardiovascular disease. Circulation. 2016;**133**:518-536

[5] Zocalli C. Traditional and emerging cardiovascular and renal risk factors: An epidemiologic perspective. Kidney International. 2006;**70**:26-33

[6] Ayodele OE, Alebiosu CO. Burden of chronic kidney disease: An inter- national perspective. Advances in Chronic Kidney Disease. 2010;**17**:215-224

[7] Coresh J, Byrd-Holt D, Astor BC et al. Chronic kidney disease awareness, prevalence, and trends among US adults, 1999-2000. Journal of the American Society of Nephrology. 2005;**16**:180-188

[8] Chadban SJ, Briganti EM, Kerr PG et al. Prevalence of kidney damage in Australian adults: The AusDiab kidney study. Journal of the American Society of Nephrology. 2003;**14**(Suppl 2):S131-S138

[9] Verhave JC, Gansevoort RT, Hillege HL et al, PREVEND Study Group. An elevated urinary albumin excretion predicts de novo development of renal function impairment in the general population. Kidney International. Supplement. 2004;**92**:S18-S21

[10] Go AS, Chertow GM, Fan D et al. Chronic kidney disease and the risks of death, cardiovascular events, and hospitalization. New England Journal of Medicine. 2004;**23**:1296-1305

[11] Lainščak M. Cardiovascular Risk in Chronic Kidney Disease - eJIFCC 20/01; 2009. http://www.ifcc.org

[12] Foley RN, Parfrey PS, Sarnak MJ. Epidemiology of cardiovascular disease in chronic renal disease. Journal of the American Society of Nephrology. 1998;**9**:S16-S23

[13] McClellan WM, Langston RD, Presley R. Medicare patients with cardiovascular disease have a high prevalence of chronic kidney disease and a high rate of progression to end-stage renal disease. Journal of the American Society of Nephrology. 2004;**15**:1912-1919

[14] Ridao N, Luno J, Garcia de Vinuesa S, Gómez, Valderrábano F. Prevalence of hypertension in renal disease. Nephrology, Dialysis, Transplantation. 2001;**16**(Suppl 1):70-73

[15] Morgado E, Neves PL. Hypertension and chronic kidney disease: cause and consequence—therapeutic considerations. In: Babaei H, editor. Antihypertensive drugs. Rijeka: InTech; 2012:45-63

[16] Lowrie EG, Huang WH, Lew NL, Liu Y. The relative contribution of measured variables to death risk among hemodialysis patients. In: Friedman E, editor, Death on Hemodialysis: Preventable or Inevitable? Hingham, MA: Kluwer Academic Publishers; 1994:121-141

[17] Agarwal R. Blood pressure components and the risk for end-stage renal disease and death in chronic kidney disease. Clinical Journal of the American Society of Nephrology. 2009;**4**:830-837

[18] Kovesdy CP, Bleyer AJ, Molnar MZ, Ma JZ, Sim JJ, Cushman WC, Quarles LD, Kalantar-Zadeh K. Blood pressure and mortality in U.S. veterans with chronic kidney disease: A cohort study. Annals of Internal Medicine. 2013;**159**:233-242

[19] Foley RN, Parfrey PS, Harnett JD, Kr GM, Murray DC, Barre PE. Impact of hypertension on cardiomyopathy, morbidity and mortality in end-stage renal disease. Kidney International. 1996;**49**:1379-1385

[20] Yuan J, Zou XR, Han SP, et al. Prevalence and risk factors for cardiovascular disease among chronic kidney disease patients: results from the Chinese cohort study of chronic kidney disease (C-STRIDE). BMC Nephrol. 2017;**18**:23

[21] Mann JF, Gerstein HC, Pogue J, Bosch J, Yusuf S. Renal insufficiency as a predictor of cardiovascular outcomes and the impact of ramipril: The HOPE randomized trial. Annals of Internal Medicine. 2001;**134**:629-636

[22] Pohl MA, Blumenthal S, Cordonnier DJ, et al. Independent and additive impact of blood pressure control and angiotensin II receptor blockade on renal outcomes in the irbesartan diabetic nephropathy trial: Clinical implications and limitations. Journal of the American Society of Nephrology. 2005;**16**:3027-3037

[23] Heerspink HJ, Ninomiya T, Perkovic V, et al, ADVANCE Collaborative Group. Effects of a fixed combination of perindopril and indapamide in patients with type 2 diabetes and chronic kidney disease. European Heart Journal. 2010;**31**:2888-2896

[24] Wright JT Jr, Williamson JD, Whelton PK, et al. A randomized trial of intensive versus standard blood-pressure control. New England Journal of Medicine. 2015;**373**:2103-2116

[25] Hirsch S. An update on proteinuric chronic kidney disease: The dual-goal approach. Cleveland Clinic Journal of Medicine. 2008;**75**:705-713

[26] Weiss J, Johnson ES, Petrick A, Smith DH, Yang X, Thorp ML. Systolic blood pressure and mortality among older community-dwelling adults with CKD. American Journal of Kidney Diseases. 2010;**56**:1062-1071

[27] KDIGO Guidelines. Clinical practice guideline for the management of blood pressure in chronic kidney disease. Kidney International. Supplement. 2012;**2**

[28] Heerspink HJ, Ninomiya T, Zoungas S, de Zeeuw D, Grobbee DE, Jardine MJ, Gallagher M, Roberts MA, Cass A, Neal B, Perkovic V. Effect of lowering blood pressure on cardiovascular events and mortality in patients on dialysis: A systematic review and meta-analysis of controlled trials. Lancet. 2009;**373**:1009-1015

[29] Agarwal R, Sinha AD. Cardiovascular protection with antihypertensive dugs in dialysis patients: Systematic review and meta-analysis. Hypertension. 2009;**53**:860-866

[30] USDRS. 2015 Annual Report. American Journal of Kidney Diseases. 2016;**67**(Suppl 1): S291-S334

[31] Afkarian M, Sachs M, Kestenbaum B, Hirsh IB, Tuttle KR, Himmelfarb J, Boer IH. Kidney disease and increased mortality risk in type 2 diabetes. Journal of the American Society of Nephrology. 2013;**24**:302-308

[32] Gleissner C, Galkina E, Nadler JL, Ley K. Mechanisms by which diabetes increases cardiovascular disease. Drug Discovery Today. Disease Mechanisms. 2007;**4**:131-140

[33] Sarnak MJ, Levey AS, Schoolwerth AC, et al. Kidney disease as a risk factor for development of cardiovascular disease a statement from the American Heart Association Councils on kidney in cardiovascular disease, high blood pressure research, clinical cardiology, and epidemiology and prevention. Circulation. 2003;**108**:2154-2169

[34] Stehouwer CDA, Smulders YM. Microalbuminuria and risk for cardiovascular disease: Analysis of potential mechanisms. Journal of the American Society of Nephrology: JASN. August 2006;**17**(8):2106-2111

[35] Schroijen MA, Dekkers OM, Grootendorst D, et al, and the NECOSAD Study Group. Survival in dialysis patients is not different between patients with diabetes as primary renal disease and patients with diabetes as a co-morbid condition. BMC Nephrology. 2011;**12**:69-76

[36] Fang W, Yang X, Kothari J, et al. Patient and technique survival of diabetics on peritoneal dialysis: One-center's experience and review of the literature. Clinical Nephrology. 2008;**69**:193-200

[37] United States Renal Data System. American Journal of Kidney Diseases. 2010;**55**(Suppl 1)

[38] Lewis EJ, Husincker LG, Bain RP, et al, for the the Collaborative Study Group. The effect of angiotensin-converting-enzyme inhibitor on diabetic nephropathy. The New England Journal of Medicine. 1993;**329**:1456-1462

[39] Lewis EJ, Hunsicker LG, Clarke WR, et al, for the Collaborative Study Group. Renoprotective effect of the angiotensin-receptor antagonist irbesartan in patients with nephropathy due to type 2 diabetes. New England Journal of Medicine. 2001;**345**:851-860

[40] Shurraw S, Tonelli M. Statins for treatment of dyslipidemia in chronic kidney disease. Peritoneal Dialysis International. 2006;**26**:523-539

[41] Tsimihodimos V, Mitrogianni Z, Elisaf M. Dyslipidemia associated with chronic kidney disease. Open Cardiovascular Medicine Journal. 2011;**5**:41-48

[42] Ross R. Atherosclerosis: An inflammatory disease. New England Journal of Medicine. 1999;**340**:115-126

[43] Mimic-Oka J, Simic T, Pljesa M. Oxidative modifications of plasma proteins in different stages of kidney failure. Medicine and Biology. 2001;**8**:1-5

[44] Stenvinkel P, Heimburger O, Lindholm B, Kaysen GA, Bergstrom J. Are two types of malnutrition in chronic renal failure? Evidence of relationship between malnutrition, inflammation and atherosclerosis (MIA syndrome). Neprol Dial Transplant. 2000;**15**:953-960

[45] Kalantar-Zadeh K, Block G, Humphreys MH, Kopple JD. Reverse epidemiology of cardiovascular risk factors in maintenance dialysis patients. Kidney International. 2003;**63**: 793-808

[46] Lowrie EG, Lew NL. Death risk in hemodialysis patients: The predictive value of commonly measured variables and an evaluation of death rate differences between facilities. American Journal of Kidney Diseases. 1990;**15**:458-482

[47] Iseki K, Yamazato M, Tozawa M, Takishita S. Hypocholesterolemia is a significant predictor of death in a cohort of chronic hemodialysis patients. Kidney International. 2002;**61**:1887-1893

[48] Koch M, Kutkuhn B, Trenkwalder E, Bach D, Grabensee B, Dieplinger H, Kronenberg F. Apolipoprotein B, fibrinogen, HDL cholesterol, and apolipoprotein(a) phenotypes

predict coronary artery disease in hemodialysis patients. Journal of the American Society of Nephrology. 1997;**8**:1889-1898

[49] Tonelli M, Isles C, Curhan GC et al. Effect of pravastatin on cardiovascular events in people with chronic kidney disease. Circulation. 2004;**110**:1557-1563

[50] Neves PL, Malho A, Cabrita A, et al. Statins and vitamin D: A friendly association in pre-dialysis patients. International Urology and Nephrology. 2010;**42**:173-179

[51] Baigent C, Landray MJ, Reith, et al. The Effects of lowering LDL cholesterol with simvastatin plus ezetimibe in patients with chronic kidney disease. (Study of Heart and Renal Protection): A randomised placebo-controlled trial. Lancet. 2011;**377**: 2181-2192

[52] Fellstrom BC, Jardine AG, Schmieder RE, et al, for the AURORA Study Group. Rosuvastatin and cardiovascular events in patients undergoing hemodialysis. New England Journal of Medicine. 2009;**360**:1395-1407

[53] Wanner C, Kane V, Marz W, et al, for German Diabetes and Dialysis Study Investigators. Atorvastatin in patients with type 2 diabetes mellitus undergoing hemodialysis. New England Journal of Medicine. 2005;**353**:238-248

[54] Guedes AM, Neves PL. Statins for renal patients: A fiddler on the roof? International Journal of Nephrology. 2012;**2012**. DOI: 10.1155/2012/806872

[55] KDIGO Guidelines. Pharmacological cholesterol-lowering treatment in adults. Kidney International Supplement. 2013;**3**:271-279

[56] Di Lullo L, Gorini A, Russo D, Santoboni A, Ronco C. Left ventricular hypertrophy in chronic kidney disease patients: From pathophysiology to treatment. Cardiorenal Medicine. 2015;**5**:254-266

[57] Levy D, Anderson KM, Savage DD, Kannel WB, Christiansen JC, Castelli WP. Echocardiographically detected left ventricular hypertrophy: Prevalence and risk factors The Framingham Heart Study. Annals of Internal Medicine. 1988;**108**:7-13

[58] Parfrey S, Foley RN, Harnett JD, Kent GM, Murray DC, Barre PE. Outcome and risk factors for left ventricular disorders in chronic uraemia. Nephrology, Dialysis, Transplantation. 1996;**11**:1277-1285

[59] Jerónimo T, Fragoso A, Mendes F, et al. Mineral metabolism and inflammation: Factors related to left ventricular hypertrophy in patients with diabetic nephropathy. Portuguese Journal of Nephrology & Hypertension. 2016;**30**:121-131

[60] Ioannou K, Stel VS, Dounousi E, et al. Inflammation, endothelial dysfunction and increased left ventricular mass in chronic kidney disease (CKD) patients: a longitudinal study. PLoS One **10**:e0138461

[61] Gutiérrez OM. Connecting the dots on fibroblast growth factor 23 and left ventricular hypertrophy. Nephrology, Dialysis, Transplantation. 2016;**31**:1031-1033

[62] Neves PL, Silva AP, Bernardo I. Elderly patients in chronic hemodialysis: Risk factors for left ventricular hypertrophy. American Journal of Kidney Diseases. 1997;**30**:224-228

[63] Ruzicka M, Leenen FHH. Hypertensive therapy in dialysis patients. Seminars in Dialysis. 1994;**3**:176-178

[64] Covic A, Mardare NG, Ardeleanu S, Prisada O, Gusbeth-Tatomir P, Goldsmith DJ. Serial echocardiographic changes in patients on hemodialysis: An evaluation of guideline implementation. Journal of Nephrology. 2006;**19**:783-793

[65] Culleton BF, Walsh M, Klarenbach SW, et al. Effect of frequent nocturnal hemodialysis vs conventional hemodialysis on left ventricular mass and quality of life: A randomized controlled trial. JAMA. 2007;**298**:1291-1299

[66] London GM, Pannier B, Guerin AP, et al. Alterations of left ventricular hypertrophy in and survival of patients receiving hemodialysis: Follow-up of an interventional study. Journal of the American Society of Nephrology. 2001;**12**:2759-2767

[67] Block G A, Hulbert-Shearon TE, Levin NW, Port FK. Association of serum phosphorus and calcium x phosphorus product with mortality risk in chronic hemodialysis patients: A national study. American Journal of Kidney Diseases. 1998;**31**:607-617

[68] Tentori F, Blayney MJ, Albert JM et al. Mortality risk for dialysis patients with different levels of serum calcium, phosphorus, and PTH: The Dialysis Outcomes and Practice Patterns Study (DOPPS). American Journal of Kidney Diseases. 2008;**52**:519-530

[69] Tonelli M, Sacks F, Pfeffer M et al. Relation between serum phosphate level and cardiovascular event rate in people with coronary disease. Circulation. 2005;**112**:2627-2633

[70] Dhingra R, Sullivan LM, Fox CS et al. Relations of serum phosphorus and calcium levels to the incidence of cardiovascular disease in the community. Archives of Internal Medicine. 2007;**167**:879-885

[71] Foley RN, Collins AJ, Ishani A, et al. Calcium-phosphate levels and cardiovascular disease in community-dwelling adults: The Atherosclerosis Risk in Communities (ARIC) Study. American Heart Journal. 2008;**156**:556-563

[72] Jung HH, Kim SW, Han H. Inflammation, mineral metabolism and progressive coronary artery calcification in patients on haemodialysis. Nephrology, Dialysis, Transplantation. 2006;**21**:1915-1920

[73] Adeney KL, Siscovick DS, Ix JH et al. Association of serum phosphate with vascular and valvular calcification in moderate CKD. Journal of the American Society of Nephrology. 2009;**20**:381-387

[74] Kannel WB, Wolf PA, Garrison RJ. Monograph Section 34: Some Risk Factors Related to the Annual Incidence of Cardiovascular Disease and Death Using Pooled Repeated Biennial Measurements: Framingham Heart Study, 30-Year Followup. Springfield, Mass: National Technical Information Service; 1987. pp. 1-459

[75] Narang R, Ridout D, Nonis C, Kooner JS. Serum calcium, phosphorus and albumin levels in relation to the angiographic severity of coronary artery disease. International Journal of Cardiology. 1997;**60**:73-79

[76] Rasouli M, Kiasari AM. Serum calcium and phosphorus associate with the occurrence and severity of angiographically documented coronary heart disease, possibly through correlation with atherogenic (apo)lipoproteins. Clinical Chemistry and Laboratory Medicine. 2006;**44**(1):43-50

[77] Ruan L, Chen, Srinivasan SR, Xu J, Toprak A, Berenson GS. Relation of serum phosphorus levels to carotid intima-media thickness in asymptomatic young adults (from the Bogalusa Heart Study). American Journal of Cardiology. 2010;**106**(6):793-797

[78] Onufrak SJ, Bellasi A, Shaw LJ, et al. Phosphorus levels are associated with subclinical atherosclerosis in the general population. Atherosclerosis. 2008;**199**:424-431

[79] Saab G, Whooley MA, Schiller NB, Ix JH. Association of serum phosphorus with left ventricular mass in men and women with stable cardiovascular disease: Data from the Heart and Soul Study. American Journal of Kidney Disease. 2010;**56**:496-505

[80] Kendrick J, Kestenbaum B, Chonchol M. Phosphate and cardiovascular disease. Advances in Chronic Kidney Disease. 2011;**18**:113-119

[81] El-Abbadi MM, Pai AS, Leaf EM, et al. Phosphate feeding induces arterial medial calcification in uremic mice: Role of serum phosphorus, fibroblast growth factor-23, and osteopontin. Kidney International. 2009;**75**:1297-1307

[82] Amann K, Ritz E, Wiest G et al. A role of parathyroid hormone for the activation of cardiac fibroblasts in uremia. Journal of the American Society of Nephrology. 1994;**4**:1814-1819

[83] Rostand SG, Drüeke TB. Parathyroid hormone, vitamin D, and cardiovascular disease in chronic renal failure. Kidney. International. 1999;**56**:383-392

[84] Jono S, Nishizawa Y, Shioi A, Morii H. Parathyroid hormone–related peptide as a local regulator of vascular calcification: Its inhibitory action on in vitro calcification by bovine vascular smooth muscle cells. Arteriosclerosis, Thrombosis, and Vascular Biology. 1997;**17**:1135-1142

[85] Jono S, McKee M, Shioi A, Nishizawa Y, Mori K, et al. Phosphate regulation of vascular smooth muscle cell calcification. Circulation Research. 2000;**87**:e10-e17

[86] Graciolli FG, Neves KR, dos Reis LM, et al. Phosphorus overload and PTH induce aortic expression of Runx2 in experimental uraemia. Nephrology, Dialysis, Transplantation. 2009;**24**:1416-1421

[87] Moe SM, O'Neill KD, Duan D, et al. Medial artery calcification in ESRD patients is associated with deposition of bone matrix proteins. Kidney International. 2002;**61**:638-647

[88] Shuto E, Taketani Y, Tanaka R, et al. Dietary phosphorus acutely impairs endothelial function. Journal of the American Society of Nephrology. 2009;**20**:1504-1512

[89] Di Marco GS, König M, Stock C, et al. High phosphate directly affects endothelial function by downregulating annexin II. Kidney International 2013;**83**:213-222

[90] Maizel J, Six I, Dupont S, et al. Effects of sevelamer treatment on cardiovascular abnormalities in mice with chronic renal failure. Kidney International 2013;**84**:491-500

[91] Mathew S, Lund RJ, Strebeck F, Tustison KS, Geurs T, Hruska KA. Reversal of the adynamic bone disorder and decreased vascular calcification in chronic kidney disease by sevelamer carbonate therapy. Journal of the American Society of Nephrology. 2007;**18**:122-130

[92] Van TV, Watari E,Taketani Y, et al. Dietary phosphate restriction ameliorates endothelial dysfunction in adenine-induced kidney disease rats. Journal of Clinical Biochemistry and Nutrition. 2012;**51**:27-32

[93] Ahn J, Yu K, Stolzenberg-Solomon R, et al. Genome-wide association study of circulating vitamin D levels. Human Molecular Genetics. 2010;**19**(13):2739-2745

[94] Bachschmid MM, Van der loo B. A new sunshine in the vasculature. Circulation. 2005;**111**:1571-1573

[95] Weishaar RE, Simpson RU. Involvement of vitamin D3 with cardiovascular function, II: Direct and indirect effects. American Journal of Physiology. 1987;**253**:E675-E683

[96] Hochhauser E, Barak J, Kushnir T, Navon G, Meyer MS, Edelstein S, Ben Bassat MB, Vidne BA. Mechanical, biochemical, and structural effects of vitamin D deficiency on the chick heart. Angiology. 1989;**40**:300-308

[97] O'Connell TD, Berry JE, Jarvis AK, Somerman MJ, Simpson RU.1,25-dihydroxyvitamin D3 regulation of cardiac myocyte proliferation and hypertrophy. American Journal of Physiology - Heart and Circulatory Physiology. 1997;**272**:H1751-H1758

[98] Wakasugi M, Noguchi T, Inoue M, Kazama Y, Tawata M, Kanemaru Y Onaya T. Vitamin D3 stimulates the production of prostacyclin by vascular smooth muscle cells. Prostaglandins. 1991;**42**:127-136

[99] Wu J, Garami M, Cao L, Li Q, Gardner DG. 1,25(OH)2D3 suppresses expression and secretion of atrial natriuretic peptide from cardiac myocytes. American Journal of Physiology. 1995;**268**:E1108-E1113

[100] Zittermann A, Schleithoff SS, Koerfer R. Putting cardiovascular disease and vitamin D deficiency into perspective. The British Journal of Nutrition. 2005;**94**:483-492

[101] Smogorzewski M, Perna AF, Borum PR, Massry SG. Fatty acid oxidation in the myocardium: Effects of parathyroid hormone and CRF. Kidney International. 1988;**34**:797-803

[102] Pfeilschifter J, Lauhuf F, Müller-Beckmann B, Blum WF, Pfistr T, Ziegler R. Parathyroid hormone increases the concentration of insulin-like growth factor-I and transforming growth factor beta 1 in rat bone. Journal of Clinical Investigation. 1995;**96**:767-774

[103] Artaza JN, Mehrotra R, Norris KC. Vitamin D and the cardiovascular system. CJASN. 2009 September;**4**(9):1515-1522

[104] Kiechl S, Werner P, Knoflach M, Furtner M, Willeit J, Schett G. The osteoprotegerin/RANK/RANKL system: A bone key to vascular disease. Expert Review of Cardiovascular Therapy. 2006;**4**:801-811

[105] Kiechl S, Schett G, Schwaiger J, et al. Soluble receptor activator of nuclear factor-ligand and risk for cardiovascular disease. Circulation. 2007;**116**:385-391

[106] Krivosíková Z, Spustová V, Stefíková K, Dzúrik R. The influence of vitamin D supplementation on OPG/RANKL/RANK system in postmenopausal women: The six month clinical study. Bone. 2006;**38**:S27

[107] HofBauer LC, Kühne CA, Viereck V. The OPG/RANKL/RANK system in metabolic bone disease. Journal of Musculoskeletal & Neuronal Interactions. 2004;**4**:268-275

[108] Scragg R. Seasonality of cardiovascular disease mortality and the possible protective effect of ultra-violet radiation. International Journal of Epidemiology. 1981;**10**:337-341

[109] Fabsitz R, Feinleib M. Geographic patterns in county mortality rates from cardiovascular diseases. American Journal of Epidemiology. 1980;**111**:315-328

[110] Smith WC, Tunstall-Pedoe H. European regional variation in cardiovascular mortality. British Medical Bulletin. 1984;**40**:374-379

[111] Giovannucci E, Liu Y, Hollis BW et al. 25-hydroxyvitamin D and risk of myocardial infarction in men: A prospective study. Archives of Internal Medicine. 2008;**168**:1174-1180

[112] Dobnig H, Pilz S, Scharnagl H et al. Independent association of low serum 25-hydroxyvitamin D and 1,25-dihydroxy VD levels with all-cause and cardiovascular mortality. Archives of Internal Medicine. 2008;**168**:1340-1349

[113] Wang L, Song Y, Manson JE et al. Circulating 25-hydroxy-vitamin D and risk of cardiovascular disease: A meta-analysis of prospective studies. Circulation. Cardiovascular Quality and Outcomes. 2012;**5**:819-829

[114] Grandi NC, Breitling LP, Brenner H. Vitamin D and cardiovascular disease: Systematic review and meta-analysis of prospective studies. Preventive Medicine. 2010;**51**:228-233

[115] Thadhani R, Appelbaum E, Pritchett Y, Chang Y, Wenger J, et al. Vitamin D therapy and cardiac structure and function in patients with chronic kidney disease: The PRIMO randomized controlled trial. JAMA. 2012;**307**:674-684

[116] Wu J, Garami M, Cheng T et al. 1,25(OH)2 VD3, and retinoic acid antagonize endothelin-stimulated hypertrophy of neonatal rat cardiac myocytes. Journal of Clinical Investigation. 1996;**97**:1577-1588

[117] Meems LM, Cannon MV, Mahmud H et al. The vitamin D receptor activator paricalcitol prevents fibrosis and diastolic dysfunction in a murine model of pressure overload. Journal of Steroid Biochemistry and Molecular Biology. 2012;**132**:282-289

[118] Oliveira RB, Moysés RMA. FGF-23: State of the art. Jornal Brasileiro de Nefrologia. 2010;**32**:323-331

[119] Quarles LD. Skeletal secretion of FGF-23 regulates phosphate and vitamin D metabolism. Nature Reviews Endocrinology. 2012;**8**:276-286

[120] Kestenbaum B, Sachs MC, Hoofnagle AN, et al. Fibroblast growth factor-23 and cardiovascular disease in the general population: The Multi-Ethnic Study of Atherosclerosis. Circulation. Heart Failure. 2014;**7**:409-417

[121] Wolf M. Forging forward with 10 burning questions on FGF23 in kidney disease. Journal of the American Society of Nephrology. 2010;**21**:1427-1435

[122] Tuñón J, Cristóbal C, Tarín N et al. Coexistence of low vitamin D and high fibroblast growth factor-23 plasma levels predicts an adverse outcome in patients with coronary artery disease. PLoS One. 2014;**9**:e95402

[123] Burnett SM, Gunawardene SC, Bringhurst FR, Jüppner H, Lee H, Finkelstein JS. Regulation of C-terminal and intact FGF-23 by dietary phosphate in men and women. Journal of Bone and Mineral Research. 2006;**21**:1187-1196

[124] Antoniucci DM, Yamashita T, Portale AA. Dietary phosphorus regulates serum fibroblast growth factor-23 concentrations in healthy men. Journal of Clinical Endocrinology and Metabolism. 2006 Aug;**91**(8):3144-3149

[125] Hasegawa H, Nagano N, Urakawa I, et al. Direct evidence for a causative role of FGF23 in the abnormal renal phosphate handling and vitamin D metabolism in rats with early-stage chronic kidney disease. Kidney International. 2010;**78**:975-980

[126] Wahl P, Wolf M. FGF23 in chronic kidney disease. Advances in Experimental Medicine and Biology. 2012;**728**:107-125

[127] Drüeke TB, Massy ZA. Circulating Klotho levels: Clinical relevance and relationship with tissue Klotho expression. Kidney International. 2013;**83**(19):13-15.

[128] Aline Martin A, Valentin David,L. Darryl Quarles. Regulation and function of the FGF23/Klotho endocrine pathways. Physiological Reviews. 2012;**92**:131-155

[129] Touchberry CD, Green TM, Tchikrizov V, et al. FGF23 is a novel regulator of intracellular calcium and cardiac contractility in addition to cardiac hypertrophy. American Journal of Physiology, Endocrinology and Metabolism. 2013;**304**:E863-E873

[130] Gutierrez OM, Mannstadt M, Isakova T, et al. Fibroblast growth factor 23 and mortality among patients undergoing hemodialysis. New England Journal of Medicine. 2008;**359**:584-592

[131] Jean G, Terrat JC, Vanel T, et al. High levels of serum fibroblast growth factor (FGF)-23 are associated with increased mortality in long haemodialysis patients. Nephrology, Dialysis, Transplantation. 2009;**24**:2792-2796

[132] Faul C, Amaral AP, Oskouei B, et al. FGF23 induces left ventricular hypertrophy. Journal of Clinical Investigation. 2011;**121**:4393-4408

[133] Wyatt CM and Drueke TB. Fibroblast growth factor receptor 4: The missing link between chronic kidney disease and FGF23-induced left ventricular hypertrophy? Kidney International. 2016;**89**:7-9

[134] Mirza MA, Hansen T, Johansson L, et al. Relationship between circulating FGF23 and total body atherosclerosis in the community. Nephrology, Dialysis, Transplantation. 2009;**24**(10):3125-3131

[135] Parker BD, Schurgers LJ, Brandenburg VM, et al. The associations of fibroblast growth factor 23 and uncarboxylated matrix Gla protein with mortality in coronary artery disease: The Heart and Soul Study. Annals of Internal Medicine. 2010;**152**(10):640-648

[136] Liabeuf S, Okazaki H, Desjardins L, et al. Vascular calcification in chronic kidney disease: Are biomarkers useful for probing the pathobiology and the health risks of this process in the clinical scenario? Nephrology, Dialysis, Transplantation. 2014;**29**(7):1275-1284

[137] Zhang M, Yan J, Zhu M , Ni Z. Fibroblast growth factor 23 predicts coronary calcification and poor prognosis in patients with chronic kidney disease stages 3-5D. Annals of Clinical and Laboratory Science. 2015;**45**(1):17-22

[138] Price PA, Lim JE. The inhibition of calcium phosphate precipitation by fetuin is accompanied by the formation of a fetuin-mineral complex. Journal of Biological Chemistry. 2003;**278**:22144-22152

[139] Roos, M, Lutz, J, Salmhofer, H, et al, Relation between plasma fibroblast growth factor-23, serum fetuin-A levels and coronary artery calcification evaluated by multislice computed tomography in patients with normal kidney function. Clinical Endocrinology. 2008;**68**:660-665

[140] Scialla JJ, Lau WL, Reilly MP, et al. Chronic Renal Insufficiency Cohort Study Investigators. Fibroblast growth factor 23 is not associated with and does not induce arterial calcification. Kidney International. 2013;**83**(6):1159-1168

[141] Fukino K, Suzuki T, Saito Y, et al. Regulation of angiogenesis by the aging suppressor gene klotho. Biochemical and Biophysical Research Communications. 2002;**293**:332-337

[142] Kurosu H, Yamamoto M, Clark JD, Pastor JV, Nandi A, Gurnani P, et al. Suppression of aging in mice by the hormone Klotho. Science. 2005 Sep 16;**309**(5742):1829-1833

[143] Matsumura Y, Aizawa H, Shiraki-Iida T, Nagai R, Kuro-o M, Nabeshima Y. Identification of the human klotho gene and its two transcripts encoding membrane and secreted klotho protein. Biochemical and Biophysical Research Communications. 1998 Jan 26;**242**(3): 626-630

[144] Kuro-o M. Overview of the FGF23-Klotho axis. Pediatric Nephrology. 2010 Apr;**25**(4): 583-590. PubMed PMID: 19626341

[145] Shroff R and Shanahan MC. Klotho: An elixir of youth for the vasculature? Journal of the American Society of Nephrology. 2011;**22**:5-7

[146] Erben RG. Update on FGF23 and Klotho signaling. Molecular and Cellular Endocrinology. 2016;**432**:56-65

[147] Kuro-o M. Klotho and aging. Biochimica et Biophysica Acta. 2009;**1790**(10):1049-1058

[148] Hu MC, Shi M, Zhang J, et al. Klotho deficiency causes vascular calcification in chronic kidney disease. Journal of the American Society of Nephrology: JASN. 2011;**22**(1):124-136

[149] Xie J, Yoon J, An SW, Kuro-o M, Huang CL. Soluble klotho protects against uremic cardiomyopathy independently of fibroblast growth factor 23 and phosphate. Journal of the American Society of Nephrology. 2015 May;**26**(5):1150-1160

[150] Xie J, Cha SK, An SW, Kuro-O M, Birnbaumer L, Huang CL, Cardioprotection by Klotho through downregulation of TRPC6 channels in the mouse heart. Nature Communications. 2012;**3**:1238

[151] Hu MC, Shi M, Cho HJ, et al. Klotho and phosphate are modulators of pathologic uremic cardiac remodeling. American Society of Nephrology. 2015;**26**(6):1290-1302

[152] Floege J, Fliser D.Klotho Deficiency and the cardiomyopathy of advanced CKD. Journal of the American Society of Nephrology. 2015;**26**:1229-1237

Chapter 5

Cardiovascular Aspects of Patients with Chronic Kidney Disease and End-Stage Renal Disease

Ali Osama Malik, Sumit Sehgal,
Hashim Hussnain Ahmed, Subodh Devabhaktuni,
Edward Co, Arhama Aftab Malik, Syed Shah and
Chowdhury Ahsan

Additional information is available at the end of the chapter

http://dx.doi.org/10.5772/intechopen.69294

Abstract

Chronic kidney disease (CKD) is a globally recognized public health concern. Multiple studies have shown the association of CKD with cardiovascular mortality that persists after adjustment for traditional cardiovascular disease (CVD) risk factors. CKD causes accelerated coronary artery disease (CAD). In this chapter, we discuss the pathophysiological mechanisms that play a role in increasing CVD risk in patients with CKD. Further we delve into some commonly encountered challenges related to CVD in patients with CKD. These include revascularization challenges, contrasted induced nephropathy and alterations in traditional risk factors for CVD in renal transplant patients.

Keywords: coronary artery disease, chronic kidney disease, mortality, morbidity, public health

1. Introduction

Chronic kidney disease (CKD) is recognized as a major global public health problem [1]. It is estimated that 10–25% of population from Asia, Australia, Europe and United States of America (USA) is affected by CKD [2–6].

Multiple studies have shown the association of CKD with cardiovascular mortality that persists after adjustment for traditional cardiovascular disease (CVD) risk factors. These include the Atherosclerosis Risk in Communities study (ARIC) and the Cardiovascular

Health Study [7–9]. The risk of developing congestive heart failure, atrial fibrillation, stroke, coronary artery disease (CAD) and peripheral artery disease (PAD) is increased twofold in patients with glomerular filtration rate (eGFR) < 70ml/min/1.73m^2 [8, 10]. Furthermore, in two separate meta-analyses of twenty-one studies from fourteen different countries eGFR and albuminuria were found to be independently associated with increased risk of all-cause and cardiovascular mortality [11, 12].

In this chapter we discuss the acute and chronic cardiovascular impact of patients with reduced kidney function. We further delve in evaluation of coronary artery disease in patients with CKD. We also address the cardiovascular aspects of patient care in renal transplant patients including modification of traditional CVD risk factors in patients taking immunosuppressive therapy.

2. Epidemiology

CKD is a globally recognized public health burden [13]. USA alone deals with a population of more than 20 million people with CKD [14]. Data from other developed and developing nations confirms the rising trend of the disease. Data from China estimates this number to be close to 100 million Chinese being affected with CKD [15].

CKD has long shared its associations with CVD. The prevalence of CVD among patients with CKD has been known across trials in USA, Japan, Spain, United Kingdom and, recently, across China. Highest prevalence was found in U.K., 47.2% followed by Spain, 39.1%, U.S., 33.4%, Japan, 26.8% and China 9.8% [16–19].

United States Renal Data System (USRDS) reports from 2016 revealed the prevalence of any cardiovascular event to be twice among those with CKD compared to those without it, 68.8% vs. 34.1% respectively.

2.1. Linear relationship of cardiovascular mortality with EGFR

CKD is an independent risk factor for progression to cardiovascular disease, known to contribute to cardiovascular morbidity and mortality [20]. Go et al., using longitudinal measurement of estimated eGFR, demonstrated the inverse relationship between eGFR and mortality rate secondary to cardiovascular events, below an eGFR of 60 ml/min per 1.73 m^2 [21]. A meta-analysis from 2011, comprising a grand total of 266,975 patients reported an exponential rise in mortality with eGFR below 60 ml/min per 1.73 m^2 [22]. (21,307,840) For cardiovascular mortality, adjusted hazard ratios at eGFR 60, 45, and 15 ml/min per 1.73 m^2 were 1.11 (0.93–1.32), 1.73 (1.49–2.00), and 3.08 (1.89–5.01), respectively [22].

Manjunath et al., also demonstrated eGFR as an independent risk factor for progression to CVD [23]. In a sample population of 4893, subjects with GFR 90 mL/min/1.73 m^2 had a 15% risk of CVD over 3 years while subjects with GFR 30 mL/min/1.73 m^2 had a 40% risk of CVD [23]. These findings were independent from traditional risk factors of cardiovascular diseases.

2.2. Albuminuria a marker of worse cardiovascular outcomes in CKD patients

Abuminuria has been proven to be a significant risk factor for all cause and CVD related mortality in patients with CKD. Pooled data from Van der Welde et al., demonstrated a significant increase in cardiovascular mortality in patients with Albumin-to-creatinine ratio of 10 mg/dl compared to 5 mg/dl [22]. Similar results demonstrating an association of CVD mortality with albuminuria have been reported in other large scale studies [11, 12].

3. Ischemic heart disease in chronic kidney disease

3.1. Background

Cardiovascular (CV) mortality is the leading cause of death in CKD patients and the risk of CV mortality increases with decrease in eGFR. Most of the burden of CV mortality in CKD patients is secondary to ischemic heart disease or complications associated with it including congestive heart failure. The severity and incidence of CAD increases as the kidney function declines with the prevalence of multi-vessel CAD and left main disease being significantly higher in the CKD population [24].

Coronary arteries in CKD patients have shown to exhibit more extensive atherosclerosis [25]. Multiple studies have shown the association of CKD with cardiovascular mortality that persists after adjustment for traditional cardiovascular disease (CVD) risk factors [26, 27]. Mineralocorticoid excess, oxidative stress and cellular inflammation are linked to plaque formation and rupture in CKD patients. Vitamin D deficiency a common sequela of CKD could explain the propensity of CKD patients to develop CAD. It has been shown that patients with Vitamin D deficiency have higher risk of myocardial infarction (MI). Similarly fibroblast growth factor 23 (FGF 23) a hormone usually elevated in CKD patients, to mitigate hyperphosphatemia was associated with increased CVD mortality in patients with CKD [28, 29].

In summation, the pathophysiological basis of increased CVD risk and severity in patients with CKD is due to a complex interplay of factors involving hormonal and immune mediated responses. However the risk of CAD in CKD has been well established. Hence in 2013 the American Heart Association (AHA) issued a statement to classify CKD as an independent risk factor for developing CVD [30].

3.2. Revascularization in CKD patients with stable CAD

Management of patients with established CAD and CKD is challenging. Medical management in patients with renal dysfunction has been based on therapy shown to be beneficial in patient population without CKD. These medications include aspirin, beta-blockers, nitrates, hydroxymethylglutaryl co-enzyme A reductase inhibitors (statins) and angiotensin converting enzyme inhibitors. However because of routine exclusion of CKD patients from clinical trials, the efficacy of these agents in patients with CKD is still unclear.

No robust evidence is yet available to ascertain whether CKD patients with chronic stable angina who undergo revascularization have a definite survival advantage compared to CKD patients on medical therapy alone. In the only randomized study of dialysis patients comparing invasive approach (PCI and coronary artery bypass graft surgery (CABG)) with medical therapy alone, the invasive approach had a clear survival benefit [31]. However medical therapy at that time only consisted of calcium channel blockers, and use of other agents proven to have survival advantage in patients with cardiovascular disease was not the norm. Furthermore, this study only included patients with diabetes mellitus. In another study done in 2002, PCI did not significantly improve survival [32].

Multiple studies have found that patients with CKD who undergo revascularization for CAD have worst outcomes compared to patients with normal kidney function [32, 33]. Patients with CKD have more cardiovascular risk factors at baseline [32]. Furthermore, CKD itself was independently associated with worst outcomes including increased all-cause mortality and subsequent cardiac events [32].

In CKD revascularization procedures including percutanous coronary intervention (PCI) and coronary artery bypass graft surgery (CABG) are complicated by risk of contrast induced nephropathy (CIN) and increased risk of bleeding due to dual antiplatelet therapy. CIN is discussed in detail in separate section.

CKD results in complex hemostatic disorder manifested by increased bleeding and thrombosis. Hence the use of antiplatelet therapy has the potential for both benefit and harm. Reduced platelet aggregation, intrinsic platelet dysfunction and abnormalities in platelet-endothelial interactions are found in CKD and may in part account for increased bleeding risk with PCI in these patients [34–36].

On the contrary, some studies have suggested the presence of pro-thrombotic state in CKD patients that manifest by an increase in serum fibrinogen, von Willibrand factor and reduction in antithrombin 3 [34, 37–39]. Therefore, it is unclear whether dual antiplatelet therapy after PCI is beneficial and safe in CKD patients. Furthermore, few studies have evaluated the appropriate dosing of antithrombotic agents or anticoagulants in patients with CKD [40].

Although clinical restenosis rates are not higher compared to patients with normal renal function, on repeated angiography restenosis rates were found to be as high as 60–81% [41, 42]. Thus, absence of symptoms of restenosis in patients with chronic renal insufficiency may lead to silent ischemia and contribute to high risk of subsequent cardiac events.

CKD patients have worse outcomes after CABG. One study found in-hospital mortality rate to be 14.6% [43]. Another study that was done on end-stage renal disease (ESRD) patients over course of 10 years found peri-operative mortality to be about 14% in cardiac surgery patients [44]. Even mild renal insufficiency is associated with double in-hospitality rates in one analysis [45]. CAD is more diffuse in patients with renal dysfunction which likely contributes higher complication rates and worst outcomes.

Szczech et al. published a study in 2001 that showed survival benefit among patients with ESRD undergoing CABG as compared to PCI, while controlling for severity of CAD, LV dysfunction and other comorbid conditions [46]. However in analysis of CREDO-Hyoto PCI/CABG registry Marui A et al. found CABG relative to PCI reduced risk of cardiac death, sudden death, myocardial infarction and need for revascularization in patients with left main disease or multi-vessel CAD only [47]. In a study by Banglore et al., revascularization with Everolimus eluting stensts was compared to CABG in patients with CKD. The authors concluded that CABG was associated with higher short term risk of death, stroke and repeat revascularization, whereas PCI with everolimus-eluting stent was associated with higher long-term risk of revascularization and perhaps MI [48]. Current American College of Cardiology (ACC) and American Heart Association (AHA) guidelines recommend CABG for patients with left main or multi-vessel disease irrespective of renal function.

3.3. Non-invasive cardiac imaging in patients with CKD

As already mentioned CKD patients are at a higher risk of CVD. Imaging plays a central role in risk stratification and assessment of severity of CAD. A range of imaging modalities have been developed to assist with diagnosis and risk stratification of CVD in patients with CKD.

Myocardial perfusion imaging (MPI) is widely used for non-invasive assessment of myocardial ischemia due to CAD [49]. MPI can be performed using single photon emission computed tomography (SPECT) as well as positron emission tomography (PET). SPECT MPI is more widely available. It can be performed with a variety of stressors such as exercise or administration of vasodilatory agents (adenosine or regadenoson) or dobutamine. SPECT detects areas of reduced perfusion by measuring and comparing the distribution of injected radioactive tracers such as 99 technetium or 201 thallium, when at rest and after stressor/vasodilator agents.

For PET MPI stress perfusion is measured in the same way as SPECT. Various agents can be used as radiotracer including H2 15 O, ammonia or rubidium. With PET absolute quantification of myocardial blood flow is possible. Although both SPECT and PET MPI have widely been studied for detection of CAD in general population, data regarding their use in CKD population in limited.

Echocardiography plays a pivotal role in assessment of cardiac dysfunction in patients with or without renal insufficiency. Various cardiac abnormalities including left ventricular hypertrophy (LVH), diastolic or systolic dysfunction are predictive of poor prognosis in CKD patients and can be rapidly diagnosed using 2 D trans-thoracic echocardiogram (TTE). Stress echocardiography is an established technique used to investigate myocardial viability and ischemia. Patients can be stressed either pharmacologically with dobutamine or with exercise [50]. However, the sensitivity and specificity of stress echocardiography is modest in patients with CKD. In a systemic review by Sharma et al. sensitivity of stress echocardiography was 80% in patients with ESRD [51]. Factors limiting the role of stress echocardiography for detecting CAD in patients with CKD include LVH and blunted chronotropic response in patients with CKD [52, 53].

CT coronary angiography (CTA) has good sensitivity and specificity for detection of CAD in non-CKD population [54]. However, data is limited in patients with CKD. Iodinated contrast agent is required that increases the risk of contrast induced nephropathy. (contrast induced nephropathy is discussed in separate section) Furthermore concerns exist that diffuse calcifications in CKD patients might render interpretation of CTA findings difficult. In patients on hemodialysis (HD) calcifications can occur in intima, where it contributes to luminal stenosis or medial where it is related to vascular stiffness. CTA might not be able to discern the difference. Despite these limitations some small studies have reported > 90% sensitivity of CTA to detect CAD in patients on HD [55]. However, coronary angiography was not used as gold standard in these studies.

Leading authors have advocated for combining functional imaging technique with anatomical imaging technique for CAD screening in clinical practice. Although these hybrid techniques are potentially useful in general population, none have been validated in patients with CKD [56, 82]. Role of non-invasive imaging for pre-transplant evaluation of CAD is addressed in a separate section.

3.4. Contrast Induced Nephropathy

PCI in patients with CKD is challenging due to presence of complex calcified lesions and the very high risk of CIN. PCI in patients with advanced CKD is associated with increased risk of CIN which is independently associated with major adverse clinical events [57]. Outcomes are even worse if renal replacement therapy is required [57].

Pathophysiologically several mechanisms are involved in acute kidney injury caused by CIN. Studies have shown evidence of acute tubular necrosis (ATN). Two mechanism of ATN have been postulated. Direct nephrotoxicity of contrast agents has been documented [58, 59]. Furthermore, it has also been hypothesized that renal vasoconstriction, mediated by endothelin and prostaglandins resulting in medullary hypoxia causes ATN [60–62].

Studies have demonstrated a dose-dependent relationship of acute kidney injury (AKI) caused by CIN [63]. The type of contrast alters the risk of CIN. The use of first generation hyperosmolar ionic agents is associated with a greater risk of CIN [64]. Prevention strategies for CIN that have been well established also apply to patients undergoing PCI. These include using minimal amount of contrast, avoiding ionic contrast and non-steroidal anti-inflammatory drugs (NSAIDs).

Most recently Galougahi et al. have described a case series of a unique approach toward revascularization in patients with CKD by sequential diagnostic angiography using ultra-low volumes of contrast followed by staged physiology and intravascular ultrasound (IVUS)-guided zero contrast PCI in three patients with severely calcified coronary lesions [65]. While such strategies have potential for more wider acceptance, at this time they are not practiced widely due to technical and procedural limitations.

4. Use of troponin concentration level in patients with chronic kidney disease

Troponin proteins are present in both cardiac and skeletal muscle [66]. Cardiac troponin C is identicial to troponin C expressed in skeletal muscle. However cardiac troponin TnT and TnI are each derived from genes that are specific to the heart [66]. Hence troponin T (cTnT) and Troponin I (cTnI) are considered the preferred biochemical markers to detect myocardial injury and to diagnose acute myocardial infarction (AMI). Since the introduction of high sensitivity cardiac troponin (hs-cTn) assays, more accurate detection of low levels of circulating cardiac troponins became feasible [67].

However the increase in sensitivity of hs-cTn for AMI is accompanied by decrease in specificity [68, 69]. In patients with chronic kidney disease elevated hs-cTn concentrations are associated with reduced renal function.

The interpretation of serum markers for myocardial injury in patients with renal insufficiency remains controversial. Large scale trials of patients with acute coronary syndrome (ACS) have documented the importance of troponin elevations in risk stratification, prognosis and therapeutic utilization. However most of these studies excluded patients with renal insufficiency.

Cardinaels et al. recently showed that in patients with acute chest discomfort hs-cTnT and hs-cTnI were strongly correlated with eGFR [70]. Although differences were small, the authors reported a greater correlation of hs-cTnT with eGFR compared to hs-cTnI. Furthermore, the association of hs-cTnT is greater with eGFR as compared to any other cardiac parameters including coronary plaque severity, coronary calcium score and left ventricular structure [70]. In contrast to hs-TnT, hs-TnI has a greater association with LV mass compared to eGFR. Hence it is possible that hs-TnT is more susceptible to renal clearance then hs-cTnI. However, these differences are yet to be completely established.

Furthermore, many investigators have hypothesized uremic-induced skeletal myopathy may be responsible for increased troponins in patients with renal failure [66]. This conclusion is centered on the notion that uremia may promote re-expression of cardiac TnT from injured or regenerating cardiac muscle fibers. Some anecdotal reports show elevated serum TnT levels in patients with skeletal muscle injury or inflammatory myopathies in the absence of any obvious myocardial ischemia [71, 72]. In marathon runners without any history of coronary artery disease cardiac TnT levels were elevated after running a marathon [73]. Hence cardiac troponin levels may be elevated in patients with renal insufficiency in the absence of AMI due to increased production from skeletal muscles and possible due to decreased renal clearance. It is imperative to evaluate troponin concentrations in patients with CKD in proper clinical context and utilization of other resources such as Electrocardiogram (EKG) to rule out AMI.

5. Cardio-renal Syndromes

The heart and kidneys work together to manage blood pressure, electrolyte and fluid excretion, but most importantly extracellular fluid balance [74]. Cardio-renal syndrome (CRS) is defined as a broad spectrum of diseases where both the heart and kidneys are involved in an acute or chronic setting [75]

There are five types of CRSs. Type I, or acute CRS, is acute heart failure leading to acute kidney injury [74] Type II, or chronic CRS, occurs in the setting of chronic heart failure which leads to kidney injury [75]. Type III or acute nephrocardiac is caused by acute kidney injury

Cardiorenal type	Inciting event	Secondary event	Example
Type I	Acute heart failure	Acute kidney injury	Acute coronary syndrome leading to decreased cardiac output and acute kidney injury
Type II	Chronic heart failure	Progressive kidney disease	Chronic heart failure leading to decreased cardiac output
Type III	Acute kidney injury	Acute cardiac disease (heart failure, arrhythmia, pulmonary edema)	Acute kidney failure (drug induced, glomerulonephritis)
Type IV	Chronic kidney disease	Decreased cardiac output, Increased blood pressure leading to cardiac hypertrophy	Chronic kidney disease due to chronic hypertension or diabetic nephropathy
Type V	Systemic disease	Both kidney and heart dysfunction and disease	diabetes mellitus, sepsis, lupus

Table 1. Classification of cardio-renal syndromes.

leading to acute heart failure, example Uremic cardiomyopathy [75]. Type IV, or chronic nephrocardiac, occurs with chronic kidney disease which causes heart failure for example diastolic heart failure and kidney failure [75]. Lastly, is type V which is secondary to systemic disease leading to heart and kidney failure [75]. **Table 1** summarizes the five types of CRSs.

Management of patients with acute decompensated heart failure and worsening renal function can be challenging. A randomized control trial compared the effect of venovenous ultrafiltration with intravenous diuretics on renal function with acute decompensated heart failure and worsening renal function [76]. This study found that there was no significant difference between diuretics and ultrafiltration in weight loss, mortality or the rate of re-hospitalization for acute decompensated heart failure during a 60 day follow-up.

6. CAD evaluation before kidney transplant

Cardiovascular disease is the leading cause of morbidity and mortality in patients with end-stage renal disease (ESRD) and in those after kidney transplant [77, 78]. Based on Medicare billing claims incidence of myocardial infarction have ranged from 8.7 to 16.7% by 3 years after kidney transplant listing and from 4.7 to 11.1% after kidney transplantation [79]. Cardiovascular disease accounts for 30% of the overall mortality especially in the peri-transplantation period [80]. So, the preoperative cardiovascular risk assessment is of high importance before the kidney transplant surgery as these patients are closely followed up for over the 3 years and events are reported to the United Network for Organ Sharing (UNOS).

Figure 1 summarizes a clinical approach to preoperative cardiovascular risk assessment before kidney transplantation.

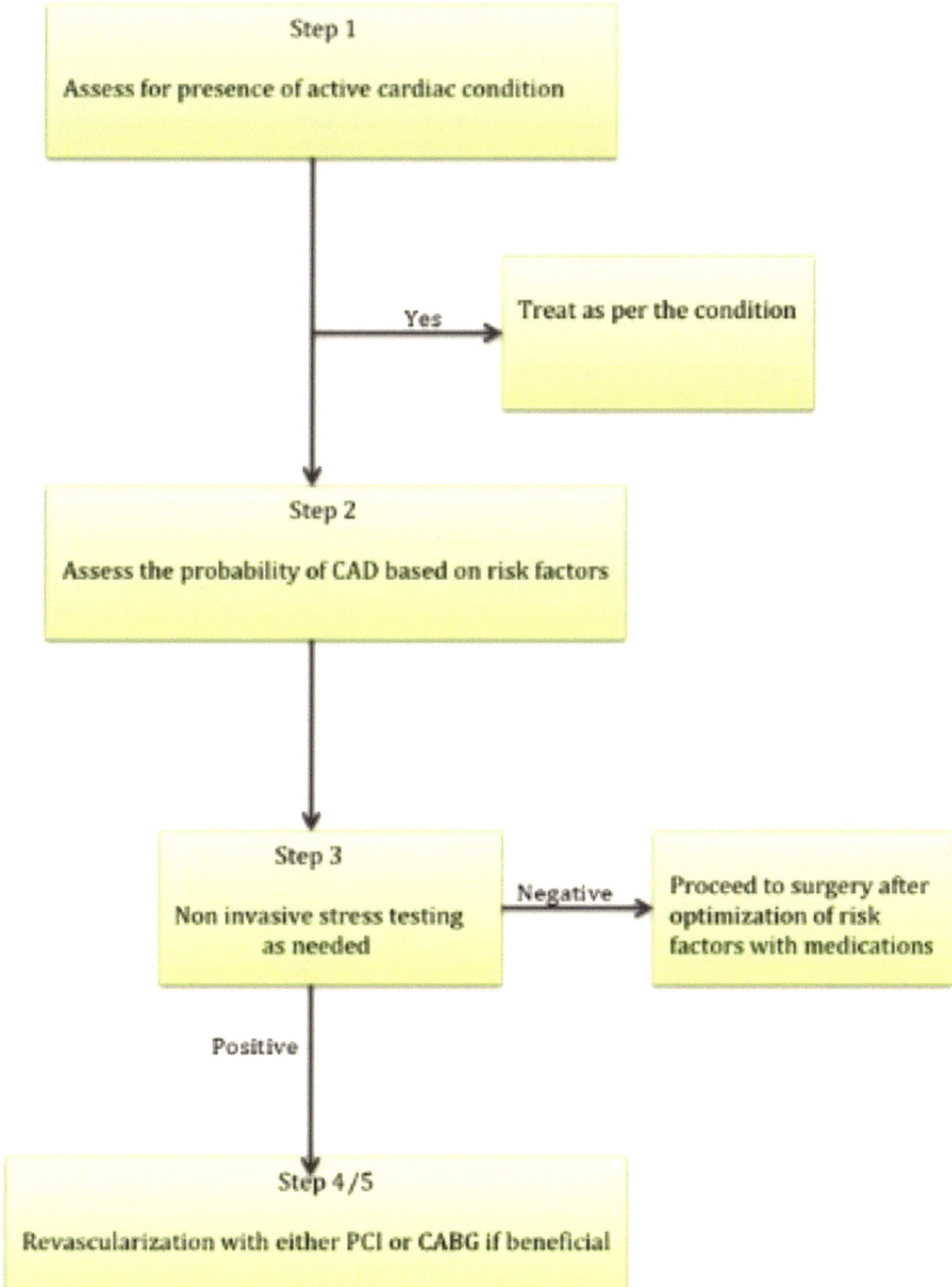

Figure 1. Pre-operative cardiovascular risk assessment before kidney transplant.

Step 1: Assess for presence of active cardiac condition:

Patients with active cardiac condition should be ruled out by detailed history and physical examination. Active cardiac conditions include- unstable coronary syndromes (e.g., unstable angina, severe angina, or recent MI), decompensated heart failure, significant arrhythmias, and severe valvular disease. The presence of one or more of these conditions is associated with high rates of perioperative cardiovascular morbidity and mortality and may require delay or cancellation of surgery.

Step 2: Assess for presence of risk factors

After excluding active cardiac condition, presence of risk factors for CAD should be assessed. Traditional Framingham risk score has modest to moderate ability to predict long-term coronary events among kidney transplantation patients. Risk stratification based on 2007 Lisbon conference [81] strategy improved the sensitivity and specificity for the identification of CAD (sensitivity, 94% vs. 77%; specificity, 33% vs. 24%) when compared to ACC/AHA recommended CAD risk stratification strategy The risk factors for CAD Aeemed relevant to transplantation candidates in the Lisbon Conference report include diabetes mellitus, prior cardiovascular disease, >1 year on dialysis, left ventricular hypertrophy, age > 60 years, smoking, hypertension, and dyslipidemia.

Currently, the preoperative assessment is done based on the ACC/AHA scientific statement [78]. As per this "Noninvasive stress testing may be considered in kidney transplantation candidates with no active cardiac conditions based on the presence of multiple coronary artery disease (CAD) risk factors regardless of functional status. Relevant risk factors among transplantation candidates include diabetes mellitus, prior cardiovascular disease, more than 1 year on dialysis, left ventricular hypertrophy, age greater than 60 years, smoking, hypertension, and dyslipidemia. The specific number of risk factors that should be used to prompt testing remains to be determined, but the committee considers 3 or more as reasonable (Class IIb; Level of Evidence C)."

Step 3: Non-invasive testing

Most common non-invasive stress testing modalities include dobutamine stress echocardiogram (DSE) and MPI. The diagnostic accuracy of these tests varies with sensitivity ranging from 0.29 to 0.92 (MPI) 0.44–0.89 (DSE) and specificity of around 0.67–0.89 (MPI) and 0.71–0.94 (DSE) [78]. MPI accuracy can be effected by presence of balanced ischemia resulting in more false negative results. Recently, coronary computed tomography angiography (CCTA) was shown to be a reliable test with high sensitivity (93%) and a high negative predictive value (97%) for diagnosing obstructive CAD before kidney transplantation. Hybrid imaging techniques like combining CCTA and SPECT have a sensitivity and specificity of 67 and 86% [82]

Step 4: Coronary angiography

Based on the noninvasive testing, coronary angiography is performed as needed to determine the presence and extent of obstructive CAD.

Step 5: Revascularization

Revascularization is done either with PCI with stent or CABG after assessment of extent of obstructive CAD and risk factors like diabetes as per the ACC/AHA guidelines for management of stable ischemic heart disease.

7. Cardiovascular risk in renal transplant patients

Renal transplant (RT) has dramatically improved the survival and quality of life for successful recipients. Despite advancements in surgical methods and medical management of RT patients, cardiovascular disease (CVD) remains the leading cause of death in patients with functional grafts.

The risk of CVD improves after RT when compared to patients with end-stage renal disease (ESRD) awaiting transplantation. However, mortality due to CVD is ten times higher in renal transplant recipients than the age and sex-matched general population [83, 84].

The increased risk of CVD cannot be explained by traditional risk factors alone.Non-traditional risk factors in RT patient population also play a pivotal role [85].

Traditional CVD risk factors include Hypertension, Diabetes Mellitus, Dyslipidemia, Tobacco use, and Obesity. In this section the effect of immunosuppressive agents on these traditional risk factors will be discussed.

7.1. Non-traditional risk factors

In addition to traditional CVD risk factors, RT patients develop specific risk factors related to ESRD including but not limited to endothelial dysfunction, electrolyte imbalances (calcium and phosphorous), anemia and variations in the plasma volume following dialysis.

A retrospective study using database from Données Informatisées et Validées en Transplantation (DIVAT) evaluated 244 RT patients post-transplant for 1 year for ST-segment elevation myocardial infarction (STEMI), non-ST-segment elevation myocardial infarction (NSTEMI), new onset atrial fibrillation or ventricular fibrillation, and death from cardiovascular diseases.

The results revealed that a past medical history of cardiovascular disease (Hazard Ratio (HR) = 2.06, p = 0.03), left ventricular hypertrophy (HR = 2.04, p = 0.04) and abnormal myocardial perfusion imaging (HR = 2.18, p = 0.05) were associated with a higher risk of early cardiovascular event [86].

7.2. Left ventricle hypertrophy

LVH is a common co-morbidity observed in chronic kidney disease (CKD) and end-stage renal disease (ESRD) patients [87]. Multiple factors have been implicated as the cause of LVH including over-activation of the sympathetic nervous system, volume overload, hypertension, inhibition of nitric oxide, arterial stiffness, diabetes, dyslipidemia, endothelial dysfunction, and anemia of chronic disease. Electrocardiographic (ECG) evidence of LVH in the first year after RT was found to be an independent risk factor for death and subsequent congestive heart failure [88]. Persistent or de novo LVH is also a strong independent risk factor for death after 5 years, confirming the continuing importance of LVH even in the late post-transplant period [88].

The presence of LVH is a important prognostic factor for CVD mortality and morbidity in RT patients. Whether a successful renal transplantation can reverse LVH still remains a debatable issue [87].

7.3. Over-activation of the sympathetic nervous system

To entertain the hypothesis that development of LVH may be connected to excessive activation of the sympathetic nervous system, the effect of pre-transplant bilateral native nephrectomy on left ventricular mass and function has been evaluated. A study group of 32 patients who had undergone pre-transplant bilateral native nephrectomy were compared to 32 control group patients and evaluated with echocardiography and/or cardiac magnetic resonance (CMR) [89].

After a 90-month follow-up, bilateral native nephrectomy before transplantation was associated with a lower left ventricular mass index (LVMI; $p = 0.001$), left atrial volume index (LAVI; $p = 0.004$), and a lower grade (grade I) of left ventricular diastolic dysfunction [89]. In comparison with controls, the study group had lower systolic blood pressure ($p = 0.04$) and required a fewer number of anti-hypertensive medications ($p = 0.001$) [89].

7.4. Inflammatory state

Pro-inflammatory markers have also been studied in RT patient population. Neopterin is synthesized by macrophages upon stimulation by interferon-gamma. Serum neopterin is a marker of a pro-inflammatory state in RT patients. Clinical trial data has revealed that Neopterin is associated with cardiovascular events and all-cause mortality in renal transplant patients.

The Assessment of LEscol in Renal Transplant (ALERT) trial prospectively analyzed RT patients with stable graft for an association between serum neopterin and subsequent clinical events: graft loss, major cardiovascular events (MACE) and all-cause mortality.The long-term follow-up suggests that neopterin-to-creatinine ratio is significantly associated with MACE ($p = 0.009$) and all-cause mortality ($p = 0.002$) [90].

7.5. Proteinuria

A prospective trial of 90 RT patients with normal graft function in the post-transplantation period (3–5 years) investigated the association between proteinuria and graft/patient survival and to determine whether proteinuria may be a predictor for cardiovascular disease. High-grade (≥500 mg/24 hours) proteinuria in RT patients is strongly associated with poor graft survival and increased risk of cardiovascular events [91]. These findings were similar to CKD patients without transplant as previously described.

7.6. Anemia

According to the follow-up data from the ALERT study, anemia is a predictor of graft loss but not associated with an increased incidence of cardiovascular morbidity and mortality or all-cause mortality in RT patients [92].

7.7. Immunosuppressive therapy

RT patients are usually on a combination of following maintenance medications:

Corticosteroids: Prednisone.

Antiproliferative agents: Mycophenolate Mofetil and Azathioprine.

Calcineurin inhibitors: Tacrolimus and Cyclosporine.

mTOR inhibitors: Sirolimus and Everolimus.

No immunosuppressive drug has been directly associated with cardiovascular events. However, immunosuppressive drugs impact the traditional risk factors and play a crucial role.

8. Hypertension

8.1. Corticosteroids

According to the historical literature, corticosteroids were believed to cause elevated blood pressure by water and salt retention via an effect on the mineralocorticoid receptor. However, recent data points that blockade of NO formation by inhibition of both inducible and endothelial nitric oxide synthase (eNOS), inhibition of transmembrane arginine transport and inhibition of the synthesis of the NOS cofactor BH4 play a prominent role [93].

8.2. Antiproliferative agents

Anti-proliferative agents were thought to worsen hypertension in RT patients. However recent studies in patients with systemic lupus erythematosus suggests an improved blood pressure control with the use of mycophenolate mofetil.

8.3. Calcineurin inhibitors

Cyclosporine monotherapy induces hypertension to the same extent as corticosteroids [94]. The mechanism by which cyclosporine and tacrolimus increase blood pressure is complex. One proposed mechanism is that cyclosporine stimulates transmembrane influxes of calcium, thereby leading to vascular smooth muscle cell contraction and vasoconstriction.

Other proposed mechanisms include increased production of endothelin 1 (ET-1), transforming growth factor (TGF), renin, and inhibition of NO production by multiple pathways.

Recent data suggests that tacrolimus results in less renal vasoconstriction than cyclosporine. RT patients being treated with tacrolimus and equivalent dosages of corticosteroids require fewer anti-hypertensive medications than patients being treated with cyclosporine [95].

9. Dyslipidemia

9.1. Corticosteroids

Corticosteroids increase total cholesterol, low-density lipoprotein (LDL), high- density lipoprotein (HDL), and hepatic synthesis of very low-density lipoprotein (VLDL) [96]. Corticosteroids lead to decreased LDL receptor synthesis and subsequent expression, thereby leading to reduced uptake and degradation of LDL [97].

9.2. Calcineurin inhibitors

Cyclosporine increases total cholesterol, LDL, and VLDL but decreases HDL. Cyclosporine decreases the activity of lipoprotein lipase (LPL) leading to hypertriglyceridemia. It also impairs the clearance of LDL by a similar mechanism to corticosteroids [98].

When comparing patients on tacrolimus versus cyclosporine, tacrolimus-treated patients have lower total cholesterol, LDL, and triglycerides. The levels of HDL are comparable. In a randomized, prospective trial evaluating RT patients with conversion from cyclosporine to tacrolimus, total cholesterol improved significantly by a mean of 0.5 mmol/L, LDL by 0.35 mmol/L and triglycerides by 0.4 mmol/L. These results were sustained up to 2 years after conversion [99].

9.3. mTOR inhibitors

Sirolimus is notorious for causing hyperlipidemia; increasing VLDL and LDL. One hypothesis is that sirolimus increases hepatic production of triglycerides and secretion of VLDL [100]. In clinical trials evaluating serum lipid profile, the addition of sirolimus 10 milligrams to cyclosporine and corticosteroids for 6 weeks increased both total cholesterol and LDL by 50% and triglycerides by almost 100%. The effects were fully reversible after discontinuation of sirolimus [100].

10. Diabetes mellitus

Post-transplantation diabetes mellitus (PTDM) has evolved into a concerning challenge in RT patients. Approximately one-third of nondiabetic kidney transplant recipients develop persistent impaired glucose metabolism by 6 months post-transplantation [101]. Risk factors for PTDM include age, obesity, African American race and Hispanic ethnicity, family history and impaired glucose tolerance. Additionally, transplant related risk factors also play a role: immunosuppressive medications, HLA mismatch, donor gender, type of underlying renal disease and viral infections (HCV and CMV) [102].

The implications of PTDM in patient outcomes are not well established, but data from the USRDS/UNOS have shown that PTDM increases the risk of post-transplant myocardial infarction [103].

10.1. Corticosteroids

Corticosteroids lead to development of PTDM by enhancing insulin resistance. PTDM is reversible by cessation of corticosteroids.

10.2. Antiproliferative agents

There is no data suggesting that mycophenolate mofetil or azathioprine play a role in development of PTDM.

10.3. Calcineurin inhibitors

RT patients receiving calcineurin inhibitors have a higher incidence of PTDM. The etiology is impairment in pancreatic beta-cell secretory function [104]. Dose reduction has been shown to reverse diabetes in majority of the affected patients. The incidence of PTDM with tacrolimus is postulated to be as high as 20%. The higher incidence of PTDM with tacrolimus versus cyclosporine is believed to be due to stronger potency of tacrolimus in calcineurin inhibition than cyclosporine [105].

Tacrolimus leads to PTDM in a dose-dependent manner. It leads to complete reversible inhibition of the insulin gene transcription with no acute effects on insulin secretion or the glucose uptake by insulin. Therefore, in majority of patients, PTDM is reversible after reducing the dose of tacrolimus and withdrawing corticosteroids.

10.4. mTOR inhibitors

There is no data suggesting that sirolimus or everolimus plays a role in development of PTDM.

11. Management of immunosuppressive agents in controlling risk factors

11.1. Corticosteroids

Corticosteroids negatively impact blood pressure, lipid profile, and glucose metabolism. Randomized trials have shown that corticosteroid withdrawal or corticosteroid-free immunosuppression improves hypertension, dyslipidemia, and glucose metabolism [106].

11.2. Calcineurin inhibitors

In patients receiving cyclosporine combined with mycophenolate mofetil, a 50% reduction in cyclosporine dose or complete cyclosporine withdrawal from a mycophenolate mofetil or sirolimus-based regimen results in fewer anti-hypertensive medications [106]. Tacrolimus increases the risk of PTDM more than cyclosporine, therefore, switching from tacrolimus to cyclosporine may lead to improvement in PTDM.

12. Conclusion

Renal transplantation is the single most effective intervention for reducing CV risk in appropriately selected patients with ESRD. Even though renal transplant has significantly improved survival for successful recipients, CVD remains the leading cause of death in patients with functional grafts [107].

In addition to traditional CVD risk factors, RT patients develop specific risk factors related to ESRD including but not limited to left ventricular hypertrophy, over-activation of the sympathetic nervous system, pro-inflammatory state, and proteinuria.

Post-transplantation, patients are maintained on a regimen of immunosuppressive medications. Even though immunosuppressive drugs have not been directly associated with cardiovascular events, they play pivotal role in risk associated with traditional risk factors of hypertension, dyslipidemia, and diabetes.

Strategies targeting transplant-specific CV risk factors should include optimization of renal function, limiting risk of rejection, avoidance of PTDM and anticipation of CV side effects of immunosuppression.

Author details

Ali Osama Malik[1], Sumit Sehgal[2], Hashim Hussnain Ahmed[3], Subodh Devabhaktuni[2], Edward Co[1], Arhama Aftab Malik[5], Syed Shah[4] and Chowdhury Ahsan[2*]

*Address all correspondence to: chahsan92@yahoo.com

1 Department of Internal Medicine, University of Nevada, School of Medicine, Reno, Nevada

2 Department of Cardiovascular Medicine, University of Nevada, School of Medicine, Reno, Nevada

3 Department of Surgery, Shaukat Khanum Memorial Cancer and Research Center, Pakistan

4 Kidney Specialist of Southern Nevada, Nevada, USA

5 Aga Khan University, Karachi, Pakistan

References

[1] Levey AS. et al. Chronic kidney disease as a global public health problem: Approaches and initiatives–A position statement from kidney disease improving global outcomes. Kidney International. 2007;**72**(3):247-259

[2] Wen CP. et al. All-cause mortality attributable to chronic kidney disease: A prospective cohort study based on 462 293 adults in Taiwan. Lancet. 2008;**371**(9631):2173-2182

[3] Chadban SJ. et al. Prevalence of kidney damage in Australian adults: The AusDiab kidney study. Journal of the American Society of Nephrology. 2003;**14**(7 Suppl 2):S131-S138

[4] Hallan SI. et al. International comparison of the relationship of chronic kidney disease prevalence and ESRD risk. Journal of the American Society of Nephrology. 2006;**17**(8):2275-2284

[5] Coresh J. et al. Prevalence of chronic kidney disease in the United States. Jama. 2007;**298**(17):2038-2047

[6] Imran S. et al. Burden of chronic kidney disease in an urban city of Pakistan, a cross-sectional study. Journal of the Pakistan Medical Association. 2015;**65**(4):366-369

[7] Manjunath G. et al. Level of kidney function as a risk factor for atherosclerotic cardiovascular outcomes in the community. Journal of the American College of Cardiology. 2003;**41**(1):47-55

[8] Fried LF. et al. Renal insufficiency as a predictor of cardiovascular outcomes and mortality in elderly individuals. Journal of the American College of Cardiology. 2003;**41**(8):1364-1372

[9] Shlipak MG. et al. Chronic renal insufficiency and cardiovascular events in the elderly: Findings from the Cardiovascular Health Study. The American Journal of Geriatric Cardiology. 2004;**13**(2):81-90

[10] Kottgen A. et al. Reduced kidney function as a risk factor for incident heart failure: The atherosclerosis risk in communities (ARIC) study. Journal of the American Society of Nephrology. 2007;**18**(4):1307-1315

[11] Matsushita K. et al. Association of estimated glomerular filtration rate and albuminuria with all-cause and cardiovascular mortality in general population cohorts: A collaborative meta-analysis. Lancet. 2010;**375**(9731):2073-2081

[12] Matsushita K. et al. Estimated glomerular filtration rate and albuminuria for prediction of cardiovascular outcomes: A collaborative meta-analysis of individual participant data. The Lancet Diabetes & Endocrinology. 2015;**3**(7):514-525

[13] Meguid El Nahas A, Bello AK. Chronic kidney disease: The global challenge. Lancet. 2005;**365**(9456):331-340

[14] Denker M. et al. Chronic Renal Insufficiency Cohort Study (CRIC): Overview and Summary of Selected Findings. Clinical Journal of the American Society of Nephrology. 2015;**10**(11):2073-2083

[15] Zhang L. et al. Prevalence of chronic kidney disease in China: A cross-sectional survey. Lancet. 2012;**379**(9818):815-822

[16] Rahman M. et al. Association between chronic kidney disease progression and cardiovascular disease: Results from the CRIC Study. American Journal of Nephrology. 2014;**40**(5):399-407

[17] Iimori S. et al. Anaemia management and mortality risk in newly visiting patients with chronic kidney disease in Japan: The CKD-ROUTE study. Nephrology (Carlton). 2015;**20**(9):601-608

[18] Martinez-Castelao A. et al. Baseline characteristics of patients with chronic kidney disease stage 3 and stage 4 in Spain: The MERENA observational cohort study. BMC Nephrology. 2011;**12**:53

[19] Yuan J. et al. Prevalence and risk factors for cardiovascular disease among chronic kidney disease patients: Results from the Chinese cohort study of chronic kidney disease (C-STRIDE). BMC Nephrology. 2017;**18**(1):23

[20] Shlipak MG. et al. Association of renal insufficiency with treatment and outcomes after myocardial infarction in elderly patients. Annals of Internal Medicine. 2002;**137**(7): 555-562

[21] Go AS. et al. Chronic kidney disease and the risks of death, cardiovascular events, and hospitalization. The New England Journal of Medicine. 2004;**351**(13):1296-1305

[22] van der Velde M. et al. Lower estimated glomerular filtration rate and higher albuminuria are associated with all-cause and cardiovascular mortality. A collaborative meta-analysis of high-risk population cohorts. Kidney International. 2011;**79**(12):1341-1352

[23] Manjunath G. et al. Level of kidney function as a risk factor for cardiovascular outcomes in the elderly. Kidney International. 2003;**63**(3):1121-1129

[24] Chonchol M. et al. Chronic kidney disease is associated with angiographic coronary artery disease. American Journal of Nephrology. 2008;**28**(2):354-360

[25] Chin CY. et al. Coronary plaque characteristics in hemodialysis-dependent patients as assessed by optical coherence tomography. American Journal of Cardiology. 2017;**119**

[26] Farzaneh-Far A. Morphology of coronary atherosclerotic lesions in patients with end-stage renal failure. Nephrology Dialysis Transplantation. 2000;**15**(10):1710

[27] Nakano T. et al. Association of kidney function with coronary atherosclerosis and calcification in autopsy samples from Japanese elders: The Hisayama study. American Journal of Kidney Diseases. 2010;**55**(1):21-30

[28] Gutierrez OM. et al. Fibroblast growth factor 23 and mortality among patients undergoing hemodialysis. The New England Journal of Medicine. 2008;**359**(6):584-592

[29] Isakova T. et al. Fibroblast growth factor 23 and risks of mortality and end-stage renal disease in patients with chronic kidney disease. Jama. 2011;**305**(23):2432-2439

[30] Sarnak MJ. et al. Kidney disease as a risk factor for development of cardiovascular disease: A statement from the American Heart Association Councils on Kidney in Cardiovascular Disease, High Blood Pressure Research, Clinical Cardiology, and Epidemiology and Prevention. Circulation. 2003;**108**(17):2154-2169

[31] Manske CL. et al. Coronary revascularisation in insulin-dependent diabetic patients with chronic renal failure. Lancet. 1992;**340**(8826):998-1002

[32] Best PJ. et al. The impact of renal insufficiency on clinical outcomes in patients undergoing percutaneous coronary interventions. Journal of the American College of Cardiology. 2002;**39**(7):1113-1119

[33] Kahn JK. et al. Short- and long-term outcome of percutaneous transluminal coronary angioplasty in chronic dialysis patients. American Heart Journal. 1990;**119**(3 Pt 1):484-489

[34] Malyszko J. et al. Hemostasis, platelet function and serotonin in acute and chronic renal failure. Thrombosis Research. 1996;**83**(5):351-361

[35] Di Minno G. et al. Platelet dysfunction in uremia. Multifaceted defect partially corrected by dialysis. American Journal of Medicine. 1985;**79**(5):552-559

[36] Soslau G. et al. Selective reduction of serotonin storage and ATP release in chronic renal failure patients platelets. American Journal of Hematology. 1990;**35**(3):171-178

[37] Gordge MP. et al. Platelet function and the bleeding time in progressive renal failure. Thromb Haemost. 1988;**60**(1):83-87

[38] Mezzano D. et al. Hemostatic disorder of uremia: The platelet defect, main determinant of the prolonged bleeding time, is correlated with indices of activation of coagulation and fibrinolysis. Thrombosis and Haemostasis. 1996;**76**(3):312-321

[39] Mezzano D. et al. Endothelial cell markers in chronic uremia: Relationship with hemostatic defects and severity of renal failure. Thrombosis Research. 1997;**88**(6):465-472

[40] Reddan D. et al. Anticoagulation in acute cardiac care in patients with chronic kidney disease. American Heart Journal. 2003;**145**(4):586-594

[41] Schoebel FC. et al. Restenosis after elective coronary balloon angioplasty in patients with end stage renal disease: A case-control study using quantitative coronary angiography. Heart. 1997;**78**(4):337-342

[42] Le Feuvre C. et al. Comparison of clinical outcome following coronary stenting or balloon angioplasty in dialysis versus non-dialysis patients. American Journal of Cardiology. 2000;**85**(11):1365-1368

[43] Labrousse L. et al. Early and long term results of coronary artery bypass grafts in patients with dialysis dependent renal failure. European Journal of Cardio-Thoracic Surgery. 1999;**15**(5):691-696

[44] Horst M. et al. Cardiac surgery in patients with end-stage renal disease: 10-year experience. The Annals of Thoracic Surgery. 2000;**69**(1):96-101

[45] Anderson RJ. et al. Renal failure predisposes patients to adverse outcome after coronary artery bypass surgery. VA Cooperative Study #5. Kidney International. 1999;**55**(3): 1057-1062

[46] Szczech LA. et al. Differential survival after coronary revascularization procedures among patients with renal insufficiency. Kidney International. 2001;**60**(1):292-299

[47] Marui A. et al. Percutaneous coronary intervention versus coronary artery bypass grafting in patients with end-stage renal disease requiring dialysis (5-year outcomes of the CREDO-Kyoto PCI/CABG Registry Cohort-2). American Journal of Cardiology. 2014;**114**(4):555-561

[48] Bangalore S. et al. Revascularization in patients with multivessel coronary artery disease and chronic kidney disease: Everolimus-eluting stents versus coronary artery bypass graft surgery. Journal of the American College of Cardiology. 2015;**66**(11): 1209-1220

[49] Raggi P, Alexopoulos N. Cardiac imaging in chronic kidney disease patients. Seminars in Dialysis. 2017

[50] Sharma R. et al. Dobutamine stress echocardiography and cardiac troponin T for the detection of significant coronary artery disease and predicting outcome in renal transplant candidates. European Journal of Echocardiography. 2005;**6**(5):327-335

[51] Wang LW. et al. Cardiac testing for coronary artery disease in potential kidney transplant recipients: A systematic review of test accuracy studies. American Journal of Kidney Diseases. 2011;**57**(3):476-487

[52] Tita C. et al. Stress echocardiography for risk stratification in patients with end-stage renal disease undergoing renal transplantation. Journal of the American Society of Echocardiography. 2008;**21**(4):321-326

[53] Parnham SF. et al. Myocardial Ischemia assessment in chronic kidney disease: Challenges and pitfalls. Frontiers in Cardiovascular Medicine. 2014;**1**:13

[54] Mowatt G. et al. 64-Slice computed tomography angiography in the diagnosis and assessment of coronary artery disease: Systematic review and meta-analysis. Heart. 2008;**94**(11):1386-1393

[55] Mao J. et al. Coronary computed tomography angiography in dialysis patients undergoing pre-renal transplantation cardiac risk stratification. Cardiology Journal. 2010;**17**(4): 349-361

[56] Chiu DY. et al. Cardiac imaging in patients with chronic kidney disease. Nature Reviews Nephrology. 2015;**11**(4):207-220

[57] Ali ZA. et al. Imaging- and physiology-guided percutaneous coronary intervention without contrast administration in advanced renal failure: A feasibility, safety, and outcome study. European Heart Journal. 2016;**37**(40):3090-3095

[58] Detrenis S. et al. Lights and shadows on the pathogenesis of contrast-induced nephropathy: State of the art. Nephrology Dialysis Transplantation. 2005;**20**(8):1542-1550

[59] Persson PB, Hansell P,Liss P. Pathophysiology of contrast medium-induced nephropathy. Kidney International. 2005;**68**(1):14-22

[60] Cantley LG. et al. Role of endothelin and prostaglandins in radiocontrast-induced renal artery constriction. Kidney International. 1993;**44**(6):1217-1223

[61] Katholi RE. et al. Nephrotoxicity from contrast media: Attenuation with theophylline. Radiology. 1995;**195**(1):17-22

[62] Russo D. et al. Early effects of contrast media on renal hemodynamics and tubular function in chronic renal failure. Journal of the American Society of Nephrology. 1995;**6**(5):1451-1458

[63] Cigarroa RG. et al. Dosing of contrast material to prevent contrast nephropathy in patients with renal disease. American Journal of Medicine. 1989;**86**(6 Pt 1):649-652

[64] Rudnick MR. et al. Nephrotoxicity of ionic and nonionic contrast media in 1196 patients: A randomized trial. The Iohexol cooperative study. Kidney International. 1995;**47**(1):254-261

[65] Karimi Galougahi K. et al. Zero-contrast percutaneous coronary intervention on calcified lesions facilitated by rotational atherectomy. Catheterization and Cardiovascular Interventions. 2017

[66] Freda BJ. et al. Cardiac troponins in renal insufficiency: Review and clinical implications. Journal of the American College of Cardiology. 2002;**40**(12):2065-2071

[67] Thygesen K. et al. Third universal definition of myocardial infarction. Circulation. 2012;**126**(16):2020-2035

[68] Alcalai R. et al. Acute coronary syndrome vs nonspecific troponin elevation: Clinical predictors and survival analysis. Archives of Internal Medicine. 2007;**167**(3):276-281

[69] Giannitsis E, Katus HA. Cardiac troponin level elevations not related to acute coronary syndromes. Nature Reviews Cardiology. 2013;**10**(11):623-634

[70] Cardinaels EP. et al. High-sensitivity cardiac troponin concentrations in patients with chest discomfort: Is it the heart or the kidneys as well? PLoS One. 2016;**11**(4):e0153300

[71] Mair J. et al. Serum cardiac troponin T after extraordinary endurance exercise. Lancet. 1992;**340**(8826):1048

[72] Kobayashi S. et al. Serum cardiac troponin T in polymyositis/dermatomyositis. Lancet. 1992;**340**(8821):726

[73] Ohba H. et al. Effects of prolonged strenuous exercise on plasma levels of atrial natriuretic peptide and brain natriuretic peptide in healthy men. American Heart Journal. 2001;**141**(5):751-758

[74] Sarraf M, Masoumi A, Schrier RW. Cardiorenal syndrome in acute decompensated heart failure. Clinical Journal of the American Society of Nephrology. 2009;**4**(12):2013-2026

[75] Ronco C, Di Lullo L. Cardiorenal syndrome. 'Heart Failure Clinics. 2014;**10**(2):251-280

[76] Bart BA. et al. Ultrafiltration in decompensated heart failure with cardiorenal syndrome. The New England Journal of Medicine. 2012;**367**(24):2296-2304

[77] Pilmore H. et al. Reduction in cardiovascular death after kidney transplantation. Transplantation. 2010;**89**(7):851-857

[78] Lentine KL. et al. Cardiac disease evaluation and management among kidney and liver transplantation candidates: A scientific statement from the American heart association and the American college of cardiology foundation. Journal of the American College of Cardiology. 2012;**60**(5):434-480

[79] Lentine KL, Brennan DC,Schnitzler MA. Incidence and predictors of myocardial infarction after kidney transplantation. Journal of the American Society of Nephrology. 2005;**16**(2):496-506

[80] Ramanathan V. et al. Screening asymptomatic diabetic patients for coronary artery disease prior to renal transplantation. Transplantation. 2005;**79**(10):1453-1458

[81] Abbud-Filho M. et al. A report of the Lisbon conference on the care of the kidney transplant recipient. Transplantation. 2007;**83**(8 Suppl):S1-S22

[82] Winther S. et al. Diagnostic performance of coronary CT aangiography and myocardial perfusion imaging in kidney transplantation candidates. JACC: Cardiovasc Imaging. 2015;**8**(5):553-562

[83] Kasiske BL, Chakkera HA,Roel J. Explained and unexplained ischemic heart disease risk after renal transplantation. Journal of the American Society of Nephrology. 2000;**11**(9):1735-1743

[84] Ducloux D, Kazory A, Chalopin JM. Predicting coronary heart disease in renal transplant recipients: A prospective study. Kidney International. 2004;**66**(1):441-447

[85] Munagala MR, Phancao A. Managing cardiovascular risk in the post solid organ transplant recipient. Medical Clinics of North America. 2016;**100**(3):519-533

[86] Marcen R. Cardiovascular risk factors in renal transplantation–current controversies. Nephrology Dialysis Transplantation. 2006;**21**(Suppl 3):iii3-iii8

[87] Dounousi E. et al. Differences in cardiac structure assessed by echocardiography between renal transplant recipients and chronic kidney disease patients. Transplantation Proceedings. 2014;**46**(9):3194-3198

[88] Rigatto C. et al. Electrocardiographic left ventricular hypertrophy in renal transplant recipients: Prognostic value and impact of blood pressure and anemia. Journal of the American Society of Nephrology. 2003;**14**(2):462-468

[89] Obremska M. et al. Beneficial effect of bilateral native nephrectomy as complete denervation on left ventricular mass and function in renal transplant recipients. Polish Archives of Internal Medicine. 2016;**126**(1-2):58-67

[90] Pihlstrom H. et al. Neopterin is associated with cardiovascular events and all-cause mortality in renal transplant patients. Clinical Transplantation. 2014;**28**(1):111-119

[91] Guliyev O. et al. High-grade proteinuria as a cardiovascular risk factor in renal transplant recipients. Transplantation Proceedings. 2015;**47**(4):1170-1173

[92] Schjelderup P. et al. Anemia is a predictor of graft loss but not cardiovascular events and all-cause mortality in renal transplant recipients: Follow-up data from the ALERT study. Clinical Transplantation. 2013;**27**(6):E636-E643

[93] Whitworth JA, Mangos GJ, Kelly JJ. Cushing, cortisol, and cardiovascular disease. Hypertension. 2000;**36**(5):912-916

[94] Chapman JR. et al. Hypertension after renal transplantation. A comparison of cyclosporine and conventional immunosuppression. Transplantation. 1987;**43**(6):860-864

[95] Radermacher J. et al. Pronounced renal vasoconstriction and systemic hypertension in renal transplant patients treated with cyclosporin A versus FK 506. Transplant International. 1998;**11**(1):3-10

[96] Hricik DE, Schulak JA. Metabolic effects of steroid withdrawal in adult renal transplant recipients. Kidney International Supplements. 1993;**43**:S26-S29

[97] Kancha RK, Hussain MM. Up-regulation of the low density lipoprotein receptor-related protein by dexamethasone in HepG2 cells. Biochimica et Biophysica Acta. 1996;**1301**(3):213-220

[98] Espino A. et al. The effect of cyclosporine and methylprednisolone on plasma lipoprotein levels in rats. Journal of Laboratory and Clinical Medicine. 1995;**125**(2):222-227

[99] Artz MA. et al. Conversion from cyclosporine to tacrolimus improves quality-of-life indices, renal graft function and cardiovascular risk profile. American Journal of Transplantation. 2004;**4**(6):937-945

[100] Morrisett JD, Abdel-Fattah G, Kahan BD. Sirolimus changes lipid concentrations and lipoprotein metabolism in kidney transplant recipients. Transplantation Proceedings. 2003;**35**(3 Suppl):143s-150s

[101] Valderhaug TG. et al. Fasting plasma glucose and glycosylated hemoglobin in the screening for diabetes mellitus after renal transplantation. Transplantation. 2009;**88**(3):429-434

[102] Sharif A, Baboolal K. Complications associated with new-onset diabetes after kidney transplantation. Nature Reviews Nephrology. 2011;**8**(1):34-42

[103] Jardine AG. et al. Fluvastatin prevents cardiac death and myocardial infarction in renal transplant recipients: Post-hoc subgroup analyses of the ALERT Study. American Journal of Transplantation. 2004;**4**(6):988-995

[104] Nam JH. et al. Beta-Cell dysfunction rather than insulin resistance is the main contributing factor for the development of postrenal transplantation diabetes mellitus. Transplantation. 2001;**71**(10):1417-1423

[105] Pirsch JD. et al. A comparison of tacrolimus (FK506) and cyclosporine for immunosuppression after cadaveric renal transplantation. FK506 kidney transplant study group. Transplantation. 1997;**63**(7):977-983

[106] Marcen R. Immunosuppressive drugs in kidney transplantation: Impact on patient survival, and incidence of cardiovascular disease, malignancy and infection. Drugs. 2009;**69**(16):2227-2243

[107] Stoumpos S, Jardine AG, Mark PB. Cardiovascular morbidity and mortality after kidney transplantation. Transplant International. 2015;**28**(1):10-21

Section 2

Inflammation and CKD

Chapter 6

Inflammation and Chronic Kidney Disease: Current Approaches and Recent Advances

Simona Mihai, Elena Codrici,
Ionela Daniela Popescu, Ana-Maria Enciu,
Laura Georgiana Necula, Gabriela Anton and
Cristiana Tanase

Additional information is available at the end of the chapter

http://dx.doi.org/10.5772/intechopen.72716

Motto: *"All disease begins in the gut." (Hippocrates)*

Abstract

Despite being a "silent epidemic" disease, chronic kidney disease (CKD) is considered one of the major causes of mortality, together with its main complication, the cardiovascular disease, which contributes to the poor prognosis of these patients. Inflammation has been recognized as an essential part of CKD and is closely linked to cardiovascular complications. The identification of novel biomarkers using omics technologies is rapidly advancing and could improve the early detection in renal diseases. Omics approaches, including proteomics, could provide novel insights into disease mechanisms, identifying at the same time accurate inflammatory biomarker panels with an essential role in disease monitoring and follow-up. Recent advances highlight the gut microbiota as an important source of inflammation in kidney diseases. An increasing body of evidence reveals the cross talk between microbiota and host in CKD; in addition, gut dysbiosis may represent an underappreciated cause of inflammation and subsequently could lead to malnutrition, accelerated cardiovascular disease and CKD progression. This chapter discusses the relationship between inflammation and CKD and highlights the novel approaches regarding microbiota involvement in CKD pathology, as well as their potential to facilitate improving the quality of life.

Keywords: chronic kidney disease, inflammation, gut microbiota, omics

1. Introduction

Chronic kidney disease (CKD) is defined, according to KDIGO 2017 Clinical Practice Guideline Update for the Diagnosis, Evaluation, Prevention, and Treatment of Chronic Kidney

Disease–Mineral and Bone Disorder (CKD-MBD), as "abnormalities of kidney structure or function, present for more than 3 months, with implications for health." CKD is classified based on pathological cause, glomerular filtration rate category (from G1, normal, to G5, kidney failure), and albuminuria category (from A1, <30 mg/g, to A3 > 300 mg/g) [1]. It will inexorably lead to end-stage renal disease, unless managed as to address treatment of the underlying condition, diagnosing and treating the pathologic manifestations and timely planning for long-term renal replacement therapy. A recent systematic review and meta-analysis of observational studies revealed that CKD has an estimated global prevalence between 11 and 13%, with the majority of cases in stage 3 [2]. The complexity of CKD pathogenesis is underlined by a plethora of risk factors: genetic and epigenetic age [3], low birth weight, socioeconomic status, obesity [1], smoking and/or hypoxia [4], and vascular factors, induced by atherosclerosis [5], hypertension [6], and diabetes mellitus [7]. Furthermore, the *complications* of this disease also impact beyond the kidney, with cardiovascular burden (such as coronary artery disease, congestive heart failure, arrhythmias, and sudden cardiac death) as a major mark [8]. CKD associates also with enhanced formation of atherosclerotic plaques [9]. Other complications include endocrine dysfunctions involving hormones that control calcium [10] and phosphate balance [11], vitamin D metabolism, and, consequently, bone mineralization defects [12]. Hemodialysis patients are further at risk for cardiovascular complications, such as vascular overload leading to arterial stiffness [13] or, apparently paradoxical, ischemia induced by repeated episodes of hypovolemic hypoperfusion during hemodialysis [9].

Inflammation has been recognized as an essential part of chronic kidney disease (CKD) since the late 1990s and is now considered a well-established risk factor for this pathology [14], as well as for other renal pathologies. In fact, inflammation is now considered a key player in different major pathologies such as cardiovascular disease [15], neurodegeneration [16], or cancer progression and survival [17]. Chronic systemic inflammation, sometimes referred to as low-grade chronic inflammation, is characterized by 2–3 fold increase of circulating inflammatory mediators (such as interleukins 1, 6 tumor necrosis factor, and their soluble receptors), slow developing, persistent and of multifactorial origin, sometimes difficult to identify [18]. Recent findings associate chronic systemic inflammation with alteration of gut microbiota, which is in permanent cross talk with the immune system. This cross talk is essential for maintenance of a tolerant immune response toward commensal flora and elimination of pathogens [19]. Intestinal dysbiosis is detrimental for health in ways overpassing the intestinal environment, from production of toxic metabolites, overconsumption of energy, and molecular mimicry of host proteins [20]. This chapter will present an up-to-date findings relating to chronic systemic inflammation and CKD, with emphasis on gut dysmicrobism involvement and whether intervention on gut microbiota could be proven beneficial for the outcome of this fatal disease.

2. Inflammation and its impact on CKD progression: an update

Persistent, low-grade inflammation is considered crucial component of CKD, having a huge contribution to the development of all-cause mortality related to renal disease. There has been an ascending growth of interest regarding the role of inflammation in CKD and end-stage renal disease (ESRD), which shifts the perception of inflammation as no longer a new, but rather a traditional risk factor for CKD morbidity and mortality [14, 21]. A challenging theory regarding the direct effect of inflammation on the progression of both CKD and cardiovascular disease came out with the assumption of association between markers of inflammation, changes in GFR and nutrition habits in elderly individuals. It was found that the deterioration in renal function (alteration of GFR, urea and creatinine) was associated with an increasing number of markers of inflammation and thrombosis [22]. Regardless of a genetic background, CKD is a condition that accelerates premature aging through diverse mechanisms in the internal milieu, counting DNA damage, inflammation, low Klotho expression, redox perturbations, toxicity, and local signaling of growth factors [23]. It is generally known that there is a heterogeneous distribution of intrarenal vasculature in normal conditions, and only medulla is under hypoxic conditions. In order to bypass energy deprivation in the deficient pO_2 parts of the kidneys, an avalanche of mediators is involved to regulate the complex processes, including hormones, autocoids, and vasoactive substances: medullipin, prostaglandins, endothelins, nitric oxide, angiotensin II, kinins, and adenosine. A state of sustained inflammation could surely alter the microvascular feedback to its regulators and could activate the reaction of an array of tubular toxins, including reactive oxygen species (ROS), generating further renal failure [24]. The highly reactive ROS could alter different structures and functional pathways in cells, and, as a repercussion, a vicious circle arises, in which the inflammatory cells are stimulated by cell damage caused by ROS, giving birth to a state of oxidative stress. The common oxidant "imbalance" theory is remarkably completed with recent advances regarding the cross talk between oxidants and antioxidants; the reasoning for antioxidant therapies consists thus in repairing the imbalances in the redox environment of cells [25]. The old theory suggesting the oxidative stress as a "unifying concept of cardiovascular disease in uremia" [26] is continuously enriched, and novel molecules, belonging to the Paraoxonase family, are suggested as potential biomarkers. Paraoxonase-1 seems to have a protective effect against lipoprotein oxidation and its expression is decreased in CKD patients, being a marker for antioxidant status [27]. The development of specific redox proteomic techniques will facilitate the implementation of new preventive and therapeutic strategies to fight against atherosclerosis and other metabolic diseases [28].

In comparison with the well-established clinical markers, proteomic biomarkers could offer an accurate and earlier detection of renal pathology. Although the "breaking point" could be various in different patients, in some populations, the circulating creatinine levels fall into normal ranges despite loss of more than 50% of renal function, so supplementary biomarkers of renal function are desired. Recent studies conclude that a cross talk between inflammation, bone, vasculature, and renal function exists in CKD. In early stage 2 of CKD, an increased expression of a panel of proteomic biomarkers was observed, including IL-6, TNF-α, osteoprotegerin, osteocalcin, osteopontin, and FGF-23, which, at a first glance, highlights the hope of improving the management of patients with CKD starting with early stages, which is an area to focus research in the near future [29]. Another study evaluating the association between kidney function, albuminuria, and biomarkers of inflammation in a large cohort of CKD patients showed that plasma levels of IL-1β, IL-1RA, IL-6, TNF-α, hs-CRP, and fibrinogen were higher among participants with lower levels of estimated glomerular filtration rate (GFR). Moreover, inflammation score was higher among patients with lower estimated GFR and higher urine albumin to creatinine ratio (UACR). These results demonstrated that biomarkers of inflammation were inversely associated with measures of kidney function and positively with albuminuria [30]. The erythrocyte sedimentation rate, a nonspecific measure of inflammation, has been shown to be predictive of end-stage renal disease in adolescents [31]. The level of pro-inflammatory cytokine IL-2 was elevated in hemodialysis patients with uremic pruritus (a common tormenting symptom among these patients) when compared to hemodialysis patient controls without pruritus [32]. The results obtained from several researches suggest that tumor necrosis factor-like weak inducer of apoptosis (TWEAK) plays an important role in kidney injury associated with inflammation and promotes acute and chronic kidney diseases [33]. There are several studies testing different nanoconjugates that could prevent TWEAK-induced cell death and inflammatory signaling in different cell types, including renal tubular cells [34]. The results obtained from a study investigating hemodialysis patients showed that the group of patients with a specific pattern of high pro-inflammatory cytokines (IL-1, IL-6, and TNF-α) had increased mortality when compared to patients with a pattern of high T-cell regulatory or anti-inflammatory parameters (IL-2, IL-4, IL-5, IL-12, CH50, and T-cell number) [35].

Availability of omics multiplex technology offered the opportunity of shifting the analysis of single individual marker toward assessing cytokine panels [36]. It was described an inflammatory panel, consisting of pro-inflammatory cytokines IL-1, IL-6, and TNF-α with anti-inflammatory ones IL-2, IL-4, IL-5, IL-12, CH50, as well, with a significant impact on CKD patients' survival [35]. Recently, significant attention has been granted to the potential role of adipokines in CKD, such as pro-inflammatory leptin, apelin, omentin, visfatin, resistin, and anti-inflammatory adiponectin. Based on the data from the National Health and Nutrition Examination Survey (NHANES), it was shown that CKD is correlated with increased leptin levels [37]. Moreover, adiponectin expression in ESRD patients was also significantly increased compared to healthy individuals [14].

Atherosclerosis is now considered a chronic inflammatory disease and, in turn, cardiovascular disease is a major complication of CKD. Thus, a vicious circle is created between inflammation and CKD. Atherosclerosis is accelerated in CKD by complex mechanisms involving a cross talk between lymphocyte T helper type 1 and subendothelial macrophages as antigen presenting cells. The triggers of this cellular response are alteration of lipid metabolism and subendothelial deposit of plasma lipoproteins. Locally recruited lymphocytes react to autoantigens from the apolipoprotein B100 protein of LDL, generating an inflammatory response [38]. Within the predialysis CKD patients, the prevalence of inflammation is increasing and represents a critical indicator of patient health and future outcome. In ESRD, the process of hemodialysis itself may contribute to the pro-inflammatory state, and different types of dialysis membrane could determine an inflammatory response. However, hemodialysis does not represent the only source of inflammation, since the predialysis CKD patients already manifest a certain inflammatory state [39]. A persistent inflammatory state in CKD is not only linked to cardiovascular complications but is also one of the key players in the development of malnutrition/protein-energy wasting, having as consequence the malnutrition-inflammation-cachexia syndrome in CKD/ESRD patients. It was also described, in a cohort of dialysis patients, that circulating levels of IL-1 and IL-6 could suppress the PTH secretion, which, in turn, may reflect the malnutrition-inflammation-cachexia syndrome, rather than the low bone turnover disease [40]. The pathophysiology of inflammation could be different with regard to different racial, ethnic, or genetic features. Recent studies specify that dietary habits could add a peculiar signature to the gut microbiota composition, and intestinal dysbiosis itself could thus interfere with the inflammatory mechanisms in CKD population.

In summary, persistent low-grade inflammation has been recognized as an important component of CKD scenario, playing major roles in the pathophysiology of the disease, with a major imprint on its complications. Nevertheless, further investigations are necessary to decipher the role of inflammation in CKD population, particularly in the early stages.

3. The role of inflammation in the development of cardiovascular diseases in CKD

Cardiovascular disease represents one of the main determinants of CKD's poor prognosis, since early stages of CKD are significantly correlated with increased risk of subsequent coronary heart disease [41]. In agreement with several clinical studies, approximately 50% of patients with CKD have a rising mortality due to the cardiovascular complications, such as advanced calcific arterial and valvular disease; however, the mechanisms that involves the accelerated calcification in CKD continue to be questionable, thus no specific therapies have emerged to target the disease prevention [42].

The current CKD guidelines are recommending the screening for vascular calcification (VC), for the reason that VC represents a cardiovascular risk factor, and it is correlated with an increased morbidity and mortality in CKD group, culminating in CKD stage 5. Vascular calcification is now considered an active process that involves many proteins, as possible candidate markers [43]. In CKD individuals, several studies have highlighted various circulating biomarkers that could play important roles in extra-skeletal calcification and mineral metabolism alterations, which are considered characteristics of CKD-mineral bone disorder (CKD-MBD) [44]. As a result, these findings have revealed that CKD-MBD comprises laboratory and bone abnormalities and vascular calcification and has deleterious consequences on clinical outcomes; however, these processes are interconnected and they have to be studied in association with cardiovascular diseases [1].

Cardiovascular calcification represents though an exceptional marker of chronic inflammatory status in CKD, strongly correlated with morbidity and mortality. Curiously, CKD accelerates the atherosclerosis evolution and it has been showed that CKD produces increasing vascular inflammation and calcification. Recent advances highlighted the potential involvement of matrix vesicles (secreted by macrophages), as key molecules in the alternative processes independent of osteogenic differentiation [45]. Deciphering the association between these mechanisms and signaling pathways could bring novel insights into the mechanistics of calcification and could possibly move forward to new therapeutic strategies aiming at cardiovascular disease in CKD [46]. These findings are in concordance with the genetics, and it was shown that 40–50% of coronary calcification cases could be linked to genetic predisposition, considering that several loci were linked to coronary arterial calcification [47]. The involvement of single polymorphisms located at 9p21 locus near the cyclin genes was proposed as a genetic mechanism of this pathology; the concerned genes could be generally associated with cellular senescence and inflammation, although the accurate causative DNA sequences continue to be uncertain [48]. Recent evidence suggests that the overlap between CKD and cardiovascular disease is due, on one hand, to the dynamic cross talk between these organs, resulting in cardio-renal syndrome, increasingly recognized [49] and, on the other hand, it could be linked to the common etiologies of these major diseases (hypertension and diabetes mellitus). It has also been investigated as a possible common disorder of the kidneys and heart whereby acute or chronic dysfunction in one organ may induce acute or chronic dysfunction in the other organ; nevertheless, a complete picture of the mechanisms implicated in these processes is still missing [49]. The highly reactive oxygen species (ROS) present the potential of disrupting different structural and functional pathways in cells. Therefore, the inflammatory cells are activated by cell damage produced by ROS; thus, a vicious circle of chronic disturbance is constantly perpetuated. The oxidant imbalance theory comprises several important pathways and cell metabolism also has been under the surveillance of the cross talk between oxidants and antioxidants. The role of oxidative stress in the pathogenesis of CKD relies though on the hypothesis that antioxidant therapies could target and reconstruct the disturbances in the redox environment of cells [50]. Different therapeutic strategies have been considered to decrease oxidative stress (OS) in models of CKD and cardiovascular disease, proposing a low oxidant intake in different dietary approaches. Oxidative stress and inflammation increase with aging, and these conditions are related to kidney failure in its early stages, as well. There are evidences that a diet supplemented with oxidants could produce increased serum levels of OS and inflammatory mediators in both normal aging and in CKD. It is mentioned that dietary intervention could offer novel therapeutic strategies by reducing OS and inflammation in patients with CKD and in aging population with decreased kidney function [51].

Due to the circulating nature of many inflammatory mediators (cytokines and immune cells), it is tempting to hypothesize that the immune system could have crucial roles in organ interactions and could mediate the reciprocal dysfunction that is experienced in cardio-renal syndromes.

4. Omics technologies and clinical relevance of proteomic biomarkers in renal diseases: rolling proteomics into clinics

Over the last decade, there has been an increasing progression of omics approaches, accompanied by remarkable improvement of methodologies and analytical instruments, based on the concept that a thorough characterization of a complex system, providing novel perceptions into functional pathways and regulatory networks, could be deciphered in frame of these omics. In the light of recent advances in bioinformatics and biostatistics on state-of-the-art platforms, the access of scientists in correlating the experimentally observed data regarding the fundamental biochemical and pathological mechanisms was facilitated [52, 53]. Proteomic biomarkers in kidney disease may represent, along with classical markers serum creatinine and urinary albumin, valuable tools in clinical diagnosis due to their accurate potential for clinical implementation. Moreover, proteomic biomarkers could also be useful in characterizing the most suitable therapeutic targets in a given patient or disease setting [54].

The huge step forward was accomplished by coupling liquid chromatography with mass spectrometry, enabling untargeted protein identification. Additionally, capillary electrophoresis had also an accelerated development in the last years, being able to rapidly separate analytes in a highly reproducible manner [55]. Also, matrix-assisted laser desorption/ionization (MALDI) platform has moved the boundaries above, being able to assess tissue specimens with high resolution in order to discriminate individual cells. This approach can provide detailed information related to CKD and the potential to detect specific biomarkers. Recent evidence suggests that MALDI could generate molecular signatures of primary and secondary kidney injury, with one particular signal, identified as serine/threonine-protein kinase MRCK gamma, being overexpressed in the glomeruli of primary membranous nephropathy (MN). These findings could be potential future targets for the further stratification of these patients [56]. Other studies emphasize the role of omics technologies, including MALDI to generate molecular signatures capable to distinguish between normal kidney and pathological kidney, with specific signals representing potential indicators of CKD development [57]. Kidney and Urinary Pathway Knowledge Base (KUPKB) represents an open source to explore multi-omics data and to generate new *in silico* theories using a novel approach based on semantic web technologies [58]. Moreover, CKDdb represents the most comprehensive molecular information resource in characterizing CKD-related experiments and model systems, potentially useful in the design of disease models, thus avoiding the challenges related with handling and integration of heterogeneous enormous data [59].

The emerging knowledge generated by the application of omics (genomics, proteomics, and metabolomics) in major diseases, including CKD, could provide new insights into the pathophysiology of the disease by identifying novel biomarkers that could improve, in real time, the early diagnostics, monitoring, and prognostics; thus, omics will provide a major impact in the field of personalized medicine [60].

5. Gut microbiota as a source of inflammation in CKD: a bidirectional relationship

Accumulating evidence over the recent years has highlighted that chronic inflammation represents a nontraditional risk factor in CKD population and was revealed that gastrointestinal tract is a major player in systemic inflammation occurring in CKD [61]. The gut microbiota preserves the symbiotic relationship with the host in normal conditions and is essential for regulation of local and systemic immunity [62], although its imbalance has latterly been related with several diseases [63]. Alteration in the functions or signaling pathways of the commensal flora contributes to the pathogenesis of diverse diseases, including chronic inflammation and renal disorders, as well; gut bacterial DNA fragments have been detected in the blood of both predialysis CKD and chronic hemodialysis patients [64]. The decisive role of the biochemical milieu in shaping the gut microbiota, in terms of structure, composition, and function, which could promote a proinflammatory activity, was also described and it could simultaneously restrict the beneficial effects offered by a balanced microbiota. Such conditions could lead to an altered status, targeting inflammation, uremic toxicity, and other complications inside the CKD patients [65]. The interactions are bidirectional: on the one hand, uremia negatively interferes with the microbiota, altering the composition and metabolism and, on the other hand, the microbiota dysbiosis releases compounds that are normally excreted by the kidneys but could be considered as potential uremic toxins, both conditions further leading to a toxin avalanche exposure, due to the disruption of the epithelial barrier with an increased intestinal permeability, often referred to as "leaky gut," a condition that has been reported in CKD [66].

Uremia status seems to impair the intestinal barrier function and promotes inflammation throughout the gastrointestinal tract. A prospective, observational study reported the baseline concentration of indoxyl sulfate, a uremic toxin that could have a predictive power in CKD progression [67]. Other uremic toxins, p-cresol sulfate and trimethylamine N-oxide (TMAO), were assessed in relation to kidney function (estimated GFR), and the results conclude that the elevated expression was associated to an increased risk for all-cause mortality in ESRD patients. [68]. Uremia represents a condition that accompanies kidney failure and CKD. Uremic toxins originated in, or inserted into, the body via the intestine, such as glycation metabolites, phenols, indoles, all may play important roles in CKD pathophysiology. Consequently, it is biologically plausible, but not well accepted, that a crucial player in the toxic scenario of the CKD resides in the gut microbiota [69].

Deciphering the role of gut microbiota in CKD progression needs a complex comprehension regarding its composition, function, and homeostasis within each individual. As expected, the gut microbiota composition shows great variations, representing a unique signature with each individual harboring, consisting mainly of Gram-negative Bacteroidetes and the Gram-positive low-GC Firmicutes [68]. Gut dysbiosis in CKD was correlated with an increase in pathogenic flora compared to symbiotic flora, which, along with enhanced intestinal permeability, increases absorption of endotoxins with harmful consequences in the organism. The gut-derived uremic toxins, along with an expanded permeability of the intestinal barrier, have been correlated with an increased inflammatory state and oxidative stress, which are constant features of advanced CKD, with a major impact on its complications [65]. The dysbiotic intestinal microflora could be correlated to the intestinal wall edema and ischemia, as well as to a defective colonic epithelial barrier [65]. Recent evidences suggested that several circulating metabolites derived from gut microbiota metabolism could be related to systemic immunoinflammatory response and kidney damage. It has been shown that short-chain fatty acids (SCFAs), which are metabolites essentially derived from dietary fiber fermentation in the gut, are significant players in modulation of immunity, blood pressure, glucose, and lipid metabolism. In addition, SCFAs also "modulate different cell signal transduction processes via G-protein–coupled receptors and act as epigenetic regulators by the inhibition of histone deacetylase and as potential mediators involved in the autophagy pathway." Though controversial, the SCFAs may be regarded as potential therapeutic targets and seem to represent the link between kidney damage and inflammatory response [70]. Gut inflammation is prevalent in CKD and is subsequently involved in systemic inflammation by disruption in the epithelial tight junction, leading to endotoxin and bacterial translocation; this state is associated with a defective Nrf2 pathway. On the basis that Nrf2 represents a protein that regulates the expression of antioxidant proteins that protect against oxidative damage triggered by injury and inflammation, oral administration of Nrf2 activator (study conducted on rats) has reestablished the epithelial tight junction protein expression, alleviating arterial hypertension and rehabilitating the markers of kidney function [71].

In conclusion, accumulating evidence recognizes that dietary fiber may reverse gut dysbiosis and abolish microinflammation, being in agreement with epidemiological evidence suggesting correlations between higher dietary fiber intake, better kidney function, and lower inflammation, at least in the general population. Many researchers accept that supporting intestinal health and restoring the integrity of the gut wall will represent one of the most important goals in improving the quality of life within CKD individuals.

6. Restoring microbiota balance: the exploration of novel therapeutic avenues in renal diseases

Intestinal inflammation and gut microbiota dysbiosis, as well, are now recognized as important contributors in chronic inflammation and other CKD complications, thus explaining the gut-therapeutic novel avenues taken into consideration in designing CKD interventions [61] .

The microbiota can be considered as a recently discovered "organ," being involved in many pathological axes, in relation with almost every organ, including kidneys; there are different metabolites derived from microbiota dysbiosis engaged in distinct physiology pathways linking to renal dysfunction [72]. The bidirectional relationship between gut microbiota and CKD is noted in many studies, and the effect of CKD on gut structure, leading further to dysbiosis (**Figure 1**) is also mentioned. The abundance of specific bacterial groups are dominated by Bacteroides, Prevotella, or Ruminococcus in normal individual gut microbiota [73], and these enterotypes are markedly correlated with long-term diets, especially the proteins and

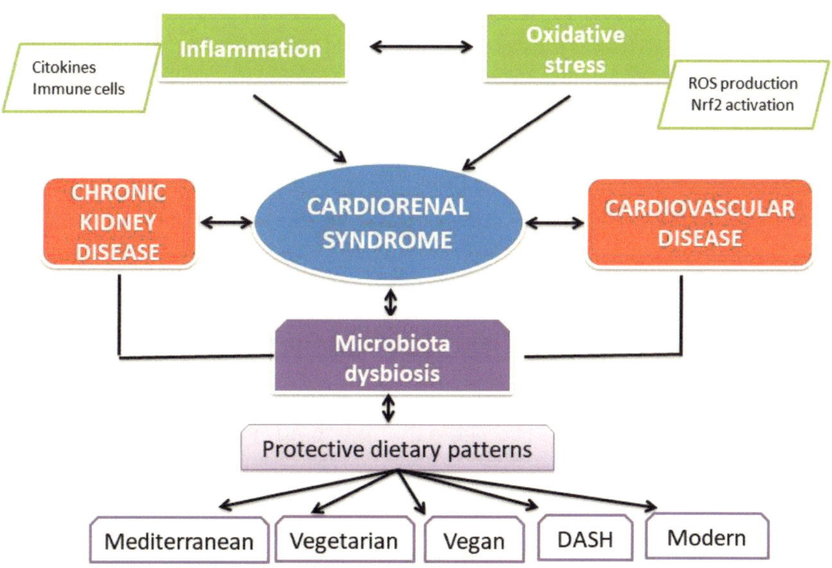

Figure 1. The crosstalk between CKD and inflammation in correlation with microbiota dysbiosis modulation.

animal-fat level (Bacteroides) versus carbohydrates (Prevotella) [74]. On the other side, the gut microbiota in CKD patients is altered, particularly with a decreased amount of Lactobacillaceae and Prevotellaceae families, and with an increased amount (more than 100 times higher) of Enterobacteria and Enterococci, species that are normally found in lower concentrations in healthy individuals [65]. The "supplementary organ" has also an important contribution to digestion, using two different catabolic pathways: saccharolytic (fermentation), with a high prevalence of Bifidobacteria and Lactobacilli, having short-chain fatty acids as end products, and the second, proteolytic (putrefaction) pathway, involving some species within Clostridium, Bacteroides, Enterobacterium, Bifidobacterium, and Lactobacillus [75] that leads to short or branched-chain fatty acids and other cometabolites, considered as microbial uremic toxins [76]. Another controversial mechanism linked to microbial dysbiosis in CKD patients involves the elevated gastrointestinal urea secretion, leading to important amounts of ammonia, which, in turn, contribute to the disturbance in the commensal bacteria [77]; therefore, targeting the gut microbiota composition could represent a promising approach in CKD monitoring and follow-up. Hence, it is considered that a balanced microbiota is mainly saccharolytic and therefore diet itself owns a beneficial role in modulating the gut microbiota composition [78].

Key mechanisms to preserve the gut microbiota balance are considered to include special diets, such as Mediterranean diet, (detailed in **Table 1**) enriched in nondigestible carbohydrates, subject to fermentation by gut microbiota, with low quantities of proteins or fats [75]. It was also revealed that dietary content and their metabolites, such as advanced glycated end products (AGEs), types of uremic toxin resulted in the glycation process, could be closely linked to CKD. Promising therapeutic targets based on nutrition approaches include uremic toxin absorbents and inhibitors of AGEs or the receptor for AGEs. Also specific types of amino acids (d-serine) or fatty acids (palmitate) have been indicated to be related with CKD progression, but they are preliminary results and further studies are needed to confirm their efficacy [79]. It is worth mentioning that dietary interventions could increase the quality of life in CKD patients, though their certain effects on mortality, cardiovascular events, and ESRD remain unclear [80]. The significance of a proper diet was settled in large retrospective cohort studies, which evidenced that the mortality occurrence in predialysis patients that were under dietitian surveillance decreased 19% compared with the patients not under any dietary treat. The conclusion that emerged is that a nutritional care in early stages of CKD could have a better prognosis on survival; however, randomized clinical trials are needed to prove this hypothesis [81].

Another area of potential beneficent therapies in CKD patients relies on the administration of prebiotics and probiotics, and the combination of both therapies into "synbiotic" preparations [81].

Probiotics are defined as "live microorganisms that when administered in adequate amounts confer a health benefit on the host" [82]. Probiotics consist of living bacteria, which can reshape gut microbiota, with impact on the inflammatory status, and are mainly represented by Bifidobacteria species, Lactobacilli, and Streptococci. A study on mice revealed that treatment with Lactobacillus acidophilus could have the potential to attenuate the development of atherosclerotic lesions in mice by reducing the oxidative stress and the inflammatory response [83]. However, the optimal dose of the bacteria essential to obtain an impeccable engraftment

Dietary type	Diet summary	Effects on CKD	References
Mediterranean diet	Carbohydrates, basically unrefined grains, fruits and vegetables, nuts, olive oil, fish, and a moderate consumption of red wine, dairy products, and red meats	PROTECTIVE: potentially restoring microbiota balance, ameliorating CKD conditions, slow down disease progression.	[78, 91, 92]
Vegetarian diet	Fruits and vegetables, olive oil	ADDITIONAL BENEFITS: reduce the burden of uremic toxins; attention must be paid to serum potassium levels.	[93, 94]
Vegan diet	Fruits and vegetables, olive oil	POSITIVE: the addition of inulin modulates microbiota metabolism and the high fiber intake of vegan diet may have favorable effects on intestinal microbiota.	[93]
DASH diet	Consistent with a dietary approach to hypertension	PROTECTIVE: decreased risk of rapid eGFR decline.	[95, 96]
Modern dietary pattern	High intake of fruit, soy milk, egg, milk, and deep-fried products	PROTECTIVE: inversely associated with CKD.	[97]
Western diet	Excessively rich in protein and low in fruit and vegetables, grains, and fibers	DETRIMENTAL: increased risk of rapid eGFR decline.	[96]
Southern diet	Fried foods, organ meats, sweetened beverages Rice, pork, and vegetables, and low intake of wheat	DETRIMENTAL: independently associated with mortality in persons with CKD.	[98] [97]
Modern dietary pattern, with increased cadmium intake	High intake of fruit, soy milk, egg, milk, and deep-fried products, with cadmium contamination in parts of the food supply	DETRIMENTAL: directly associated with CKD.	[97]
DGA diet	Diet based on Dietary Guidelines for Americans (DGA)	DETRIMENTAL: rapid kidney function decline.	[99]
DAL diet	Diet enriched in dietary acid load	DETRIMENTAL: increased risk of ESRD and mortality.	[100–103]

Table 1. Different dietary patterns assessed in association with CKD.

and the suspicion whether these bacteria will resist in the uremic habitat remain questionable [84]. A multinational trial involving patients with CKD stage 3 and 4 has described that half year treatment with proprietary formulation of *S. thermophilus*, *L. acidophilus*, and *B. longum* over has induced a significant decline in urea nitrogen circulating levels and has also enhanced the quality of life scores in these patients. It still remains unclear whether the described interventions may alter the integrity of gut tight junction barrier; thus, more studies are needed to enlarge the knowledge in this area [85].

Prebiotics, specialized plant fibers that promote the growth of healthy bacteria in the gut, have also an important role in preventing CKD progression [84]. The candidate prebiotics comprise inulin, fructo-oligosaccharides, galacto-oligosaccharides, soya-oligosaccharides, xylo-oligosaccharides, and pyrodextrins and have potential in promoting the growth of Bifidobacteria and *Lactobacilli* species [86]. Recent evidence indicates that prebiotic oligofructose-enriched inulin (p-inulin) improves metabolic function, reduces inflammation, and mediates also weight loss [79]. Other prebiotic studies have described the role of supplements containing fructo-oligosaccharides (FOS) and/or inulin and their potential role in modulating the gut microbiota [75]. Prebiotic supplementation with FOS was correlated with a decline in proteolytic metabolites; thus, potential prebiotics such as AXOS could significantly imbalance the protein/carbohydrate fermentation ratio, resulting in alterations in the profile of fermentation metabolites, but the modifications related to microbiota composition remain ambiguous [87, 88].

Synbiotics represent the dual approach of combining a probiotic with a prebiotic and were the subject of several studies. The Synbiotics Easing Renal Failure by Improving Gut Microbiology (SYNERGY) Study was a single-center, double-blind, placebo-controlled, randomized cross-over trial that tested the effects of synbiotics in CKD patients with moderate to severe stages [89]. In this study, preliminary results highlighted that administration of synbiotic therapy did result in appreciable decreasing in circulating levels of nephrovascular uremic toxins, being accompanied by a significant modulation of the stool microbiome (especially with enhancement of Bifidobacterium and deficiency of Ruminococcaceae) in CKD patients, not under antibiotics prescription [89]. The gut microbiota alteration in CKD produces the release of indoxyl sulfate and p-cresyl sulfate, which represent key uremic nephrovascular toxins. Emerging evidence reveals that gut microbiota modulation through diet supplementation with pre- and/probiotics could have an important role in inhibiting the generation of key nephrovascular toxins [90].

Considering the potential of all these preparations in shifting the uremic toxin expression and also in delaying the CKD progression, the exploration of these novel therapeutic avenues could provide vital insights into this inoffensive nutritional therapy.

7. Conclusions and future endeavors

Persistent, low-grade inflammation has been recently accepted as a potential hallmark of CKD, playing an essential role in its pathophysiology and being involved as well in the cardiovascular complications and all-cause poor prognosis in these patients. There has been an ascending growth of interest regarding the role of inflammation in CKD and end-stage renal disease, which shifts the perception of inflammation as no longer a new, but rather a traditional risk factor for CKD morbidity and mortality.

The increasing evidence regarding the tight cross talk between inflammation and kidney function became pathophysiologically relevant in patients with CKD, due to the development of proteomics, genomics, and other omics, and the advancements in state-of-the-art technologies for identification of novel biomarkers in renal diseases. The complex mechanisms in CKD development and progression would require not a single marker, but assessment of a panel of biomarkers in order to enhance all types of alterations that characterize such a complex and insidious disease.

A variety of novel interventions have been recently proposed to target inflammation in CKD, and it seems that, in the near future, the conventional biomarkers could be proficiently improved, or even replaced with novel ones; however, confirmation of their efficacy, sensitivity, and specificity will definitely require randomized controlled and adequately interventional clinical trials.

Growing evidence indicates that gut microbiota can be considered as a recently discovered "organ," being involved in different pathological axes, in relation with almost every organ, including kidneys. Recent advances indicate that gut dysbiosis confers unexpected health risks. The gut-kidney axis has imposed itself in the renal diseases scenario as a novel therapeutic avenue with great potential in the forthcoming future. Emerging evidences highlight the possible correlation between dysbiosis and a wide range of diseases. The gut microbiota imbalance represents though the plausible missing link between nutrition and health, focusing on CKD. Alterations in gut microbiota and a myriad of host responses have been involved in CKD prognosis, high risk of cardiovascular complications, uremic toxicity, and inflammation. There is a vicious circle in CKD, in which, on one hand, toxic gut microbiota metabolites are the major circulating uremic toxins and, on the other hand, their aggregation deteriorates gut dysbiosis and promotes CKD progression.

This novel promising field of research could lead, in the near future, to the design of remarkably personalized nutritional procedures, in order to design the most convenient dietary strategy for each individual.

Acknowledgements

All authors contributed equally to this work. This work was partially supported by the grants COP A 1.2.3., ID: P_40_197/2016 and PN 16.22.05.03.

Author details

Simona Mihai[1]*, Elena Codrici[1], Ionela Daniela Popescu[1], Ana-Maria Enciu[1,2], Laura Georgiana Necula[3], Gabriela Anton[3] and Cristiana Tanase[1,4]

*Address all correspondence to: simona.mihai21@gmail.com

1 Biochemistry-Proteomics Department, Victor Babes National Institute of Pathology, Bucharest, Romania

2 Cellular and Molecular Medicine Department, Carol Davila University of Medicine and Pharmacy, Bucharest, Romania

3 Molecular Virology Department, Stefan S. Nicolau Institute of Virology, Bucharest, Romania

4 Faculty of Medicine, Titu Maiorescu University, Bucharest, Romania

References

[1] Isakova T, Nickolas TL, Denburg M, Yarlagadda S, Weiner DE, Gutierrez OM, et al. KDOQI US Commentary on the 2017 KDIGO clinical practice guideline update for the diagnosis, evaluation, prevention, and treatment of chronic kidney disease-mineral and bone disorder (CKD-MBD). American Journal of Kidney Diseases: The Official Journal of the National Kidney Foundation. 2017;**70**(6):737-751. [Epub 2017/09/25]

[2] Hill NR, Fatoba ST, Oke JL, Hirst JA, O'Callaghan CA, Lasserson DS, et al. Global prevalence of chronic kidney disease—A systematic review and meta-analysis. PLoS One. 2016;**11**(7):e0158765. Epub 2016/07/08

[3] Smyth LJ, Duffy S, Maxwell AP, McKnight AJ. Genetic and epigenetic factors influencing chronic kidney disease. American Journal of Physiology. Renal Physiology. 2014;**307**(7):F757-F776. Epub 2014/08/01

[4] Fu Q, Colgan SP, Shelley CS. Hypoxia: The force that drives chronic kidney disease. Clinical Medicine & Research. 2016;**14**(1):15-39. Epub 2016/02/06

[5] Vassallo D, Kalra PA. Progress in the treatment of atherosclerotic renovascular disease: The conceptual journey and the unanswered questions. Nephrology, Dialysis, Transplantation: Official Publication of the European Dialysis and Transplant Association-European Renal Association. 2016;**31**(10):1595-1605. Epub 2015/07/19

[6] Griffin KA. Hypertensive kidney injury and the progression of chronic kidney disease. Hypertension. 2017;**70**(4):687-694. Epub 2017/08/02

[7] Spoto B, Pisano A, Zoccali C. Insulin resistance in chronic kidney disease: A systematic review. American Journal of Physiology. Renal Physiology. 2016;**311**(6):F1087-FF108. Epub 2016/10/22

[8] Di Lullo L, House A, Gorini A, Santoboni A, Russo D, Ronco C. Chronic kidney disease and cardiovascular complications. Heart Failure Reviews. 2015;**20**(3):259-272. Epub 2014/10/26

[9] Honore PM, Jacobs R, De Waele E, Van Gorp V, De Regt J, Joannes-Boyau O, et al. A fresh look into the pathophysiology of ischemia-induced complications in patients with chronic kidney disease undergoing hemodialysis. International Journal of Nephrology and Renovascular Disease. 2015;**8**:25-28. Epub 2015/03/21

[10] Hill Gallant KM, Spiegel DM. Calcium balance in chronic kidney disease. Current Osteoporosis Reports. 2017;**15**(3):214-221. Epub 2017/05/06

[11] Toussaint ND, Holt SG. Is serum phosphate a useful target in patients with chronic kidney disease and what is the role for dietary phosphate restriction? Nephrology. 2017;**22**(Suppl 2):36-41. Epub 2017/04/22

[12] Pimentel A, Urena-Torres P, Zillikens MC, Bover J, Cohen-Solal M. Fractures in patients with CKD-diagnosis, treatment, and prevention: A review by members of the European Calcified Tissue Society and the European Renal Association of Nephrology Dialysis and Transplantation. Kidney International. 2017. Epub 2017/10/02

[13] Czyzewski L, Wyzgal J, Czyzewska E, Sierdzinski J, Szarpak L. Contribution of volume overload to the arterial stiffness of hemodialysis patients. Renal Failure. 2017;**39**(1):333-339. Epub 2017/01/26

[14] Akchurin OM, Kaskel F. Update on inflammation in chronic kidney disease. Blood Purification. 2015;**39**(1-3):84-92. Epub 2015/02/11

[15] Golia E, Limongelli G, Natale F, Fimiani F, Maddaloni V, Pariggiano I, et al. Inflammation and cardiovascular disease: From pathogenesis to therapeutic target. Current Atherosclerosis Reports. 2014;**16**(9):435. Epub 2014/07/20

[16] Sankowski R, Mader S, Valdes-Ferrer SI. Systemic inflammation and the brain: Novel roles of genetic, molecular, and environmental cues as drivers of neurodegeneration. Frontiers in Cellular Neuroscience. 2015;**9**:28. Epub 2015/02/24

[17] Roxburgh CS, McMillan DC. Cancer and systemic inflammation: Treat the tumour and treat the host. British Journal of Cancer. 2014;**110**(6):1409-1412. Epub 2014/02/20

[18] Calcada D, Vianello D, Giampieri E, Sala C, Castellani G, de Graaf A, et al. The role of low-grade inflammation and metabolic flexibility in aging and nutritional modulation thereof: A systems biology approach. Mechanisms of Ageing and Development. 2014;**136-137**:138-47. Epub 2014/01/28

[19] Koh JH, Kim WU. Dysregulation of gut microbiota and chronic inflammatory disease: From epithelial defense to host immunity. Experimental & Molecular Medicine. 2017;**49**(5):e337. Epub 2017/05/27

[20] Chassaing B, Gewirtz AT. Gut microbiota, low-grade inflammation, and metabolic syndrome. Toxicologic Pathology. 2014;**42**(1):49-53. Epub 2013/11/29

[21] Kochi M, Kohagura K, Shiohira Y, Iseki K, Ohya Y. Chronic kidney disease, inflammation, and cardiovascular disease risk in rheumatoid arthritis. Journal of Cardiology. 2017. Epub 2017/10/04

[22] Fried L, Solomon C, Shlipak M, Seliger S, Stehman-Breen C, Bleyer AJ, et al. Inflammatory and prothrombotic markers and the progression of renal disease in elderly individuals. Journal of the American Society of Nephrology: JASN. 2004;**15**(12):3184-3191. Epub 2004/12/08

[23] Stenvinkel P, Larsson TE. Chronic kidney disease: A clinical model of premature aging. American Journal of Kidney Diseases: The Official Journal of the National Kidney Foundation. 2013;**62**(2):339-351. Epub 2013/01/30

[24] Qian Q. Inflammation: A key contributor to the genesis and progression of chronic kidney disease. Contributions to Nephrology. 2017;**191**:72-83. Epub 2017/09/15

[25] Small DM, Gobe GC. Oxidative stress and antioxidant therapy in chronic kidney and cardiovascular disease. Biochemistry, Genetics and Molecular Biology. May 22, 2013. ISBN: 978-953-51-1123-8

[26] Himmelfarb J, Stenvinkel P, Ikizler TA, Hakim RM. The elephant in uremia: Oxidant stress as a unifying concept of cardiovascular disease in uremia. Kidney International. 2002;**62**(5):1524-1538. Epub 2002/10/10

[27] Scholze A, Jankowski J, Pedraza-Chaverri J, Evenepoel P. Oxidative stress in chronic kidney disease. Oxidative Medicine and Cellular Longevity. 2016;**2016**:8375186. Epub 2016/09/01

[28] Short JD, Downs K, Tavakoli S, Asmis R. Protein thiol redox signaling in monocytes and macrophages. Antioxidants & Redox Signaling. 2016;**25**(15):816-835. Epub 2016/06/12

[29] Mihai S, Codrici E, Popescu ID, Enciu AM, Rusu E, Zilisteanu D, et al. Proteomic biomarkers panel: New insights in chronic kidney disease. Disease Markers. 2016;**2016**:3185232. Epub 2016/09/27

[30] Gupta J, Mitra N, Kanetsky PA, Devaney J, Wing MR, Reilly M, et al. Association between albuminuria, kidney function, and inflammatory biomarker profile in CKD in CRIC. Clinical Journal of the American Society of Nephrology: CJASN. 2012;**7**(12):1938-1946. Epub 2012/10/02

[31] Sundin PO, Udumyan R, Sjostrom P, Montgomery S. Predictors in adolescence of ESRD in middle-aged men. American Journal of Kidney Diseases: The Official Journal of the National Kidney Foundation. 2014;**64**(5):723-729. Epub 2014/08/16

[32] Fallahzadeh MK, Roozbeh J, Geramizadeh B, Namazi MR. Interleukin-2 serum levels are elevated in patients with uremic pruritus: A novel finding with practical implications. Nephrology, Dialysis, Transplantation. 2011;**26**(10):3338-3344. Epub 2011/03/05

[33] Sanz AB, Izquierdo MC, Sanchez-Nino MD, Ucero AC, Egido J, Ruiz-Ortega M, et al. TWEAK and the progression of renal disease: Clinical translation. Nephrology, Dialysis, Transplantation. 2014;**29**(Suppl 1):i54-i62. Epub 2014/02/05

[34] Ucero AC, Berzal S, Ocana-Salceda C, Sancho M, Orzaez M, Messeguer A, et al. A polymeric nanomedicine diminishes inflammatory events in renal tubular cells. PLoS One. 2013;**8**(1):e51992. Epub 2013/01/10

[35] Cohen SD, Phillips TM, Khetpal P, Kimmel PL. Cytokine patterns and survival in haemodialysis patients. Nephrology, Dialysis, Transplantation. 2010;**25**(4):1239-1243. Epub 2009/12/17

[36] Pistol-Tanase C, Raducan E, Dima SO, Albulescu L, Alina I, Marius P, et al. Assessment of soluble angiogenic markers in pancreatic cancer. Biomarkers in Medicine. 2008;**2**(5):447-455. Epub 2008/10/01

[37] Shankar A, Syamala S, Xiao J, Muntner P. Relationship between plasma leptin level and chronic kidney disease. International Journal of Nephrology. 2012;**2012**:269532. Epub 2012/06/06

[38] Gistera A, Hansson GK. The immunology of atherosclerosis. Nature Reviews. Nephrology. 2017;**13**(6):368-380. Epub 2017/04/11

[39] Dungey M, Hull KL, Smith AC, Burton JO, Bishop NC. Inflammatory factors and exercise in chronic kidney disease. International Journal of Endocrinology. 2013;**2013**:569831. Epub 2013/06/06

[40] Feroze U, Molnar MZ, Dukkipati R, Kovesdy CP, Kalantar-Zadeh K. Insights into nutritional and inflammatory aspects of low parathyroid hormone in dialysis patients. Journal of Renal Nutrition. 2011;**21**(1):100-104. Epub 2011/01/05

[41] Gluba-Brzozka A, Michalska-Kasiczak M, Franczyk B, Nocun M, Toth P, Banach M, et al. Markers of increased atherosclerotic risk in patients with chronic kidney disease: A preliminary study. Lipids in Health and Disease. 2016;**15**:22. Epub 2016/02/05

[42] Aikawa E, Aikawa M, Libby P, Figueiredo JL, Rusanescu G, Iwamoto Y, et al. Arterial and aortic valve calcification abolished by elastolytic cathepsin S deficiency in chronic renal disease. Circulation. 2009;**119**(13):1785-1794. Epub 2009/03/25

[43] Ford ML, Smith ER, Tomlinson LA, Chatterjee PK, Rajkumar C, Holt SG. FGF-23 and osteoprotegerin are independently associated with myocardial damage in chronic kidney disease stages 3 and 4. Another link between chronic kidney disease-mineral bone disorder and the heart. Nephrology, Dialysis, Transplantation. 2012;**27**(2):727-733. Epub 2011/07/14

[44] Liabeuf S, Okazaki H, Desjardins L, Fliser D, Goldsmith D, Covic A, et al. Vascular calcification in chronic kidney disease: Are biomarkers useful for probing the pathobiology and the health risks of this process in the clinical scenario? Nephrology, Dialysis, Transplantation. 2014;**29**(7):1275-1284. Epub 2013/09/07

[45] Rogers M, Goettsch C, Aikawa E. Medial and intimal calcification in chronic kidney disease: Stressing the contributions. Journal of the American Heart Association. 2013;**2**(5):e000481. Epub 2013/09/26

[46] Rutsch F, Nitschke Y, Terkeltaub R. Genetics in arterial calcification: Pieces of a puzzle and cogs in a wheel. Circulation Research. 2011;**109**(5):578-592. Epub 2011/08/20

[47] Hofmann Bowman MA, McNally EM. Genetic pathways of vascular calcification. Trends in Cardiovascular Medicine. 2012;**22**(4):93-98. Epub 2012/10/09

[48] Evrard S, Delanaye P, Kamel S, Cristol JP, Cavalier E, SSJWGOV calcifications . Vascular calcification: From pathophysiology to biomarkers. Clinica Chimica Acta. 2015;**438**:401-414. Epub 2014/09/23

[49] Ronco C, McCullough P, Anker SD, Anand I, Aspromonte N, Bagshaw SM, et al. Cardio-renal syndromes: Report from the consensus conference of the acute dialysis quality initiative. European Heart Journal. 2010;**31**(6):703-711. Epub 2009/12/29

[50] Gomes P, Simao S, Silva E, Pinto V, Amaral JS, Afonso J, et al. Aging increases oxidative stress and renal expression of oxidant and antioxidant enzymes that are associated with an increased trend in systolic blood pressure. Oxidative Medicine and Cellular Longevity. 2009;**2**(3):138-145. Epub 2010/07/02

[51] Vlassara H, Torreggiani M, Post JB, Zheng F, Uribarri J, Striker GE. Role of oxidants/inflammation in declining renal function in chronic kidney disease and normal aging. Kidney International. Supplement. 2009;**114**:S3-11. Epub 2009/12/01

[52] Hanna MH, Dalla Gassa A, Mayer G, Zaza G, Brophy PD, Gesualdo L, et al. The nephrologist of tomorrow: Towards a kidney-omic future. Pediatric Nephrology. 2017;**32**(3):393-404. Epub 2016/03/11

[53] Popescu ID, Codrici E, Albulescu L, Mihai S, Enciu AM, Albulescu R, et al. Potential serum biomarkers for glioblastoma diagnostic assessed by proteomic approaches. Proteome Science. 2014;**12**(1):47. Epub 2014/10/10

[54] Mischak H, Delles C, Vlahou A, Vanholder R. Proteomic biomarkers in kidney disease: Issues in development and implementation. Nature Reviews. Nephrology. 2015; **11**(4):221-232. Epub 2015/02/04

[55] Albalat A, Franke J, Gonzalez J, Mischak H, Zurbig P. Urinary proteomics based on capillary electrophoresis coupled to mass spectrometry in kidney disease. Methods in Molecular Biology. 2013;**919**:203-213. Epub 2012/09/15

[56] Smith A, L'Imperio V, Ajello E, Ferrario F, Mosele N, Stella M, et al. The putative role of MALDI-MSI in the study of membranous nephropathy. Biochimica et Biophysica Acta. 2017;**1865**(7):865-874. Epub 2016/11/29

[57] Smith A, L'Imperio V, De Sio G, Ferrario F, Scalia C, Dell'Antonio G, et al. α-1-Antitrypsin detected by MALDI imaging in the study of glomerulonephritis: Its relevance in chronic kidney disease progression. Proteomics. 2016;**16**(11-12):1759-1766

[58] Klein J, Jupp S, Moulos P, Fernandez M, Buffin-Meyer B, Casemayou A, et al. The KUPKB: A novel web application to access multiomics data on kidney disease. FASEB Journal. 2012;**26**(5):2145-2153. Epub 2012/02/22

[59] Fernandes M, Husi H. Establishment of a integrative multi-omics expression database CKDdb in the context of chronic kidney disease (CKD). Scientific Reports. 2017;**7**:40367. Epub 2017/01/13

[60] Joshi MS, Montgomery KA, Giannone PJ, Bauer JA, Hanna MH. Renal injury in neonates: Use of "omics" for developing precision medicine in neonatology. Pediatric Research. 2017;**81**(1-2):271-276. Epub 2016/10/11

[61] Lau WL, Kalantar-Zadeh K, Vaziri ND. The gut as a source of inflammation in chronic kidney disease. Nephron. 2015;**130**(2):92-98. Epub 2015/05/15

[62] Ramezani A, Raj DS. The gut microbiome, kidney disease, and targeted interventions. Journal of the American Society of Nephrology: JASN. 2014;**25**(4):657-670. Epub 2013/11/16

[63] Cigarran Guldris S, Gonzalez Parra E, Cases Amenos A. Microbiota intestinal en la enfermedad renal cronica (Gut microbiota in chronic kidney disease. Nefrologia). 2017;**37**(1):9-19. Epub 2016/08/25

[64] Wang F, Jiang H, Shi K, Ren Y, Zhang P, Cheng S. Gut bacterial translocation is associated with microinflammation in end-stage renal disease patients. Nephrology. 2012; **17**(8):733-738. Epub 2012/07/24

[65] Vaziri ND, Wong J, Pahl M, Piceno YM, Yuan J, De Santis TZ, et al. Chronic kidney disease alters intestinal microbial flora. Kidney International. 2013;**83**(2):308-315. Epub 2012/09/21

[66] Evenepoel P, Poesen R, Meijers B. The gut-kidney axis. Pediatric Nephrology. 2016; **32**(11):2005-2014. Epub 2016/11/17

[67] Wu IW, Hsu KH, Lee CC, Sun CY, Hsu HJ, Tsai CJ, et al. p-Cresyl sulphate and indoxyl sulphate predict progression of chronic kidney disease. Nephrology, Dialysis, Transplantation. 2011;**26**(3):938-947. Epub 2010/10/05

[68] Al Khodor S, Shatat IF. Gut microbiome and kidney disease: A bidirectional relationship. Pediatric Nephrology. 2017;**32**(6):921-931. Epub 2016/05/01

[69] Vitetta L, Gobe G. Uremia and chronic kidney disease: The role of the gut microflora and therapies with pro- and prebiotics. Molecular Nutrition & Food Research. 2013;**57**(5):824-832. Epub 2013/03/02

[70] Huang W, Zhou L, Guo H, Xu Y, Xu Y. The role of short-chain fatty acids in kidney injury induced by gut-derived inflammatory response. Metabolism, Clinical and Experimental. 2017;**68**:20-30. Epub 2017/02/12

[71] Lau WL, Liu SM, Pahlevan S, Yuan J, Khazaeli M, Ni Z, et al. Role of Nrf2 dysfunction in uremia-associated intestinal inflammation and epithelial barrier disruption. Digestive Diseases and Sciences. 2015;**60**(5):1215-1222. Epub 2014/11/17

[72] Briskey D, Tucker P, Johnson DW, Coombes JS. The role of the gastrointestinal tract and microbiota on uremic toxins and chronic kidney disease development. Clinical and Experimental Nephrology. 2017;**21**(1):7-15. Epub 2016/03/12

[73] Arumugam M, Raes J, Pelletier E, Le Paslier D, Yamada T, Mende DR, et al. Enterotypes of the human gut microbiome. Nature. 2011;**473**(7346):174-180. Epub 2011/04/22

[74] Wu GD, Chen J, Hoffmann C, Bittinger K, Chen YY, Keilbaugh SA, et al. Linking long-term dietary patterns with gut microbial enterotypes. Science. 2011;**334**(6052):105-108. Epub 2011/09/03

[75] Scott KP, Gratz SW, Sheridan PO, Flint HJ, Duncan SH. The influence of diet on the gut microbiota. Pharmacological Research. 2013;**69**(1):52-60. Epub 2012/11/14

[76] Evenepoel P, Meijers BK, Bammens BR, Verbeke K. Uremic toxins originating from colonic microbial metabolism. Kidney International. Supplement. 2009;**114**:S12-S19. Epub 2009/12/01

[77] Koppe L, Mafra D, Fouque D. Probiotics and chronic kidney disease. Kidney International. 2015;**88**(5):958-966. Epub 2015/09/17

[78] Montemurno E, Cosola C, Dalfino G, Daidone G, De Angelis M, Gobbetti M, et al. What would you like to eat, Mr CKD microbiota? A Mediterranean diet, please! Kidney & Blood Pressure Research. 2014;**39**(2-3):114-123. Epub 2014/08/15

[79] Hasegawa S, Jao TM, Inagi R. Dietary metabolites and chronic kidney disease. Nutrients. 2017;**9**(4). pii: E358, Epub 2017/04/05

[80] Palmer SC, Maggo JK, Campbell KL, Craig JC, Johnson DW, Sutanto B, et al. Dietary interventions for adults with chronic kidney disease. The Cochrane Database of Systematic Reviews. 2017;**4**:CD011998. Epub 2017/04/24

[81] Rysz J, Franczyk B, Cialkowska-Rysz A, Gluba-Brzozka A. The effect of diet on the survival of patients with chronic kidney disease. Nutrients. 2017;**9**(5). pii: E495, Epub 2017/05/16

[82] Mutsaers HA, Engelke UF, Wilmer MJ, Wetzels JF, Wevers RA, van den Heuvel LP, et al. Optimized metabolomic approach to identify uremic solutes in plasma of stage 3-4 chronic kidney disease patients. PLoS One. 2013;**8**(8):e71199. Epub 2013/08/13

[83] Chen L, Liu W, Li Y, Luo S, Liu Q, Zhong Y, et al. Lactobacillus acidophilus ATCC 4356 attenuates the atherosclerotic progression through modulation of oxidative stress and inflammatory process. International Immunopharmacology. 2013;**17**(1):108-115. Epub 2013/06/12

[84] Nallu A, Sharma S, Ramezani A, Muralidharan J, Raj D. Gut microbiome in chronic kidney disease: Challenges and opportunities. Translational Research. 2017;**179**:24-37. Epub 2016/05/18

[85] Ranganathan N, Ranganathan P, Friedman EA, Joseph A, Delano B, Goldfarb DS, et al. Pilot study of probiotic dietary supplementation for promoting healthy kidney function in patients with chronic kidney disease. Advances in Therapy. 2010;**27**(9):634-647. Epub 2010/08/20

[86] Devuyst O, Beaujean V, Crabbe J. Effects of environmental conditions on mitochondrial-rich cell density and chloride transport in toad skin. Pflügers Archiv/European Journal of Physiology. 1991;**417**(6):577-581. Epub 1991/02/01

[87] De Preter V, Vanhoutte T, Huys G, Swings J, De Vuyst L, Rutgeerts P, et al. Effects of Lactobacillus casei Shirota, Bifidobacterium breve, and oligofructose-enriched inulin on colonic nitrogen-protein metabolism in healthy humans. American Journal of Physiology. Gastrointestinal and Liver Physiology. 2007;**292**(1):G358-G368. Epub 2006/09/23

[88] Sanchez JI, Marzorati M, Grootaert C, Baran M, Van Craeyveld V, Courtin CM, et al. Arabinoxylan-oligosaccharides (AXOS) affect the protein/carbohydrate fermentation balance and microbial population dynamics of the simulator of human intestinal microbial ecosystem. Microbial Biotechnology. 2009;**2**(1):101-113. Epub 2009/01/01

[89] Rossi M, Johnson DW, Morrison M, Pascoe EM, Coombes JS, Forbes JM, et al. Synbiotics easing renal failure by improving gut microbiology (SYNERGY): A randomized trial. Clinical Journal of the American Society of Nephrology: CJASN. 2016;**11**(2):223-231. Epub 2016/01/17

[90] Rossi M, Johnson DW, Morrison M, Pascoe E, Coombes JS, Forbes JM, et al. SYNbiotics easing renal failure by improving gut microbiologY (SYNERGY): A protocol of placebo-controlled randomised cross-over trial. BMC Nephrology. 2014;**15**:106. Epub 2014/07/06

[91] Romagnolo DF, Selmin OI. Mediterranean diet and prevention of chronic diseases. Nutrition Today. 2017;**52**(5):208-222. Epub 2017/10/21

[92] Huang X, Jimenez-Moleon JJ, Lindholm B, Cederholm T, Arnlov J, Riserus U, et al. Mediterranean diet, kidney function, and mortality in men with CKD. Clinical Journal of the American Society of Nephrology: CJASN. 2013;**8**(9):1548-1555. Epub 2013/06/08

[93] Cupisti A, D'Alessandro C, Gesualdo L, Cosola C, Gallieni M, Egidi MF, et al. Non-traditional aspects of renal diets: Focus on fiber, alkali and vitamin K1 intake. Nutrients. 2017;**9**(5). Epub 2017/05/05

[94] Chauveau P, Combe C, Fouque D, Aparicio M. Vegetarianism: Advantages and drawbacks in patients with chronic kidney diseases. Journal of Renal Nutrition: The Official Journal of the Council on Renal Nutrition of the National Kidney Foundation. 2013;**23**(6):399-405. Epub 2013/09/28

[95] Asghari G, Yuzbashian E, Mirmiran P, Azizi F. The association between dietary approaches to stop hypertension and incidence of chronic kidney disease in adults: The Tehran lipid and glucose study. Nephrology, Dialysis, Transplantation: Official Publication of the European Dialysis and Transplant Association—European Renal Association. 2017;**32**(Suppl_2):ii224-ii30. Epub 2017/02/16

[96] Lin J, Fung TT, Hu FB, Curhan GC. Association of dietary patterns with albuminuria and kidney function decline in older white women: A subgroup analysis from the Nurses' Health Study. American Journal of Kidney Diseases: The Official Journal of the National Kidney Foundation. 2011;**57**(2):245-254. Epub 2011/01/22

[97] Shi Z, Taylor AW, Riley M, Byles J, Liu J, Noakes M. Association between dietary patterns, cadmium intake and chronic kidney disease among adults. Clinical Nutrition. 2017. Epub 2017/01/18

[98] Gutierrez OM, Muntner P, Rizk DV, McClellan WM, Warnock DG, Newby PK, et al. Dietary patterns and risk of death and progression to ESRD in individuals with CKD: A cohort study. American Journal of Kidney Diseases: The Official Journal of the National Kidney Foundation. 2014;**64**(2):204-213. Epub 2014/04/01

[99] Foster MC, Hwang SJ, Massaro JM, Jacques PF, Fox CS, Chu AY. Lifestyle factors and indices of kidney function in the Framingham Heart Study. American Journal of Nephrology. 2015;**41**(4-5):267-274. Epub 2015/05/23

[100] Banerjee T, Crews DC, Wesson DE, Tilea AM, Saran R, Rios-Burrows N, et al. High dietary acid load predicts ESRD among adults with CKD. Journal of the American Society of Nephrology: JASN. 2015;**26**(7):1693-1700. Epub 2015/02/14

[101] Kanda E, Ai M, Kuriyama R, Yoshida M, Shiigai T. Dietary acid intake and kidney disease progression in the elderly. American Journal of Nephrology. 2014;**39**(2):145-152. Epub 2014/02/12

[102] Scialla JJ, Appel LJ, Astor BC, Miller ER, 3rd, Beddhu S, Woodward M, et al. Net endogenous acid production is associated with a faster decline in GFR in African Americans. Kidney International. 2012;**82**(1):106-112. Epub 2012/04/06

[103] Tyson CC, Lin PH, Corsino L, Batch BC, Allen J, Sapp S, et al. Short-term effects of the DASH diet in adults with moderate chronic kidney disease: A pilot feeding study. Clinical Kidney Journal. 2016;**9**(4):592-598. Epub 2016/08/02

Chapter 7

Inflammation in Nonimmune-Mediated Chronic Kidney Disease

Camilla Fanelli, Ayman Noreddin and Ane Nunes

Additional information is available at the end of the chapter

http://dx.doi.org/10.5772/intechopen.70611

Abstract

Regardless of its etiology, chronic kidney disease (CKD) is characterized by proteinuria, serum creatinine retention, glomerulosclerosis (GS), and tubulointerstitial damage. Notably, the last one has been correlated more closely with the evolution to kidney failure than the extent of glomerular injury. Tubulointerstitial inflammation comprises the activation of tubular epithelial cells, which release inflammatory mediators and chemokines promoting the influx of leukocytes in the renal parenchyma and the activation/proliferation of resident fibroblasts, leading to excessive production of extracellular matrix (EM), fibrosis, and renal function loss. Therefore, inflammation exerts a key role in the pathogenesis of CKD, although the mechanisms by which this process is activated and perpetuated, even when the initial insult is not immune-mediated, such as in the hypertensive nephrosclerosis, in the diabetic nephropathy, and in the crystal-induced renal disease, remain unclear. This chapter provides an overview on inflammation and CKD development not related to autoimmunity or caused by presence of foreign antigens. Cellular and molecular mechanisms involved in different pathways and its potential therapeutic targets to detain the progression of inflammation and fibrosis in CKD are also presented ahead as a contribution in this book.

Keywords: chronic kidney disease, inflammation, immune system, innate immunity, adaptive immunity

1. Introduction

Chronic kidney disease (CKD) is considered a global health problem that motivates life science researchers and physicians to investigate the mechanisms beyond its development, and to seek for new therapeutic strategies to detain the evolution of renal function loss [1].

Progressive CKD may be initiated by several conditions of different etiological basis; however, in almost all cases, renal disease progresses with the development of a chronic and self-sustained inflammatory reaction, which involves both innate and adaptive arms of immune response and leads to kidney fibrosis. Reasons why inflammation parallels CKD progression even when the initial renal injury does not involve autoimmune disorders or infection episodes remain unclear [2]. In the following sections, we are going to discuss some epidemiological data on CKD in the United States (US) and in the World, as well as briefly review the pathophysiological mechanisms involved in CKD development and progression, with special attention to the participation of inflammatory components in this process.

2. Chronic kidney disease and inflammation: definition and numbers

CKD is a general term used to define a group of heterogeneous disorders that structurally compromise the kidneys, resulting in reduction or insufficiency of renal function. CKD is one of the major degenerative conditions that lead to progressive disability, and is the ninth cause of death in the US [3]. Every year, kidney disease kills more people than breast or prostate cancer. According to the National Kidney Foundation, CKD assumed epidemic proportions in the last decades and meets all the required criteria to be considered as a major public health concern [3–8]. The 2016 Annual Data Report of the US Renal Data System (USRDS) showed that around 26 millions of American adults have some degree of kidney disease, of which, more than 661,000 have end-stage renal disease (ESRD), defined by the requirement of renal replacement therapy (RRT) for life-saving [4, 5]. Accordingly, there were 468,000 Americans on dialysis and approximately 193,000 individuals living with a transplanted kidney, in the last year [5].

This reality is also true for the other countries around the world. The Bulletin of the World Health Organization estimated the global number of patients receiving RRT to be higher than 1.4 million, with incidence of growing by around 8% annually [6]. This high prevalence and mortality, allied to the elevated costs of treating this growing epidemic represents a big burden on healthcare systems worldwide, especially in low and middle income countries, where long term dialysis is financially unaffordable [7–9]. This dramatic scenario motivates the medical community to intensify the efforts in preventing kidney injury and to improve the early detection of this condition. Moreover, scientific investigation to elucidate the pathophysiological mechanisms involved in the evolution of chronic nephropathies is of paramount importance to the development of more effective therapeutic strategies to slow or even stop the progression of CKD.

Gradual renal function deterioration is generally caused by an initial kidney injury, which acutely or chronically affects both the glomerular filtration rate (GFR) and/or the tubular reabsorption/excretion [2, 10]. The decrease of renal blood flow and the blockage of the urinary tract are the main causes of acute kidney injury (AKI). Kidneys' hypoperfusion can be caused by hypovolemia, septic shock, bleeding, hypotension, or due to renal ischemia, caused by abnormal vasoconstriction, or by the presence of blood clots, arteriosclerosis or other renal blood flow blocking agents. Bladder and/or ureteral obstruction, in turn, can occur due to anatomic alterations, prostate hypertrophy, and cancer, or by the presence of kidney/ureteral stones. AKI can be additionally caused by some specific health conditions such as the multiple myeloma or the tubular necrosis, which can result from the administration of nephrotoxic drugs and compounds. In general, these conditions reduce the GFR, promoting a sharp decrease of renal function, that can be transitory; if the renal blood hypoperfusion or the obstruction of the urinary tract is rapidly corrected, or permanent, if the regular renal blood flow and the urinary output are not restored. There are actually growing evidence that, even when an AKI episode is properly solved, and there is a complete reestablishment of renal function, the patients should be closely followed for a long period, since this population is more prone to manifest CKD in the future [10, 11].

Although acute renal lesions may lead to the development of progressive kidney insufficiency, the two main causes of CKD are still diabetes and hypertension [3–6]. Such insidious diseases are, together, responsible for up to two-thirds of the cases of CKD in the American population [3–5]. If poorly or inefficiently controlled, both diabetes and hypertension may cause significant damage to human body, especially when it is exposed to these conditions for a long period. Many organs and systems can be affected, such as the blood vessels, the central nervous system (CNS), the eyes and, finally, the kidneys [2, 10]. The exact pathophysiological mechanisms through which sustained high serum glucose concentration and blood pressure lead to renal injury have not yet been fully elucidated. Proposed theories and mechanisms based on experimental studies, clinical trials, and medical observation will be discussed further on.

The third more common cause of CKD in the US is a group of autoimmune disorders, generally designated by Glomerulonephritis (GN) [3–5]. There are a number of different kinds of GN, which differ one from the other by the type of local renal infiltrating cells, by the presence and subtyping of autoantibodies, by the accumulation of complement system components, by the specific antigens that starts the renal local immune response, and also by some differential clinical and laboratorial features, including proteinuria, hematuria, and edema [12]. Although GN is an important cause of CKD, the molecular and cellular mechanisms involved in their onset and progression are beyond the scope of this revision, since GN is considered an immune-mediated kidney condition.

In a less extent, inherited diseases like different forms of polycystic kidney disease (PKD) and genetic syndromes, such as Von Hippel-Lindau, Alport's, and Bartter's can also lead to CKD, as well as congenital malformations of the urinary system and repeated urinary tract infections (UTI) [3–6, 13].

3. Overview of CKD pathophysiology

Regardless of the nature of the initial renal insult, CKD is characterized by proteinuria, serum urea and creatinine retention, blood pressure rising, and imbalance in renal perfusion, which lead to the development of glomerular hypertension and hypertrophy, mesangial cells proliferation, and extracellular matrix (EM) overproduction, culminating in irreversible changes in glomerular and tubular architecture that impairs the function of the nephron [2, 9]. Notably, the involvement of the tubulointerstitial compartment has been correlated more closely with the evolution to kidney failure than the extent of glomerular injury per se [2, 9, 14]. The more filtering units are injured, the more overburdened the remaining nephrons become, which in turn end up succumbing due to overload in a vicious cycle of positive feedback. This process leads to global glomerulosclerosis (GS), tubular atrophy (TA), interstitial fibrosis, peritubular capillary rarefaction, and progressive renal function loss [2, 9, 14, 15], as illustrated in **Figure 1**.

The inordinate activation of the renin-angiotensin-aldosterone system (RAAS) is one of the major factors that can stimulate CKD progression [9]. Traditionally, RAAS used to be considered only as an endocrine system, whose major function was to maintain the blood pressure, even in situations of hypovolemia [16]. In the traditional description of RAAS, Renin, a hormone synthesized by the renal juxtaglomerular cells, promotes the conversion of angiotensinogen, produced in the liver, into angiotensin I (Ang I). This peptide is further cleaved by angiotensin-converting enzyme (ACE) into its active form, the Angiotensin II (Ang II), which, in turn, binds to its specific receptors (AT1) in the adrenal cortex, resulting in the release of aldosterone. Once released in the blood stream this

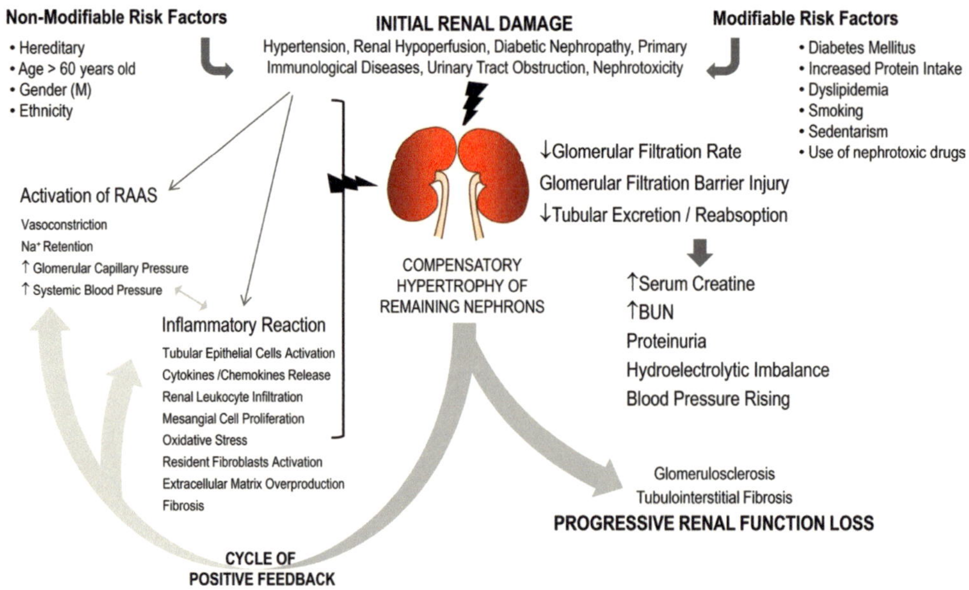

Figure 1. CKD pathophysiology. Different immune and nonimmune conditions may cause the initial renal insult that is been influenced by both modifiable and non-modifiable risk factors. This original damage causes several changes on renal function reducing the glomerular filtration rate, impairing the renal tubular hydroelectrolytic balance and damaging the glomerular filtration barrier. In a forward positive feedback, these events are able to lead to glomerulosclerosis, renal fibrosis and progressive loss of function.

mineralocorticoid steroid promotes renal and systemic vasoconstriction and tubular sodium conservation, leading to the elevation of blood pressure [9, 16]. In spite of its first description, RAAS became much more complex in the recent years, after the identification of many novel components, such as the enzyme chymase, which exerts the same function of ACE, the biologically active peptides angiotensin III, IV, 1–9 and 1–7, and a number of different Ang II receptors (AT2, AT4, among others) [16]. Moreover, depending on which intracellular downstream system is activated by Ang II, different physiological responses can be triggered [16, 17].

Ang II has been related to inflammation followed to chronic nephropathy developed by the enhancing of the immune response and favoring renal infiltration by leukocyte [18, 19]. Additionally, there are growing *in vitro* and *in vivo* evidence that Ang II promotes cell proliferation and fibroblast activation, worsening the accumulation of EM and contributing to the development of renal fibrosis [18, 20, 21]. Furthermore, a variety of studies showed the presence of both Ang II and the receptor AT1 in the renal parenchyma of animals submitted to experimental models of CKD, leading to the discovery of a complex intrarenal pro-inflammatory RAAS that seems to become overactivated under kidney injury [18–22]. Accordingly, suppression of RAAS with both ACE inhibitors (ACEi) and/or AT1 receptor blockers (ARB) become a mainstay of treatment of progressive nephropathies and, although several innovative therapeutic measures have been recently proposed for the treatment of CKD, RAAS blockage, associated to diuretics or not, remains the best available resource in this regard [9, 16, 23, 24].

In 1984, Schwartz and collaborators demonstrated for the first time an increase in fibroblast and the appearance of macrophages and lymphocytes in the renal parenchyma of rabbits submitted to a sterile model of renal ischemia/reperfusion [25]. This was one of the first studies suggesting that the inflammatory process, including mononuclear cell infiltration and fibroblast proliferation was a final pathway common to different forms of renal injury, independent of its etiology. We currently know that inflammation exerts a key role in the pathogenesis of CKD, although the mechanisms by which this process is activated and perpetuated, even when the initial insult is not immune-mediated, remain unclear.

There is growing evidence that the activation of both cellular and humoral immunity is related to the progression of renal insufficiency and a worse prognosis in nonimmune-mediated CKD. Renal infiltration by macrophages has been demonstrated in a variety of human nonimmune-mediated renal diseases, such as diabetic nephropathy (DN) [26] and hypertensive nephrosclerosis (HN) [27]. Moreover, this phenomenon was also observed in different experimental models of CKD over the last years. Accordingly, the number of inflammatory cells in the renal *interstitium* closely correlates with the severity of nephropathy and with glomerular and tubulointerstitial lesions in these experimental models [28–30]. The increase of dendritic cells (DCs) in the renal parenchyma, in turns, is believed to indicate the spreading of inflammation from glomerular to the tubulointerstitial compartment, playing a pivotal role in the progression of both AKI and CKD [31, 32]. Finally, cortical

T-lymphocyte infiltration is a common finding in both genetic [33] and pharmacologically induced [34] DN in rodents. Moreover, it has also been described in the 5/6 renal ablation model (NX) [35] and in the chronic inhibition of nitric oxide synthase model (L-NAME) [29], among others [19]. In most of these studies, the amount of T-cells in the renal *interstitium* correlates positively with the progression of albuminuria, creatinine retention, and renal structural damage, as shown in **Table 1** [36–43]. Corroborating these findings, a number of experimental studies showing significant evidence that anti-inflammatory treatment, as well as the knockout (KO) of specific pro-inflammatory genes can be effective to detain the evolution of nephropathy in different animal models of CKD, have been recently published, as shown in **Table 2** [44–52].

Although the exact sequence of the inflammatory events in progressive CKD has not been completely elucidated yet, we are currently aware that, the activation of tubular epithelial cells, inordinate production of cytokines, activation of resident phagocytes and fibroblasts, as well as the transdifferentiation of these last into pro-fibrotic myofibroblasts, parallels renal leukocyte infiltration, from the early beginning of renal disease. Furthermore, these processes follow the evolution of CKD, becoming autonomic and leading to excessive production of EM and fibrosis [9, 14, 32, 53].

Authors (first, last) and year	Ref.	Species	CKD studied	Molecules/cells studied
Gong W, Zhang A. 2016	[36]	Mouse	5/6 nephrectomy (NX)	NLRP3
Souza AC, Star RA. 2015	[37]	Mouse	5/6 nephrectomy (NX)	TLR4
D'Apolito M, Giardino I. 2015	[38]	Mouse	5/6 nephrectomy (NX)	Urea as a DAMP
Lehners A, Wenzel UO. 2014	[39]	Mouse	5/6 nephrectomy (NX)	Myeloperoxidase (MPO)
Correa-Costa, Camara NOS. 2011	[40]	Mouse	Adenine-induced tubule interstitial nephritis	TLR2, TLR4, MYD88, ASC, CASP1
Fanelli C, Zatz R. 2011	[19]	Rat	CKD caused by AT1 blockade during nephrogenesis	T-lymphocytes
Vilaysane A, Muruve DA. 2010	[41]	Mouse	Unilateral ureteral obstruction (UUO)	NLRP3
Rodriguez-Iturbe, Vaziri ND. 2004	[42]	Rat	Spontaneously hypertensive rats (SHR)	NFKB system, T-cells
Utimura R, Zatz R. 2003	[28]	Rat	ST-induced DN	T-lymphocytes
Fujihara CK, Zatz R. 2001	[29]	Rat	L-NAME-induced nitric oxide synthase inhibition	T-lymphocytes
Donadelli R, Zoja C. 2000	[43]	Rat	5/6 nephrectomy (NX)	NFKB system
Fujihara CK, Noronha IL. 1998	[35]	Rat	5/6 nephrectomy (NX)	T-lymphocytes

Table 1. Evidences of innate and adaptive immunity activation in nonimmune-mediated CKD.

Authors (first, last) and year	Ref.	Species	CKD studied	Target cell/molecule	Drug/compound	Related improvements
Ludwig-Portugall I, Kurts C. 2016	[44]	Mouse	Adenine/oxalate-induced nephritis	NLRP3	CP-456,773	CP-456,773 prevented kidney fibrosis in a murine model of crystal nephropathy induced by diets rich in oxalate or adenine.
Okabe C, Fujihara CK. 2013	[45]	Rat	Adenine-induced nephritis	NFKB system	PDTC	PDTC prevented p65 nuclear translocation, limited formation of renal interstitial foreign body granulomas, reduced the expression of Ifng, Il6, Fsp1, Mcp1 genes, and strongly attenuated interstitial fibrosis/inflammation
Kim JE, Cha DR. 2013	[46]	Mouse	db/db genetically-induced DN	NFKB system	Celastrol	Celastrol not only improved insulin resistance, glycemic, control, and oxidative stress, but also improved renal functional and structural changes through both metabolic and anti-inflammatory effects in the kidney
Gilbert RE, Kelly DJ. 2012	[47]	Rat	5/6 nephrectomy (NX) and ST-induced DN	TGFβ	FT011	FT011 attenuated hypertension, GS, and renal macrophage infiltration in Nx, as well as reduced albuminuria, GS, renal interstitial fibrosis, and inflammation in ST-DN
Ding W, Gu Y. 2012	[48]	Rat	Aldosterone/salt-induced renal injury	NFKB system	PDTC	PDTC significantly decreased the percentage of $CTGF^+$ cells, the mRNA for TGF-β, CTGF, TGF-β, ICAM-1 and collagen IV, and protein levels of CTGF and ICAM-1
Kaneyama T, Ehara T. 2010	[49]	Rat	Unilateral ureteral obstruction (UUO)	TGFβ	Tranilast	Fibrosis and tubular injuries were attenuated in UUO rats treated with tranilast compared with untreated UUO animals
Fujihara CK, Zatz R. 2007	[50]	Rat	5/6 nephrectomy (NX)	NFKB system	PDTC	PDTC attenuated renal injury and inflammation, as well as the density of cells staining positively for the phospho p65 subunit

Authors (first, last) and year	Ref.	Species	CKD studied	Target cell/molecule	Drug/compound	Related improvements
Utimura R, Zatz R. 2003	[28]	Rat	ST-induced DN	T-lymphocytes	MMF	MMF prevented albuminuria, GS, and renal cortical macrophage infiltration in DN
Shihab FS, Andoh Tf. 2002	[51]	Human	Human DN	TGFβ, TNFa	Pirfenidone	Treatment with pirfenidone, which has been shown to inhibit renal fibrosis in experimental models, prolonged the period of conservative treatment of CKD in patients with ND, delaying the need for dialysis
Fujihara CK, Zatz R. 2001	[29]	Rat	L-NAME-induced NO inhibition	T-lymphocytes	MMF	MMF significantly reduced glomerulosclerosis, renal interstitial expansion, macrophage and lymphocyte infiltration
Romero F, Tapia E. 1999	[52]	Rat	5/6 nephrectomy (NX)	T-lymphocytes	MMF	Segmental sclerosis, interstitial fibrosis, and renal infiltration by $CD43^+$ and $ED1^+$ cells were significantly reduced with MMF
Fujihara CK, Noronha IL. 1998	[35]	Rat	5/6 nephrectomy (NX)	T-lymphocytes	MMF	MMF significantly prevented GS and interstitial expansion in NX rats

Table 2. Studies using experimental CKD development and its renoprotective effects.

4. The immune system and kidney disease

The immune system (IS) is composed by a set of structures, cells, and processes that together enable an organism to recognize their self-elements from the foreign and potentially pathogenic ones, producing then, a physiological response consistent with the nature of the recognized element, which can be either a self-harmless protein or a dangerous bacterium [54]. As part of these systems, there are the so-called nonimmunological physical, chemical, and biological barriers and the immunological components itself, represented by innate and adaptive mechanisms of cellular and humoral immune response [54, 55].

In a simplistic way, the IS is responsible for four different body functions. The first one is the immune tolerance, the property that allows the body to recognize self-cells, proteins, and other constitutive elements, producing a response of tolerance and preventing autoimmune reactions. This particular state of IS unresponsiveness is also essential to ensure the regular fetal development during pregnancy and to allow the colonization of human skin, digestive tract, and vagina by beneficial microorganisms referred as microbiota [56, 57].

The second and most well-known function of IS is the immunity itself. It is the ability to recognize foreign proteins and molecules, which may indicate the presence of invading microorganisms, such as bacteria or other parasites, and respond to these foreign elements with both cellular and humoral defenses, protecting the organism against infection [54]. Additionally, through its third property, immune surveillance, the IS patrols the body to recognize and destroy self-cells infected by virus or even constitutive cells that become cancerous or suffer phenotype alterations due to genetic mutations [54, 55]. For immune surveillance to work, cancer and/or mutated cells must express specific antigens that are not frequently found on normal cells, otherwise the IS would recognize them as "self" and be tolerant of them [58, 59].

Finally, the last property of IS is the ability of self-controlling the immune response. Through a complex mechanism of feedback and cell-to-cell communication, involving a number of cytokines and cell-cytokine receptors, IS modulates its response, which can be either tolerance or immunity, according to the specific stimulus to which the organism is subjected to [54]. This property is known as immunoregulation and is of paramount importance, not only for the kidneys but also for the whole organism. Failures on the immunoregulation may lead either to the development of autoimmune diseases that can impair renal function, such as systemic lupus erythematosus (SLE), whose renal involvement is a severe type of GN called lupus nephritis or to the vulnerability to opportunistic infections, leading to repeated episodes of pyelonephritis and/or immune-mediated GN due to the accumulation of antigen-antibody complexes in the glomerular filtration barrier (GFB) [12].

The integrity of the epithelial tissue can be listed as one of the most important nonimmunological physical barriers against infection. The skin represents the largest organ of the human body and its main function is to delimit the organism, separating it and protecting it from the environment that surrounds it. Of course, it is not an insurmountable insulation, since this would be incompatible with the maintenance of life: water, atmospheric gases, and ions are able to cross the epithelial barrier simply due to passive processes such as osmosis and diffusion or through active transmembrane transport.

However, macromolecules, such as high-weight proteins or even whole cells are not able to transpose the barrier formed by epithelial tissue in a normal physiological situation, making the area covered by the intact epithelium protected from invasive pathogens. Accordingly, epithelial injury and/or scarification provide the invasive parasites a chance to enter into their future host [54, 55]. Some virulent microorganisms can produce elements capable of puncturing or injuring the epithelial tissue, opening a gateway to the host organism. Certain strains of uropathogenic *Escherichia coli* (UPEC), for instance, produce proteolytic enzymes, cytotoxic necrotizing factors, and numerous adhesive molecules (adhesins) as part of their invasion arsenal [60].

UTI is a worldwide health problem that affects over 13 million of people each year in the US. It is currently the most common infection in adult females and, in nearly all cases, it is caused by a few strains of UPEC. Although the symptoms of an uncomplicated UTI can be relatively mild, it can progress to pyelonephritis, leading to fever, nausea, vomiting, and, in about 30% of cases, bacteremia and risk of sepsis. Moreover, recurrent UTI may contribute to additional problems, including renal scarring, CKD, and an increased risk for developing bladder cancer [60]. Besides the presence of UPEC and the toxins produced by them in the urinary tract, there are evidence that proteinuria can itself cause injury to the renal and urinary epithelium. Since proteins are expected to be retained in the GFB, increased protein concentration in the urinary fluid is considered an irritating and pro-inflammatory factor for the tubular, ureteral, and bladder epithelium, leading to enhanced protein reabsorption by the tubular epithelial cells, overload of their catabolic capacity, leukocytes infiltration, and corruption of the integrity of the urinary epithelial barrier [54].

The intestinal and ureteral peristaltic movement and the flow of fluids like vomiting, diarrheal, or the urinary stream itself are also important physical barriers against infection, preventing the onset and permanence of microorganisms in the digestive system and in the lower urinary tract. In addition to these physical barriers, the maintenance of low pH in some body fluids is one of the chemical physiological strategies of greater prominence to avoid infections. Accordingly, low stomach and urinary pH can destroy most of the parasitic organisms which, by chance, succeed in penetrating these systems [55]. The last, but not least, of the "nonimmunological" barriers that protect our body from infection is the biological barrier, represented by the normal microbiota, a complete ecosystem composed by harmless microorganisms that live in balance with our body. The benefits of having the intestines, skin, and vagina occupied by specific strains of innocuous bacteria were once thought to be limited to the reduction of pathological colonization, due to the competition among the invaders and the resident flora. Nowadays, we know that the microbiota lives in fact in a mutualistic symbiosis with our body, benefiting themselves and the host [54, 55, 61].

The integrity of our intestinal microbiota, for instance, is essential to the digestion of a number of food components, making the absorption of important nutrients easier. Moreover, the anaerobic bacilli that inhabit the vaginal cavity are responsible for the maintenance of acid pH in that region, since they produce lactic acid as an anaerobic respiration metabolite, keeping the vagina free of fungal colonization. It is of note that the resident microbiota lives in a delicate balance with our IS. Its growth is controlled and limited by phagocytic cells and other elements of the IS, and the occurrence of imbalances in the property of immunoregulation, such as immunity reduction due to illness, immunosuppression, stress, or malnutrition, may lead to an exacerbated growth of microbiota population, which is potentially harmful for the human organism and should be controlled [54, 61].

5. Inflammation and innate immune response

When the above mentioned nonimmunological natural barriers are overcome by pathogens or other irritative elements, the immune response is initiated through the inflammatory reaction, as an attempt to restore tissue integrity. In case of infection, for instance, the elimination of invading microorganisms becomes a necessary condition for tissue repair. Inflammatory reaction depends on the action of specific blood cells called leucocytes. Under normal physiological conditions, there are around 5000 and 10,000 leukocytes per blood microliter, but these numbers significantly rise in the presence of an infection. Mature leukocytes can be classified both according to their original lineage (myeloid or lymphoid cells) and/or to the number of cellular nuclei they appear to have under light microscopy (mononuclear or polymorphonuclear cells), as illustrated in **Figure 2** [32, 54].

Mononuclear cells represent 35% of the total peripheral blood leukocytes. This broadest category is composed by monocytes: phagocytic cells that give rise to both macrophages and dendritic cells; mast cells, which are mainly responsible for vasodilation on inflammatory processes; lymphocytes, the effectors of our specific immune response, and finally, the natural killer cells (NK). The remaining 65% of blood leukocytes are represented by the polymorphonuclear cells, which are didactically subdivided into three different groups, according to their affinity with acid (eosinophils), alkaline (basophils) or both (neutrophils) histological dyes; these last being the first cell type to reach an injured area of the organism and initiating the inflammatory response. Leukocytes whose cytoplasm is rich in granules of enzymes and cytotoxic substances, such as reactive oxygen species, are generally called granulocytes. Basophils, eosinophils, and neutrophils can be called granulocytes. Macrophages and dendritic cells also have a considerable amount of granules in their cytoplasm; however, they are described as phagocytes, due to their ability to phagocyte invading microorganisms. All leukocytes are capable of producing a broad range of chemical mediators involved in the immune response (generally called cytokines) in response to lesions or to the presence of microorganisms. In addition to being responsible for the synthesis of these cytokines, leukocytes are also responsive to the action of these mediators, which promote, among other biological effects, leukocyte chemotaxis toward the inflammatory focus as well as its activation [32, 54, 55]. Cytokines are soluble glycoproteins, which may have autocrine, paracrine, or endocrine action. A fraction of these mediators have been at least partially described, however, there is still an almost infinite range of little known pro-inflammatory cellular signaling molecules, whose activity has not yet been fully established.

As far as we currently know, once the nonimmune body barriers are overcome by a pathogen or a dangerous substance, a microscopic battle begins in the injured tissue. The first line of defense of our immune system is the innate immunity, which comprises a group of cells, intracellular mechanisms, and chemical mediators, extremely conserved evolutionarily. Long before vertebrates first appeared on Earth, their primitive ancestors already had effective systems of immune cells recruitment, production of cytokines, activation of the complement cascade, identification of foreign elements through transmembrane and intracellular molecular pattern recognition receptors (MPRR), inactivation of pathogens through the production of reactive oxygen species (ROS), antimicrobial peptides and lytic enzymes, and, finally, removal of invader microorganisms through phagocytosis. Although innate immune system is a nonspecific evolutionarily older defense strategy, it is a fast mechanism that comes into play immediately or within hours of the appearance of a foreign element in the body, initiating the inflammatory process [32, 37–42, 54].

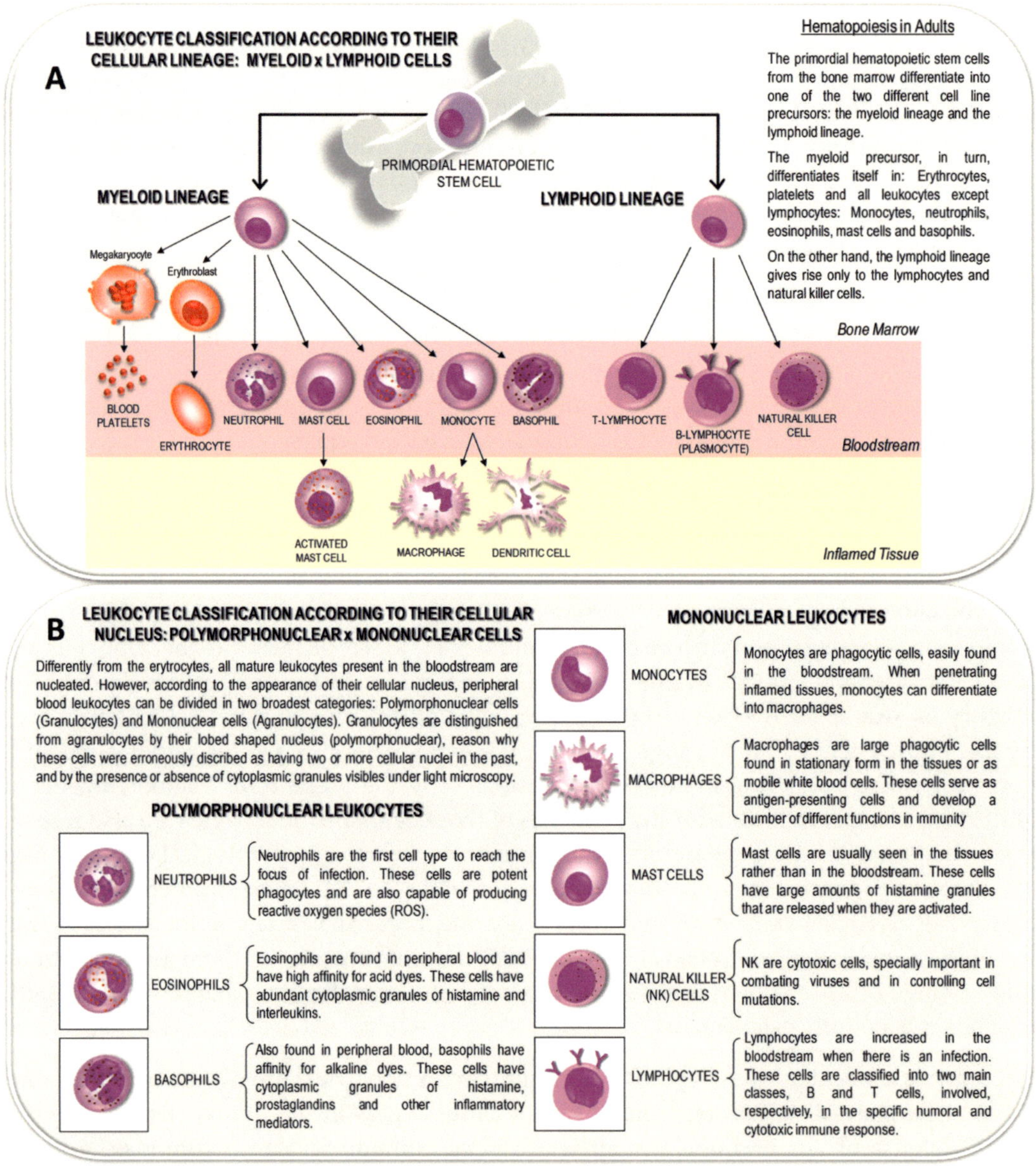

Figure 2. Leukocyte classification. Leukocytes can be classified as myeloid or lymphoid cells, according to their hematopoietic origin, or as mononuclear or polymorphonuclear cells, according to the number of cellular nuclei and cytoplasmic granules they appear to have, in their mature circulating form, under light microscopy.

Right after tissue aggression, the MPRRs of injured cells, which may be epithelial, endothelial, or mesangial cells, as well as resident phagocytes and fibroblasts, recognize pathogen-associated molecular patterns (PAMPs) that may indicate the presence of invading microorganisms and damage-associated molecular patterns (DAMPs), released by self-cells under cellular

http://dx.doi.org/10.5772/intechopen.70611

suffering. Bacterial lipopolysaccharide (LPS), flagellin, peptidoglycans, glycolipids, zymosan, and profilin, as well as single-stranded DNA (ssDNA) and double-stranded RNA are examples of PAMPs. In turn, Interleukines IL-1β and IL-18, extracellular HMGB1, ATP, and DNA, as well as uric acid crystals can be considered DAMPs [37–42].

After this first identification, local cells synthesize and release vasoactive mediators that promote vasodilatation and increase the local blood supply, causing heat and flushing; common features of inflammation. The concomitant activation of resident innate immune cells also takes part in the process. Under physiological conditions, the most common kidney resident immune cells are tissue macrophages and dendritic cells. It is of note that these last acts as sentinels in homeostasis, local injury, and infection, rapidly producing neutrophil-recruiting chemokines. In a less extent, mast cells are also seen in renal tissue and have been pointed out as local renal producers of RAAS components [14, 18]. Once activated, in addition to increasing the renal production of Ang II, mast cells release the content of their cytoplasmic granules of histamine; a biogenic amine that promotes increased vascular permeability by distancing endothelial cells (enlargement of endothelial fenestrae) near the injured region. As a result, there is a blood plasma extravasation from local blood vessels to the injured region, diluting eventual toxins produced by invading microorganisms, and bringing the proteins of complement system to the inflammation site [54, 55]. This interstitial accumulation of plasma promotes both edema and local pain, due to the compression of nerve endings. The next step is the diapedesis, or transendothelial migration, which is the leukocyte outflow from the bloodstream toward the focus of inflammation. This process is only possible due to a complex chemical communication system between the injured local tissue, the endothelial cells and the leukocytes itself, as illustrated in **Figure 3**.

The first cell types to reach the inflammatory focus are neutrophils, followed by circulating monocytes, which upon reaching the tissues become macrophages. Phagocytes also are able to reach the inflammatory spot and recognize PAMPs and DAMPs through two potential strategies: (1) phagocytosis followed by digestion of the microorganism and (2) production and excretion of anti-microbial compounds, as nitric oxide (NO), and ROS such as superoxide anion (O_2^-) and hydrogen peroxide (H_2O_2). The acute phase of inflammation can promote systemic effects. Activated macrophages, for example, release IL-1β and tumor necrosis factor (TNFα), cytokines that bind to our thermoregulatory receptors causing body temperature rising (fever), and stimulate the hypothalamic-pituitary-adrenal axis, leading to increased production of corticoid hormones, including renin, by the adrenal gland [54, 55]. Moreover, TNFα acts on the bone marrow, accelerating leukocyte proliferation. At this initial nonspecific phase of inflammatory response, the phagocytic capacity of neutrophils, monocytes, and macrophages does not depend on specific antigenic recognition, on neither the immune memory nor the presence of antibodies. Resistant microorganisms, as well as remaining phagocytes, are then drained through the lymphatic vessels to the nearest lymph node, where the antigens will be presented to the lymphocytes, initiating a more complex and long-lasting reaction, the adaptive immune response [32, 54, 55].

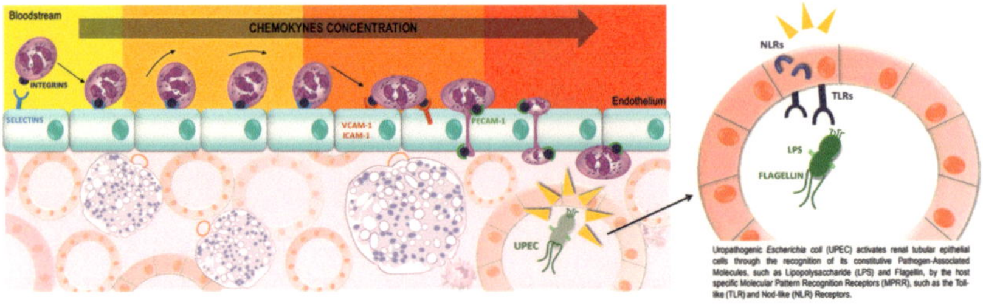

Figure 3. Diapedesis. Inflammatory response initiates right after the recognition of a foreign element by the MPRRs of host cells, particularly the toll-like (TLRs) and NOD-like receptors (NLRs). Damaged cells release specific chemokines (CCL-2, -3, -4, -5, -11, -20 and CXCL10), which attract the circulating leukocytes, guiding their migration through a gradient of concentration in the bloodstream toward the inflamed area. When these cells reach the blood vessels with the highest concentration of chemokines, they firmly adhere to the endothelium and initiate a rolling process, getting closer to the inflamed region. Once near from the inflammation site, leukocytes stop rolling, change their shape by spreading on the endothelium, and finally pass through the enlarged endothelial fenestrae, reaching the potentially infected tissue. This process is called diapedesis and it is only possible due to the chemical affinity between the constitutive integrins, present on the surface of leukocyte cellular membrane, and some specific endothelial adhesion molecules, such as selectins E and P, which stimulate leukocyte rolling, vascular cell adhesion molecule 1 (VCAM-1), intercellular adhesion molecule 1 (ECAM-1) and platelet and endothelial cell adhesion molecule 1 (PECAM-1), which contribute to the attachment of leukocytes to the endothelial membrane and to their transmigration through the endothelial barrier.

6. Innate immune response and nonimmune-mediated CKD

In the past years, renal activation of innate immune mechanisms by sterile elements has been demonstrated in nonimmune-mediated human nephropathies. Moreover, such activation of innate immunity seems to be positively correlated with the progression of renal injury in a variety of experimental models of CKD (**Table 1**). Our understanding of the mechanisms underlying the triggering of sterile inflammation was largely enhanced after the discovery of specific MPRRs: the toll-like receptors' (TLRs) and the NOD-like receptors' (NLRs) families; primarily found in leukocytes, but also present in epithelial and endothelial cells. Once activated, transmembrane and cytoplasmic TLRs trigger multiple intracellular events, involving adaptor proteins, such as MyD88, Mal/TIRAP, and TRAM, leading to nuclear translocation of transcription factors such as IRF3, IRF7, and NFKB, known to induce a variety of pro-inflammatory genes [32, 40]. On the other hand, NLRs are another class of intracellular MPRRs, very responsive to the presence of DAMPs. Their activation promotes the assembly of molecular complexes known as inflammasomes, such as the NOD2, NLRP1, NLRP3, NLRC4, etc. Inflammasomes assembly also promotes NFKB and MAPK activation, as well as the conversion of the inactive Pro-caspase 1 into the pro-inflammatory enzyme Caspase 1 (CASP1), which in turn, promotes the maturation of interleukins IL1β and IL18, thus amplifying the inflammatory response [36–41]. As mentioned above, the activation of these two main families of MPRRs, as well as, the components related to their intracellular signaling pathway were already described to be present in both human and experimental CKD. A proposed mechanism for sterile activation of immune response in nonimmune-mediated CKD is illustrated in **Figure 4**.

http://dx.doi.org/10.5772/intechopen.70611

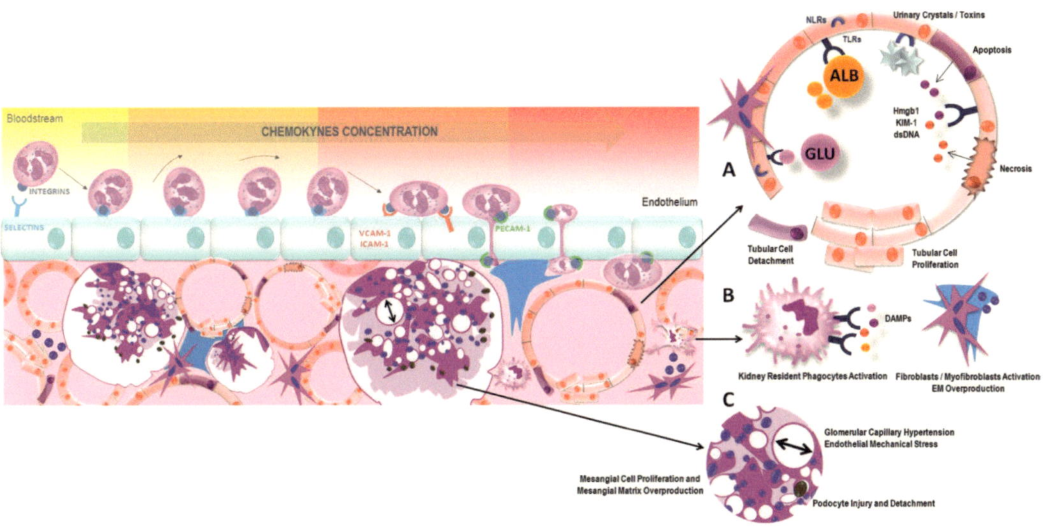

Figure 4. Renal sterile inflammation. Beyond to be activated by pathogens, MPRRs are also sensible to molecules currently related to cell damage (DAMPs). These sterile stimuli may represent the link between the initial features of nonimmune renal aggression and the establishment of chronic kidney inflammation. It is currently known that different renal cells present the intracellular machinery necessary to activate innate immune response, from endothelial to resident dendritic cells. TLRs and NLRs are stimulated in tubular epithelial cell exposed to DAMPs starting an intracellular intricate response that leads to the release of pro-inflammatory interleukins and chemokines (A). These intercellular signaling compounds are capable of recruiting circulating leukocytes to the renal parenchyma, as well as to activate resident interstitial macrophages, dendritic and mast cells, similarly to what occurs in an infection episode (B). Moreover pro-inflammatory interleukins released by both epithelial cells and renal immune sentinels can activate resident fibroblasts leading to their transdifferentiation into profibrotic myofibroblasts; cells specialized in producing large amounts of EM proteins and further pro-inflammatory signaling molecules. Additionally, glomerular sterile damage can also trigger leukocyte recruitment through the activation of innate immunity pathways. Endothelial cells of glomerular capillaries potentially react to mechanical stress caused by tissue stretching due to glomerular hypertension and hypertrophy by releasing DAMPs. This possible event promotes mesangial cells proliferation and EM overproduction, which may lead to glomerulosclerosis and the activation of further pro-inflammatory mechanisms (C).

Accordingly, experimental studies have been shown that chemical blockage of inflammasome NLRP3, NFKB system, and IL1β, limits blood pressure rising, albuminuria, creatinine retention, and renal histological alterations in different murine CKD models. Moreover, *Tlr2*, *Tlr4*, and *Nod2* knockout (KO) mice develop less tubulointerstitial nephritis and renal fibrosis when submitted to kidney injury [40]. The activation of innate immunity pathways in nonimmune-mediated CKD may represent an important link between nonspecific insults; such as glomerular wall stretching, due to glomerular hypertension and hypertrophy, tubular exposure to high protein, glucose or uremic toxins concentration, tissue damage by the presence of crystals; and late events, such as GS and interstitial fibrosis. Innate immune intracellular mechanisms are represented in detail in **Figure 5** [2, 18, 21, 54]. Since cell damage may further stimulate innate immunity, a positive feedback may establish, leading to the engagement of adaptive immunity, perpetuating inflammation, and culminating in the establishment of end-stage renal disease (ESRD).

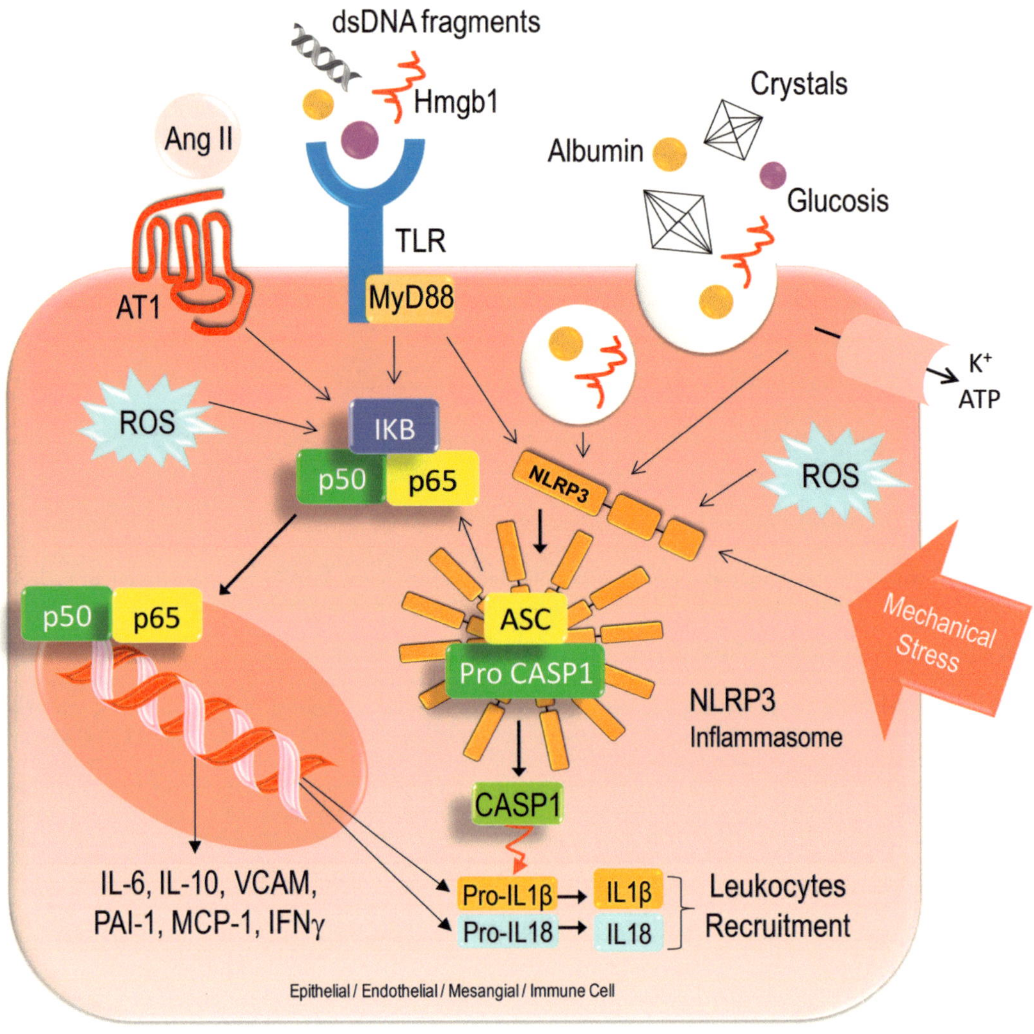

Figure 5. Some intracellular mechanisms of sterile innate immune reaction. Many different sterile stimuli can be identified as DAMPs by epithelial, endothelial, mesangial cells and also by renal resident leukocytes. Once a DAMP is recognized by a TLR, for instance, it leads to the activation of NFKB system, one of the most important intracellular pro-inflammatory pathways. The NFKB system is composed by the subunits p50 and p65, which in physiological conditions are maintained in their inactive form in the cytoplasm due to binding to the inhibitory protein IKB. Under stimulation, IKB is degraded, releasing the p50/p65 heterodimer, which penetrates into the cell nucleus to bind to DNA and act as a transcription factor, promoting the synthesis of a bunch of pro-inflammatory proteins, including the immature interleukins pro-IL1β and pro-IL18 and the active IL-6, VCAM, PAI-1, MCP-1 and IFNγ. It is of note that the NFKB system is not exclusively activated by TLRs signaling, but also by oxidative stress, Ang II and other pro-inflammatory mediators. On the other hand, the identification of intracellular DAMPs by a NLR, such as the NLRP3 for instance, promote the assembly of a molecular complex known as NLRP3 inflammasome, that also promotes NFKB system activation, as well as the conversion of the inactive pro-caspase 1 into the pro-inflammatory Caspase 1 (CASP1), promoting IL1β and IL18 maturation, thus amplifying the inflammatory response.

7. Adaptive immune response

As previously mentioned, in the presence of an infection the microorganisms, which were not eliminated by the innate immune response, are drained together with remaining phagocytes through the lymphatic vessels to the nearest lymph node, where a most specific and long lasting reaction begins: the adaptive immune response. It is important to emphasize that macrophages, dendritic cells, and other innate phagocytes represent the link between the nonspecific and the specific immune response. These leukocytes are designated as antigen presenting cells (APCs), since they have the ability of presenting foreign molecules to the lymphocytes in the lymph nodes, thereby activating and stimulating these specific cells. Lymphocytes are mononuclear leukocytes involved with the specific immune response. They originate from a lymphoid progenitor cell in the bone marrow, and may undergo differentiation in the bone marrow itself, been called B-lymphocytes or simply B-cells, or in the thymus, called T-lymphocytes or T-cells [54, 55]. Once the APCs phagocyte an invading microorganisms, they digest their proteins (antigen processing) and migrate to the lymph nodes, where they expose small peptide portions of the invader in the surface of their cellular membrane, associated with their molecules of the major histocompatibility complex of class II (MHC II). Both types of lymphocytes are able to recognize processed antigens associated with molecules of the MHC II of APCs through their membrane receptors (TCR of T-lymphocytes or BCR of B-lymphocytes). Unstimulated B or T lymphocytes, also called "naive" cells are generally small and present scarce cytoplasm. However, once stimulated, they became "effector lymphocytes," increase in size, have the cytoplasm hypertrophied and suffer mitosis, promoting clonal amplification, thus increasing the number of cells that would be sensitive to that specific activating antigen [32, 54].

In an extremely simplified view, when an antigen is recognized by the TCR of a naive T-cell, this leukocyte is activated, initiating the cellular adaptive response. First of all, the effector t-cell give rise to two different cell types through cell division: the T-Helper lymphocyte, that have the CD4 glycoprotein on the surface of their cell membrane ($CD4^+$ T-cell), and the Cytotoxic T lymphocyte, characterized by the presence of CD8 in its membrane ($CD8^+$ T-cell). Both $CD4^+$ and $CD8^+$ T-cell will be sensitive to the same antigen that promoted the activation of the T-Helper cells migrate to the inflamed area and, according to the type of stimulus they receive, these cells differentiate into one of the five known phenotypes: Th1, Th2, Th17, Tfh, and Treg [55]. Most of these subtypes of T-cells produce pro-inflammatory cytokines that acts especially upon macrophages, attracting them close to the target antigen, giving them increased membrane mobility and increasing their phagocytic and microbicidal potential. Only the Treg phenotype is described to release anti-inflammatory mediators, thus contributing to immunotolerance.

Cytotoxic T lymphocytes, in turn, can directly lysate bacteria, virus-infected cells, as well as self-cells that have suffered genetic mutation. Once the cytotoxic T-lymphocyte gets in touch with the target microorganism or antigen, a series of granzymes, perforins, and other cytotoxic molecules are released from within their cytoplasmic granules directly into the extracellular medium. Perforins are molecules that promote the formation of pores in the plasma membrane of target cells, causing abrupt entry of liquid, due to osmotic pressure, into the cytoplasm of these cells, leading to its apoptosis. Furthermore, both T-Helper and Cytotoxic lymphocytes give rise to memory $CD4^+$ and $CD8^+$ cells, respectively. This process is illustrated in **Figure 6**. Unlike the other populations of T-lymphocytes, memory T-cells may be inactive for years in the bloodstream, generating copies of themselves; thus, maintaining the memory of the recognition of the antigen that caused the activation of its precursor. Such cells are readily activated in the presence of a reinfection, being extremely important to defend our body from recurrent infections.

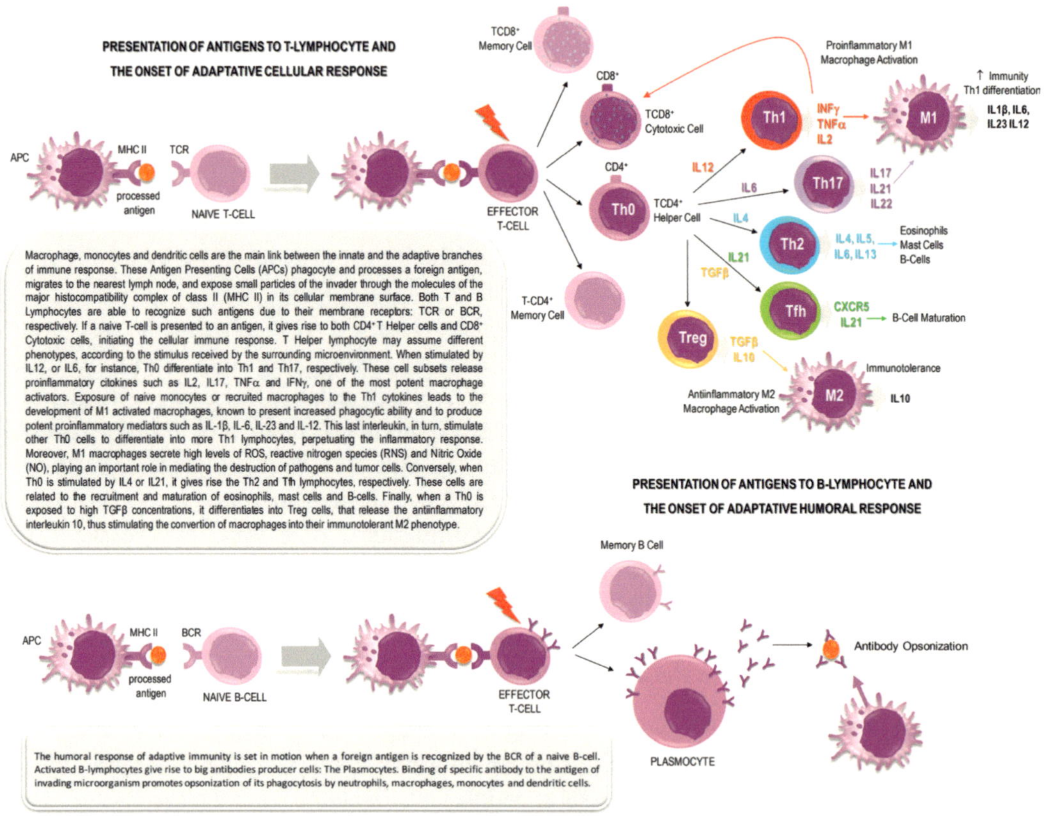

Figure 6. Presentation of antigens to lymphocytes and the onset of adaptive immune response. Mechanisms that link innate and adaptive immunity and the onset of the activation of lymphocytes.

On the other hand, when a foreign antigen is recognized by the BCR of a naive B cell, the humoral branch of adaptive immune response sets in motion. Activated B lymphocytes, or plasmocytes, synthesize specific antibodies against the invading microorganism. The antibodies produced by plasma cells may remain adhered to the cellular membrane of B-cells, promoting the binding of the cell as a whole to the parasite antigen, or be released to the bloodstream. In both cases, binding of the specific antibody to the antigen of invading microorganism promotes opsonization of its phagocytosis by neutrophils, macrophages, monocytes, and dendritic cells, besides promoting the neutralization of microbial toxins. Activated B-cells also produce memory B-cells, important to generate an accelerated and more robust antibody-mediated immune response in the case of re-infection by the same antigen [54].

8. Adaptive immune response in nonimmune-mediated CKD

Similar to the innate arm of immune response, adaptive immunity seems to be activated in both human and experimental CKD, even when the initial renal injury is not caused by infection or by any autoimmune condition. Moreover, the recruitment of lymphocytes to the renal parenchyma often correlates positively with worsening of renal function loss. T-lymphocytes are commonly seen in the kidneys of rats submitted to NX, streptozotocin-induced (ST) DN, chronic nitric oxide inhibition, among others. Accordingly, the treatment of these animals with mycophenolate mofetil (MMF), a lymphocytic inhibitor, was shown to reduce albuminuria, hypertension, glomerular, and interstitial damage. Although the exact mechanisms by which adaptive response is triggered in such "sterile" conditions are presently unclear, some hypotheses have gained strength with the development of experimental studies over the last decades [28, 29, 35, 52].

One of these hypotheses points to Ang II as a pivotal element to stimulate the activation of specific cellular immunity in nonimmune-mediated nephropathies. The role of Ang II in the activation of adaptive immunocompetent cells *in vivo* is increasingly recognized by the beneficial effects of ARBs and ACE is in several models of immune-mediated diseases and even as an adjuvant in avoiding allograft rejection after kidney transplantation. It was widely demonstrated that experimental venal infusion of Ang II in rodents induces T lymphocyte migration to specific target organs, such as the kidneys and the spleen. Moreover, these infiltrating lymphocytes assume mainly Th1 and Th17 pro-inflammatory phenotypes, increasing the release of IFN-γ and decreasing IL4 concentration in these organs, thus participating in the mechanism that drives to inflammation and hypertension. Accordingly, *in vitro* studies showed Ang II to act as an "antigen" upon cultured mouse spleen lymphocytes, promoting their activation and further clonal proliferation. T-cells have been shown to be also activated in the murine model of DOCA-salt hypertension, supposedly a nonimmune-mediated condition, in which Ang II plays an important role. In this model, pharmacological inhibition of the T-lymphocyte CD28 receptor and of its co-stimulatory protein CD80 prevented the development of hypertension and consequent renal injury. Corroborating these findings, further studies showed that *Cd80* KO mice are renoprotected when submitted to the Ang II-induced hypertension model [35, 52].

Curiously, Ang II was shown to be released by activated T cells during the blood-stage of plasmodium infection in an experimental model of malaria. Once T-cells are described to have the complete intracellular machinery to synthesize all RAAS components, including transmembrane AT1 receptors, Ang II produced by the infected cells may promote the recruitment and activation of further naive lymphocytes. According to this study, Ang II binding to the AT1 receptors of cultured T-cells leads to: upregulation of CD69 and CD25, increased cellular adhesion, and migration due to overexpression of CCR2 and CCR5 chemokine receptors and LFA-1 adhesion molecule, as well as T-cell differentiation, observed by the increased production of IL17 and IFN-γ and by the presence of cell perforins. However, the reasons why intracellular RAAS seems to be overactivated in T-cells exposed to inflammation, remains unknown.

Besides Ang II, advanced glycation end products (AGEs), represent another possible sterile "antigen" which may activate adaptive immunity in nonimmune-mediated CKD. AGEs are proteins or lipids that become glycated as a result of exposure to high glucose levels. Under some pathologic conditions, such as DM, sustained hyperglycemia and ROS production lead to increased AGE formation. Excessive AGE production is involved with the development and worsening of many degenerative diseases; including DN. Human AGE receptor (RAGE) is a multiligand cell surface MPRR that also binds Hmgb1, S100, and other DAMPs. Highly expressed in macrophages, T-, and B lymphocytes, RAGE contributes to inflammatory mechanisms, including the differentiation of Th0 in Th1 cells. RAGE-mediated leukocyte recruitment is particularly important in conditions associated with higher RAGE expression, such as DM. In these cases, when overexpressed in the surface of endothelial cells, RAGE directly mediate leukocyte recruitment, acting as a cell adhesive receptor. Moreover, AGE binding to RAGE result in overexpression of cytokines and pro-inflammatory molecules.

As illustrated in **Figure 7**, it is finally possible that the sterile DAMPs, which were, recognized by the innate MPRR of APCs, processed as antigens and presented to naive t-cells

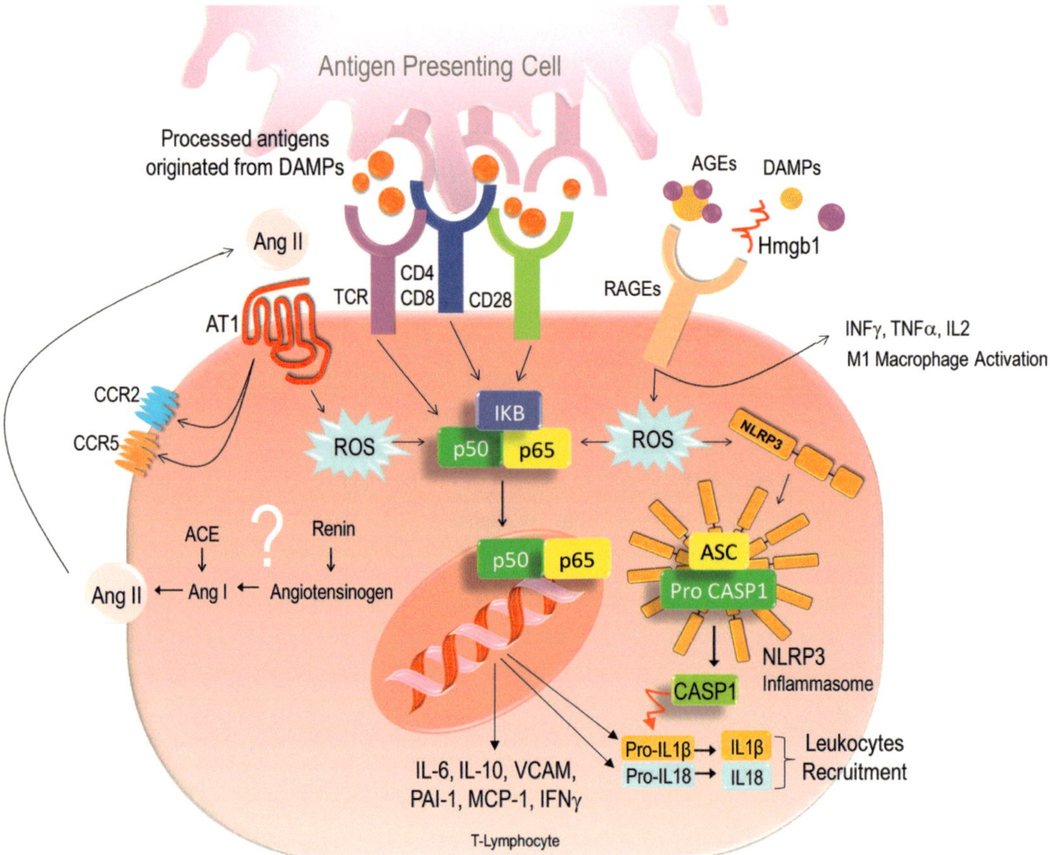

Figure 7. Some mechanisms of adaptive T-cell sterile activation. Through the binding of processed antigens to the T-lymphocyte receptors TCR, CD4, CD8 and CD28, an intracellular mechanism is set in motion, leading to the activation of NFKB system, with further production of immature interleukins pro-IL1β and pro-IL18 among other mediators. Such sterile antigens particles are believed to be originated from phagocyted DAMPs, recognized by the innate immune APCs, as previously described. Ang II also exerts a pivotal role in the activation of T cells. Although the mechanism that leads activated T cells to overproduce intracellular RAAS components remains unclear, it is well known that, in addition to enhance Ang II production, when subjected to inflammatory stimuli, T cells also expose more AT1 receptors, making themselves more responsive to Ang II produced by other leukocytes or by the cells of injured tissue. Through the binding of Ang II to its AT1 receptor, T-cells become more active, thus expressing a greater number of CCR2 and CCR5 chemokine receptors. Finally, T-lymphocytes have constitutively high expression of the advanced glycation end products receptor (RAGE). Once it binds to its specific ligand (AGE), or to other DAMPs, such as Hmgb1 or S100 proteins, it starts the conversion of Th0 lymphocyte toward the pro-inflammatory Th1 phenotype, which in turn, produces some of the most potent pro-inflammatory mediators that will further increase M1 macrophage population.

are able to trigger adaptive immune response in the same way PAMPs would be. However, further studies are required for the complete elucidation of the mechanisms involved in this process.

9. Conclusion

Sterile inflammation exerts a key pathogenic role to the development and evolution of CKD. Although all the mechanisms involved in the activation of immune response in nonimmune-mediated kidney conditions are not yet fully elucidated, some of the main assumptions for this phenomenon were discussed here. Based on our review of the literature and on the proposed integrative schemes, we can conclude that both innate and adaptive arms of immunity can be activated in CKD, with no pathological stimulus needed. Moreover, chronic inflammation contributes to CKD worsening and progression, leading to GS and renal fibrosis. The use of anti-inflammatory drugs, chemical blockers of innate immunity and anti-lymphocyte drugs have been shown to be partially effective to decelerate the chronic inflammatory process that accompanies nephropathy in experimental models of CKD (**Table 2**). However, to date, blockade of systemic and intrarenal RAAS by ACEis and/or ARBs remains the most effective treatment for delaying renal function loss.

Author details

Camilla Fanelli[1], Ayman Noreddin[2] and Ane Nunes[3]*

*Address all correspondence to: nunes.acf@gmail.com

1 Faculty of Medicine, University of São Paulo (USP), São Paulo, Brazil

2 College of Pharmacy, University of Sharjah (UOS), Sharjah, United Arab Emirates

3 School of Medicine, University of California Irvine (UCI), Irvine, United States

References

[1] El Nahas M. The global challenge of chronic kidney disease. Kidney International. 2005;**68**(6):2918-2929

[2] Anderson S, et al. Mechanisms of injury in progressive renal disease. Experimental Nephrology Supplement. 1996;**1**:34-40

[3] National Kidney Foundation. A to Z Health Guide About Chronic Kidney Disease [Internet]. 2017. Available from: https://www.kidney.org/atoz/content/about-chronic-kidney-disease#ckd [Accessed: 15 February 2017]

[4] Saran R, et al. US renal data system 2016 annual data report: Epidemiology of kidney disease in the United States. American Journal of Kidney Diseases. 2017;**69**(3S1):A7-A8

[5] United States Renal Data System, USRDS. 2016 Annual Data Report: Epidemiology of Kidney Disease in the United States. Bethesda, MD: National Institutes of Health, National Institute of Diabetes and Digestive and Kidney Diseases; 2016

[6] Mayo Foundation for Medical Education and Research (MFMER). Chronic Kidney Disease [Internet]. 2017. Available from: http://www.mayoclinic.org/diseases-conditions/chronic-kidney-disease/home/ovc-20207456 [Accessed: 10 February 2017]

[7] Couser WG, et al. The contribution of chronic kidney disease to the global burden of major noncommunicable diseases. Kidney International. 2011;**80**(12):1258-1270

[8] Schieppati A, et al. Chronic renal disease as a public health problem: Epidemiology, social, and economic implications. Kidney International. 2005;**68**(Suppl):7-10

[9] White SL, et al. How can we achieve global equity in provision of renal replacement therapy? Bulletin of the World Health Organization. 2008;**86**(3):229-237

[10] Zatz R. Bases Fisiológicas da Nefrologia. Atheneu; 2012. 394 p

[11] Thakar CV, et al. Acute kidney injury episodes and chronic kidney disease risk in diabetes mellitus. Clinical Journal of the American Society of Nephrology. 2011;**6**:2567-2572

[12] Floege J. Primary glomerulonephritis: A review of important recent discoveries. Kidney Research and Clinical Practice. 2013;**32**:103-110

[13] Chapman AB, et al. Autosomal-dominant polycystic kidney disease (ADPKD): Executive summary from a kidney disease: Improving global outcomes (KDIGO) controversies conference. Kidney International. 2015;**88**(1):17-27

[14] Noronha IL, et al. The inflammatory component in progressive renal disease—Are interventions possible? Nephrology, Dialysis, Transplantation. 2002;**17**(3):363-368

[15] Zeisberg M, et al. Mechanisms of tubulointerstitial fibrosis. Journal of the American Society of Nephrology. 2010;**21**:1819-1834

[16] Rüster C, et al. Renin-angiotensin-aldosterone system and progression of renal disease. Journal of the American Society of Nephrology. 2006;**17**:2985-2991

[17] Machado FG, et al. AT1 blockade during lactation as a model of chronic nephropathy: Mechanisms of renal injury. American Journal of Physiology. Renal Physiology. 2008;**294**:F1345-F1353

[18] Graciano ML, et al. Intrarenal renin-angiotensin system is upregulated in experimental model of progressive renal disease induced by chronic inhibition of nitric oxide synthesis. Journal of the American Society of Nephrology. 2004;**15**:1805-1815

[19] Fanelli C, et al. Effects of losartan, in monotherapy or in association with hydrochlorothiazide, in chronic nephropathy resulting from losartan treatment during lactation. American Journal of Physiology. Renal Physiology. 2011;**301**:F580-F587

[20] Wolf G, et al. Angiotensin II and cell cycle regulation. Hypertension. 2004;**43**:693-698

[21] LL W, et al. Macrophage and myofibroblast proliferation in remnant kidney: Role of angiotensin II. Kidney International. Supplement. 1997;**63**:S221-S225

[22] Siragy HM, et al. Role of the intrarenal renin-angiotensin-aldosterone system in chronic kidney disease. American Journal of Nephrology. 2010;**31**:541-550

[23] Gagliardini E, et al. Drugs to Foster kidney regeneration in experimental animals and humans. Nephron. Experimental Nephrology. 2014;**126**:91-96

[24] Arias SC, et al. Regression of albuminuria and hypertension and arrest of severe renal injury by a losartan-hydrochlorothiazide association in a model of very advanced nephropathy. PloS One. 2013;**8**(2):e56215

[25] Schwartz D, DeSchryver-Kecskemeti K, Needleman P. Renal arachidonic acid metabolism and cellular changes in the rabbit renal vein constricted kidney: Inflammation as a common process in renal injury models. Prostaglandins. 1984;**27**(4):605-613

[26] Yuan F, Kolb R, Pandey G, Li W, et al. Involvement of the NLRC4-inflammasome in diabetic nephropathy. PloS One. 2016;**11**(10):e0164135

[27] Imakiire T, Kikuchi Y, Yamada M, et al. Effects of renin-angiotensin system blockade on macrophage infiltration in patients with hypertensive nephrosclerosis. Hypertension Research. 2007;**30**(7):635-642

[28] Utimura R, Fujihara CK, Mattar AL, et al. Mycophenolate mofetil prevents the development of glomerular injury in experimental diabetes. Kidney International. 2003;**63**(1):209-216

[29] Fujihara CK, Malheiros DMAC, Noronha IL, et al. Mycophenolate mofetil reduces renal injury in the chronic nitric oxide synthase inhibition model. Hypertension. 2001;**37**(1):170-175

[30] Fujihara CK, Noronha IL, Malheiros DMAC, et al. Combined mycophenolate mofetil and losartan therapy arrests established injury in the remnant kidney. Journal of the American Society of Nephrology. 2000;**11**(2):283-290

[31] Hochheiser K, Tittel A, Kurts C. Kidney dendritic cells in acute and chronic renal disease. International Journal of Experimental Pathology. 2011;**92**:193-201

[32] Kurts C, Panzer U, Anders HJ, et al. The immune system and kidney disease: Basic concepts and clinical implications. Nature Reviews Immunology. 2013;**13**:738-753

[33] Seo JW, Kim YG, Lee SH, et al. Mycophenolate mofetil ameliorates diabetic nephropathy in db/db mice. BioMed Research International 2015;**2015**:301627.

[34] Mensah-Brown EPK, Obineche EN, Galadari S, et al. Streptozotocin-induced diabetic nephropathy in rats: The role of inflammatory cytokines. Cytokine. 2005;**31**:180-190

[35] Fujihara CK, Malheiros DMAC, Zatz R, et al. Mycophenolate mofetil attenuates renal injury in the rat remnant kidney. Kidney International. 1998;**54**:1510-1519

[36] Gong W, et al. NLRP3 deletion protects against renal fibrosis and attenuates mitochondrial abnormality in mouse with 5/6 nephrectomy. American Journal of Physiology. Renal Physiology. 2016;**310**:F1081-F1088

[37] Souza ACP, et al. TLR4 mutant mice are protected from renal fibrosis and chronic kidney disease progression. Physiological Reports. 2015;**3**(9)

[38] D'Apolito M, et al. Urea-induced ROS cause endothelial dysfunction in chronic renal failure. Atherosclerosis. 2015;**239**(2):393-400

[39] Lehners A, et al. Myeloperoxidase deficiency ameliorates progression of chronic kidney disease in mice. American Journal of Physiology. Renal Physiology. 2014;**307**(4):F407-F417

[40] Correa-Costa M, et al. Pivotal role of toll-like receptors 2 and 4, its adaptor molecule MyD88, and inflammasome complex in experimental tubule-interstitial nephritis. PloS One. 2011;**6**(12):e29004

[41] Vilaysane A, et al. The NLRP3 inflammasome promotes renal inflammation and contributes to CKD. Journal of the American Society of Nephrology. 2010;**21**:1732-1744

[42] Rodríguez-Iturbe B, et al. Evolution of renal interstitial inflammation and NF-kappaB activation in spontaneously hypertensive rats. American Journal of Nephrology. 2004; **24**(6):587-594

[43] Donadelli R, et al. Protein traffic activates NF-kB gene signaling and promotes MCP-1-dependent interstitial inflammation. American Journal of Kidney Diseases. 2000;**36**(6): 1226-1241

[44] Ludwig Portugall I, et al. An NLRP3-specific inflammasome inhibitor attenuates crystal-induced kidney fibrosis in mice. Kidney International. 2016;**90**:525-539

[45] Okabe C, et al. NF-kB activation mediates crystal translocation and interstitial inflammation in adenine overload nephropathy. American Journal of Physiology. Renal Physiology. 2012;**305**(2):F155-F163

[46] Kim JE, et al. Celastrol, an NF-kB inhibitor, improves insulin resistance and attenuates renal injury in db/db mice. PloS One. 2013;**8**(4):e62068

[47] Gilbert RE, et al. A purpose-synthesised anti-fibrotic agent attenuates experimental kidney diseases in the rat. PloS One. 2012;**7**(10):e47160

[48] Ding W, et al. Chronic inhibition of nuclear factor kappa B attenuates aldosterone/salt-induced renal injury. Life Sciences. 2012;**90**(15-16):600-606

[49] Kaneyama T, et al. Tranilast modulates fibrosis, epithelial-mesenchymal transition and peritubular capillary injury in unilateral ureteral obstruction rats. Pathology. 2010;**42**(6): 564-573

[50] Fujihara CK, et al. Chronic inhibition of nuclear factor-kappaB attenuates renal injury in the 5/6 renal ablation model. American Journal of Physiology. Renal Physiology. 2007;**292**(1):F92-F99

[51] Shihab FS, et al. Pirfenidone treatment decreases transforming growth factor-beta1 and matrix proteins and ameliorates fibrosis in chronic cyclosporine nephrotoxicity. American Journal of Transplantation. 2002;**2**(2):111-119

[52] Romero F, et al. Mycophenolate mofetil prevents the progressive renal failure induced by 5/6 renal ablation in rats. Kidney International. 1999;**55**(3):945-955

[53] Imig JD, Ryan MJ. Immune and inflammatory role in renal disease. Comprehensive Physiology. 2013;**3**(2):957-976

[54] Abbas AK, Lichtman AHH, Pillai S. Cellular and Molecular Immunology. 7th ed. Elsevier Health Sciences; 2012. 560p

[55] Murphy KM. Janeway's Immunobiology. Revised ed. Taylor & Francis Group; 2011. 888p

[56] Christiansen OB. Reproductive immunology. Molecular Immunology. 2013;**55**(1):8-16

[57] Round JL, O'Connell RM, Mazmanian SK. Coordination of tolerogenic immune responses by the commensal microbiota. Journal of Autoimmunity. 2010;**34**(3):J220-J225

[58] Dunn GP, Bruce AT, Ikeda H, et al. Cancer immunoediting: From immuno-surveillance to tumor escape. Nature Immunology. 2002;**3**(11):991-998

[59] Swann JB, Smyth MK. Immune surveillance of tumors. The Journal of Clinical Investigation. 2007;**117**(5):1137-1146

[60] Bower JM, Eto DS, Mulvey MA. Covert operations of uropathogenic *Escherichia coli* within the urinary tract. Traffic. 2005;**6**(1):18-31

[61] Reid G, Younes JA, Van der Meiet HC, et al. Microbiota restoration: Natural and supplemented recovery of human microbial communities. Nature Reviews. Microbiology. 2011;**9**:27-38

Section 3

Nutrition in CKD

The Roles of Indoxyl Sulphate and p-Cresyl Sulphate in Patients with Chronic Kidney Disease: A Review of Therapeutic Options

Melissa Nataatmadja, Yeoungjee Cho,
Katrina Campbell and David W. Johnson

Additional information is available at the end of the chapter

http://dx.doi.org/10.5772/intechopen.69325

Abstract

Indoxyl sulphate (IS) and p-cresyl sulphate (PCS) are products of proteolytic bacterial fermentation by gut microbiota. They accumulate in the sera of patients with chronic kidney disease (CKD) and have been associated with CKD progression and cardiovascular and all-cause mortality. Therapeutic strategies for lowering IS and PCS include increased clearance (enhanced dialysis), gastrointestinal sequestration (oral adsorbents), reduced synthesis (dietary protein restriction, dietary fibre augmentation and pre-, pro- or synbiotics), antioxidants and organic anion transporter modulators. This review will discuss the roles of IS and PCS as therapeutic targets and examine the clinical evidence for different treatment options and their effects on CKD and cardiovascular disease risk. We will include our group's research with pre-, pro- and synbiotic interventions to mitigate serum uraemic toxin accumulation and modify cardiovascular and renal risk.

Keywords: indoxyl sulphate, p-cresyl sulphate, uraemic toxins, chronic kidney disease, gut microbiome

1. Introduction

The reciprocal relationship observed between gut microbiota and chronic kidney disease (CKD) has led to the recent recognition of the 'gut-kidney axis'. Patients with CKD, including those with end-stage kidney disease (ESKD), often experience impaired uraemic toxin clearance, salt and water retention, dietary restrictions, anorexia, dysgeusia and malnutrition, which in turn leads to quantitative and qualitative alterations in gut microbiome composition (gut dysbiosis). Further effects include gut wall oedema, intestinal barrier impairment, translocation of bacteria and endotoxins across the intestinal wall and resultant systemic inflammation [1–3]. Gut dysbiosis may in turn lead to the production of various toxins and metabolites that contribute to uraemic toxicity, cardiovascular disease and progressive kidney scarring and failure [4–6]. The central role of the gut microbiome in kidney health therefore makes it an appealing therapeutic target in patients with CKD [7, 8].

Two key nephrovascular toxins produced by proteolytic bacterial fermentation in the gut are indoxyl sulphate (IS) and p-cresyl sulphate (PCS). IS is produced by tryptophan metabolism facilitated by *Escherichia coli* and *Clostridium sporogenes*, while PCS is generated by break down of tyrosine and phenylalanine by intestinal anaerobes, such as *Clostridium difficile, Faecalibacterium prausnitzii, Subdoligranulum* and selected strains within the *Bifidobacterium* and *Lactobacillus genus* [8]. IS and PCS are both solely produced by the gut microbiota [9–12] and accumulate in the serum of patients with CKD due to both increased intestinal production and reduced glomerular filtration and proximal tubular secretion [12–14]. Elevated serum levels of IS and PCS have been reported to be associated with CKD progression [13] and increased risks of cardiovascular events and all-cause mortality [15].

Although IS and PCS levels can be lowered with various therapeutic modalities, how this impacts on the risks of mortality and cardiovascular outcomes remains unclear. This review will discuss the roles of IS and PCS as therapeutic targets and examine the clinical evidence for different treatment options and their effects on CKD and cardiovascular disease risk.

2. Serum IS and PCS levels are elevated in CKD

Serum IS and PCS levels have been demonstrated to be elevated in patients with CKD, where IS levels may be more than 50 times and PCS levels more than 15 times the levels of those found in healthy people [12, 14]. Our group has demonstrated that IS and PCS levels are significantly elevated in patients with early-stage CKD compared with control subjects. These levels were seen to be progressively more elevated with advancing severity of CKD [13]. Increased circulating levels of IS and PCS have also been observed in living kidney donors, which were sustained at 2 years post-surgery [16]. Levels of IS and PCS appear to be most elevated in ESKD and are not effectively removed by haemodialysis [14]. In a sample of 45 haemodialysis patients, Itoh et al. observed IS and PCS levels were markedly elevated (2.99 ± 0.18 mg/dL and 3.71 ± 0.28 mg/dL, respectively) compared with the healthy subjects (0.05 ± 0.01 mg/dL and 0.22 ± 0.99 mg/dL, respectively), and these levels were only lowered by approximately 30% post-dialysis (2.02 ± 0.12 mg/dL and 2.60 ± 0.21 mg/dL, respectively). This degree of elevation and inefficient removal warrants exploration of the potential impact of these toxins in CKD.

3. Serum IS and PCS levels are associated with adverse renal, metabolic and cardiovascular effects

3.1. Renal effects

Elevation of serum IS and PCS levels in patients with CKD is associated with CKD progression [17]. The mechanisms underpinning the adverse renal effects of IS and PCS are thought to be at least partly mediated by the production of reactive oxygen species, which in turn activate the nuclear factor kappa B pathway (NFκB) (**Figure 1**) [18]. *In vitro* studies have demonstrated that pro-inflammatory cytokine release and plasminogen activator inhibitor-1 upregulation via the NFκB pathway subsequently led to inhibition of cell proliferation and induction of renal tubulointerstitial fibrosis [4, 5]. These observations have been similarly replicated in animal models, whereby oral administration of IS [6, 19] and PCS [20] caused renal function impairment, glomerular sclerosis and tubulointerstitial fibrosis. IS and PCS have also been shown both *in vitro* and *in vivo* to activate the intrarenal renin-angiotensin-aldosterone system and promote renal tubular epithelial-to-mesenchymal transition, possibly via increased expression of transforming growth factor-β and Snail [21].

In a prospective, observational study of 268 patients with varying stages of CKD, Wu and colleagues demonstrated a significant association between higher IS (hazard ratio [HR] 1.06, 95% confidence interval [CI] 1.04–1.09, $p < 0.001$) and PCS levels (HR 1.09, 95% CI 1.06–1.13, $p < 0.001$) and CKD progression, defined as greater than 50% reduction in estimated glomerular filtration rate (eGFR) or progression to ESKD [17]. Serum PCS and IS remained independently associated with CKD progression after adjustment for patient demographic characteristics (age, gender, diabetes mellitus, $p < 0.001$) or baseline renal function ($p < 0.001$). Additionally, IS and PCS levels at baseline were significantly higher in those patients who died during follow-up (serum PCS 12.07 [<1–42.06] mg/L vs. 4.1 (<1–36.24) mg/L in survivors, $p = 0.002$; serum IS 4.78 [0.7–12.54] mg/L vs. 2.07 [<0.225–53.58] mg/dL, $p = 0.05$). Elevated serum total PCS was also found to be significantly associated with all-cause mortality on univariable analysis (HR 1.10, 95% CI 1.05–1.15, $p < 0.001$) and remained a predictor of mortality independent of other risk factors on multivariable analysis adjusted for patient demographic characteristics, baseline renal function and biomarkers including highly sensitive C-reactive protein [17].

3.2. Metabolic effects

Elevated PCS has been associated with insulin resistance and may therefore predispose to the metabolic syndrome and its complications. In mouse models, the administration of PCS for 4 weeks has been observed to induce hyperglycaemia, insulin resistance, hypercholesterolaemia and fat redistribution to muscle and liver, similar to the metabolic derangements observed in CKD [22] (**Figure 1**). These metabolic effects appeared to be ameliorated by uraemic toxin-reducing therapy, as the use of the prebiotic agent, arabino-xylo-oligosaccharide, reduced serum PCS concentration and improved glucose tolerance, insulin resistance, dyslipidaemia and ectopic fat distribution in uraemic, subtotal nephrectomised mice [22].

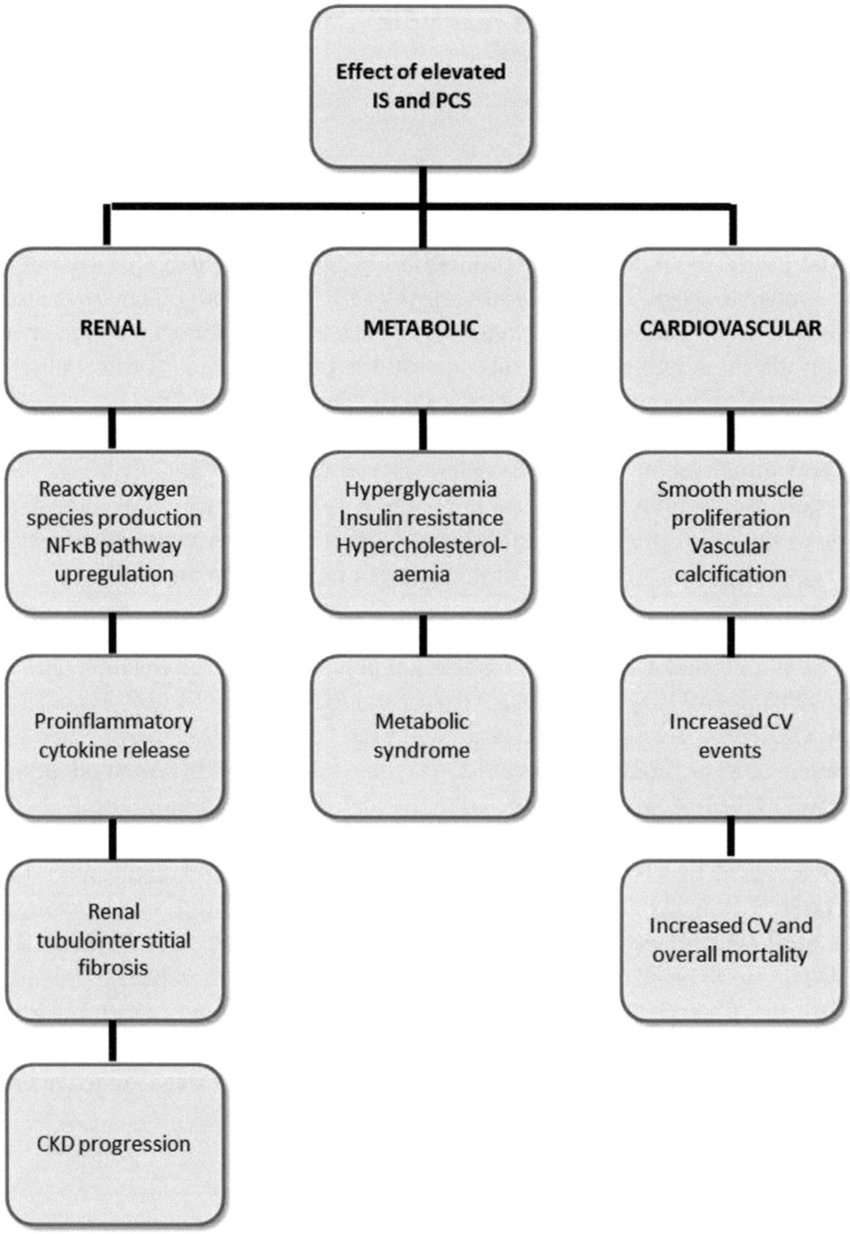

Figure 1. Mechanisms and potential effects of indoxyl sulphate (IS) and p-cresyl sulphate (PCS) on renal, metabolic and cardiovascular outcomes.

3.3. Cardiovascular effects and mortality

IS has been demonstrated to cause concentration-dependent vascular smooth muscle cell proliferation [23] and aortic calcification with aortic wall thickening in rats [6]. This appears to apply similarly to humans, such that elevated serum IS levels have been shown to be associated with aortic calcification measured by multislice spiral computed tomography [24]. Likewise, total and free PCS levels have been linked with vascular disease [25]. Not surprisingly, elevated serum levels of both toxins have been reported to be predictors of cardiovascular events and mortality. Higher serum IS levels independently predicted overall mortality (HR 2.47, 95% CI 1.62–3.77), but not CV mortality, in 139 patients with stage 2–5 CKD participating in a study performed by the European Uraemic Toxin Work Group (EUTox) [24]. Similar results were reported in a prospective, observational cohort study of 521 US incident haemodialysis patients whereby serum IS concentrations above the median value of 1.6 mg/dL were independently associated with all-cause mortality (HR 1.30, 95% CI 1.01–1.69) after adjustment for age, sex, race, comorbidity score, baseline serum albumin, obesity and serum creatinine [26]. Elevated free PCS concentration has also been demonstrated to be an independent predictor of cardiovascular events [27, 28] and overall cardiovascular mortality [25] in CKD patients, including those ESKD receiving dialysis.

A meta-analysis by Lin and colleagues of 11 observational studies involving 1572 patients with stages 1–5 CKD followed for 0.83 to 5 years found that all-cause mortality was significantly associated with both free PCS (pooled odds ratio [OR] 1.16, 95% CI 1.03–1.30, $p = 0.013$) and free IS levels (pooled OR 1.10, 95% CI 1.03–1.17, $p = 0.03$) [15]. However, there was a moderate level of heterogeneity with I^2 values of 71.5% ($p = 0.004$), and 74.2% ($p = 0.004$) for PCS and IS, respectively. Furthermore, there was a concern about publication bias based on an asymmetrical funnel plot and significant Egger's test ($p = 0.005$). Following subsequent adjustment for the effect of publication bias, the adjusted point estimate of the OR reduced from 1.16 to 1.03 (95% CI 0.93–1.16), thereby raising concern about exaggeration of the observed effect size in the primary analysis. The study also reported a significantly increased risk of cardiovascular events with elevated levels of free PCS (pooled OR 1.28, 95% CI 1.10–1.50, $p = 0.002$), although this result was again limited by a high level of heterogeneity ($I^2 = 80.7\%$, $p < 0.001$). Furthermore, there was evidence of publication bias, such that when analysis was repeated using Duval and Tweedie's trim-and-fill method, the estimate was no longer statistically significant with an adjusted OR of 1.10 (95% CI 0.93–1.27).

4. Therapeutic opportunities for reducing serum IS and PCS levels

Given the numerous deleterious, multi-system effects that have been associated with elevated serum IS and PCS concentrations, much interest has been generated in developing therapeutic options to reduce the levels of these nephrovascular toxins with the aim of improving clinical outcomes in patients with CKD. Potential therapeutic strategies to reduce IS and PCS levels in patients with CKD may involve reducing gut synthesis, gastrointestinal sequestration, reduced proximal tubular retention and increased dialytic clearance (**Table 1**).

4.1. Reduced gut synthesis

Since increased dietary protein load can result in heightened generation of uraemic toxins by the gut microbiota, prescription of very low-protein diets has experienced a resurgence of interest. Marzocco and colleagues performed a post-hoc analysis of a very low vs. low-protein

Strategy	Intervention	Outcome
Reduced gut synthesis	Very low-protein diet [29]	Reduced serum IS levels
	Dietary fibre [10, 33, 34]	Reduced serum IS and PCS levels
	Pre-, pro- and synbiotics [35–41]	Reduced IS and PCS levels
Gastrointestinal sequestration	AST-120 (Kremezin) [51–56]	Reduced renal disease progression
	Ai Xi Te [54]	Reduced renal disease progression
	Niaoduqing granules [54]	Reduced renal disease progression
Reduced proximal tubular retention	OAT^ modulators [11, 58, 61]	Reduced proximal tubular uptake of IS
Increased dialytic clearance	Extended dialysis (long dialysis, short daily dialysis) [65, 66]	No clear benefit
	Haemodiafiltration [67, 68]	Reduced serum IS and PCS levels
	Super-flux cellulose triacetate membranes [69]	Reduced serum IS levels
	Nanoporous monolith dialysis [70]	Reduced serum IS and PCS levels

^OAT: organic anion transporters

Table 1. Potential therapeutic interventions targeting indoxyl sulphate (IS) and p-cresyl sulphate (PCS).

diet cross-over study [29]. Thirty-two patients with a creatinine clearance between 20 and 55 ml/min were included and randomized to receive either a very low-protein diet (VLPD; 0.3 g/kg/day) or a low-protein diet (LPD; 0.6 g/kg/day) in the first week, then switched to the other in the second week. There was no wash-out period. The authors found that patients treated with a VLPD experienced a significant 36% reduction in serum IS levels compared with those treated with a LPD (7.12 ± 3.89 μM during VLPD vs. 11.1 ± 6.6 μM during LPD, $p < 0.0001$). Although a meta-analysis has identified reduction in the occurrence of renal death with a low-protein intake in CKD patients, the overall value of these diets remains a subject of debate, given that the risks of malnutrition may present a greater danger [30–32]. Furthermore, poor compliance is also likely to be an issue, as participants often did not meet dietary targets even with the intensive support provided within a trial setting.

There is newer evidence to suggest that dietary fibre may in fact be more important than dietary protein intake in terms of managing uraemic toxin levels. A single-centre, cross-sectional study of 40 patients with CKD measured baseline total and free serum IS and PCS levels and correlated this with dietary factors including dietary fibre, protein and protein-fibre index [10]. In this study, dietary fibre was found to be inversely associated with free and total serum PCS ($r = -0.42$ and $r = -0.44$, both $p < 0.01$) whereas dietary protein was not ($r = -0.14$, $p = 0.38$). Protein-fibre index was significantly associated with both total PCS ($r = 0.43$, $p = 0.005$) and total IS ($r = 0.40$, $p = 0.012$) levels. Increased dietary fibre as an intervention has been shown to result in significantly reduced free plasma IS in haemodialysis patients [33]. Moreover, a prospective cohort study of 390 Swedish men between the age of 70 and 71 years found an association between protein-fibre intake ratio and cardiovascular events (adjusted HR 1.33, 95% CI 1.08–1.64). These findings suggest that dietary intervention focusing on protein-fibre ratio has the potential to influence clinical outcomes [34], mediated via uraemic toxin production.

Probiotics and prebiotics represent another strategy for reducing uraemic toxin synthesis. Preparations of lactic-acid bacteria, simulating a probiotic, have been shown to decrease serum IS concentrations by 30% and also reverse aerobic bacterial overgrowth [35]. Their use has been demonstrated to result in a significant decrease in urinary PCS and an increase in faecal bifidobacteria [36]. Synbiotics, which represent a combination of pre- and probiotics, have similarly been demonstrated to reduce serum IS and PCS levels in CKD and haemodialysis patients [37–39]. More recently, the use of synbiotics for reducing uraemic toxin levels has been evaluated in the SYNbiotics Easing Renal failure by improving Gut microbiologY (SYNERGY) trial [40, 41]. In this single-centre, double-blind, placebo-controlled, cross-over trial, 37 pre-dialysis patients with stage 4 or 5 CKD were randomized to receive either synbiotic supplements or placebo for 6 weeks, followed by a 4-week wash-out period, followed by treatment with the alternative therapy for a further 6 weeks. Thirty-one participants completed both treatments. Although the study failed to demonstrate a significant change in total serum IS levels (−2 mmol/L, 95% CI −5 to 1 mmol/L, $p = 0.12$), the change in serum PCS levels did reach a level of statistical significance, with a 13% reduction in the treatment group (−14 mmol/L, 95% CI −27 to −2 mmol/L, $p = 0.03$). Furthermore, after excluding the 10 participants who had received antibiotic therapy during the trial, which is known to affect the balance of bacterial species in the gut [8, 42], the changes in serum levels with synbiotic therapy for both total IS (−5 mmol/L, 95% CI −8 to −1 mmol/L, $p = 0.03$) and PCS (−25 mmol/L, 95% CI −38 to −12 mmol/L, $p = 0.001$) were significant. The changes in free IS and PCS levels were also significant amongst antibiotic-free completers. Synbiotic therapy additionally had an effect on the stool microbiome, with significantly increased abundance of *Bifidobacterium* spp. (3.2%, $p = 0.003$) and *Lachnospiraceae* (2.1%, $p = 0.01$) and decreased abundance of *Ruminococcaceae* (4.3%, $p = 0.01$). Interestingly, albuminuria was observed to significantly increase with synbiotic therapy, which contradicted the reports of a beneficial effect on proteinuria from animal studies using other uraemic toxin-lowering therapies, such as AST-120 [43, 44]. Due to the short duration and small participant numbers of synbiotic trials to date, the effects of treatment on patient-level clinical outcomes remain unknown [2].

Lastly, the use of acarbose for lowering serum levels of gut-derived uraemic toxins has been investigated. Acarbose, an alpha-glucosidase inhibitor, causes increased delivery of undigested carbohydrate to the colon, which may drive gut bacterial fermentation towards a saccharolytic pathway and away from proteolytic fermentation and toxin production. In a pilot pre-test/post-test study involving nine healthy volunteers, Evanepoel et al. demonstrated that treatment with oral acarbose 300 mg per day for 3 weeks resulted in significant reductions in both serum p-cresol concentration (1.14–1.11 mg/L, $p = 0.047$) and urinary excretion of p-cresol (29.93–10.54 mg/day, $p = 0.03$), suggesting reduced colonic generation of p-cresol, the precursor of PCS [45]. Further studies confirming this finding are required.

4.2. Gastrointestinal sequestration

IS and PCS absorption from the gut may also be prevented by the use of oral intestinal adsorbents, such as AST-120 (Kremezin), which bind uraemic toxins and their precursors thereby sequestering them in the gut and allowing them to be excreted via the faeces. Oral administration of AST-120 has been shown to result in a dose-dependent decrease in serum IS and PCS in both human [46–48] and animal studies [19, 49], and its use is associated with slower progression of renal dysfunction [44, 50] and reduction of proteinuria [43, 44] in animal models of CKD. It has also been demonstrated to slow progression of renal dysfunction in early non-randomized and randomized studies in pre-dialysis patients [51–53]. In a subsequent Cochrane systematic review and meta-analysis of eight randomized controlled trials (RCTs) of AST-120 plus routine care compared with routine care alone in patients with stages 1–5 (non-dialysis) CKD, Wu et al. [54] reported that AST-120 treatment resulted in a significant reduction in the rate of decline in creatinine clearance (2 studies, 486 participants; standardized mean difference [SMD] 0.39, 95% CI 0.21–0.57; $I^2 = 0\%$), but did not significantly affect reciprocal serum creatinine slope over time (2 studies, 76 participants; mean difference [MD] 0.07 dL/mg/month, 95% CI −0.12 to 0.26; $I^2 = 69\%$), doubling of serum creatinine concentration (1 study, 460 participants; relative risk [RR] 0.55, 95% CI 0.19 to 1.62), ESKD incidence (3 studies, 504 participants; RR 0.70, 95% CI 0.15–3.35; $I^2 = 11\%$) or all-cause mortality (1 study, 460 participants; RR 0.70, 95% CI 0.19–1.62). In three separate placebo-controlled RCTs, AST-120 treatment did not significantly affect changes in serum creatinine, slope of reciprocal serum creatinine over time or creatinine clearance [54].

In the following year, the Evaluating Prevention of Progression in CKD (EPPIC)-1 and EPPIC-2 trials [55] reported on the effects of AST-120 (9 g/day) or placebo on CKD progression in 2035 patients with non-dialysis-dependent CKD treated at 239 sites in 13 countries. No significant difference was observed in time to primary end point (composite of doubling of serum creatinine, dialysis initiation and kidney transplantation) between treatment arms (pooled analysis HR 0.97, 95% CI 0.83–1.12, $p = 0.64$). Furthermore, the treatment group did not experience any difference in proteinuria or quality of life compared with the placebo group. Similarly, a subsequent prospective, open-label, randomized controlled trial of 579 patients with stage 3 or 4 CKD from 11 Korean centres reported that oral administration of AST (6 g/day of AST-120 in 3 divided daily doses) did not significantly affect time to the primary composite outcome of doubling of serum creatinine, eGFR decrease >50%, or initiation of renal replacement therapy (HR 1.12, 95% CI 0.85–1.48) [56]. There was no significant difference in change in serum IS levels over time between the intervention and control group ($p = 0.29$). The treatment also did not result in a significant difference in mortality, health-related quality of life or serious adverse effects.

A Cochrane systematic review of alternative oral adsorbents, Ai Xi Te and Niaoduqing granules, reported positive effects on CKD progression, but were limited by small samples sizes and poor methodologic quality with unclear or high risks of bias [54].

4.3. Reduced proximal tubular retention

Renal proximal tubular cells contain multiple transporters that perform basolateral uptake or luminal excretion of various substances, including uraemic toxins. Such transporters include the organic anion transporters (OAT)1, OAT3 and OATP4C1, as well as the organic cation transporter (OCT)2, the multidrug and toxin extrusion proteins (MATEs), the breast cancer resistance protein (BCRP) and the adenosine triphosphate (ATP)-binding cassette transporter family [57]. Anionic substances, such as IS, enter renal proximal tubule cells via basolateral

OAT, particularly OAT1 and OAT3, and are excreted into the tubular lumen by luminal OATs [58, 59]. Using cultured kidney tubule cells (LLC-PK1) and rat kidney slices, Deguchi et al. demonstrated that p-aminohippurate (OAT1 inhibitor), pravastatin (OAT3 inhibitor) and benzylpenicillin (OAT3 inhibitor) inhibited the renal tubular uptake of indoxyl sulphate to comparable extents [60]. In a 5/6-nephrectomized rat model of CKD, Enomoto et al. demonstrated that administration of IS resulted in IS accumulation in proximal tubule cells expressing OAT1 and OAT3, and was associated with more rapid CKD progression, as measured by creatinine clearance [58]. Furthermore, addition of IS to cultured rat proximal tubule (S2) cells reduced their viability, although this nephrotoxicity was abrogated by administration of the OAT1 inhibitor, probenecid [58]. Thus, OAT inhibitors, such as probenecid and statins, might be a potential strategy for preventing proximal tubule cell accumulation of IS and ensuing nephrotoxicity and CKD progression. In addition, as OATs are expressed widely throughout the body, these transporters may play a role in uraemic toxin-induced pathology in various organs. For example, Liu and colleagues demonstrated that administration of 10 μM IS to cultured Sprague-Dawley cardiac myocytes and fibroblasts stimulated myocyte hypertrophy and collagen synthesis, which was abrogated by probenecid (OAT1 antagonist) and cilastatin (OAT3 antagonist) [61].

Therapeutic manipulation of efflux transporters, such as OAT polypeptide 4C1 (SCLO4C1), may also lead to enhanced excretion of uraemic retention solutes into the urine [62]. For example, Toyohara et al. demonstrated that overexpression of SLCO4C1 in rat kidney decreased plasma levels of uraemic toxins and reduced inflammation, hypertension and cardiomegaly [11]. Moreover, renal clearance of uraemic toxins was also increased by pravastatin, which is known to upregulate proximal tubular SLCO4C1 [11].

The activities of multidrug resistance protein (MRP) 4 and BRCP efflux transporters have also been demonstrated to be downregulated by PCS *in vitro* [63] and may be potential therapeutic targets.

4.4. Increased dialytic clearance

IS and PCS are highly (>90%) protein bound and are therefore not easily removed with conventional haemodialysis and peritoneal dialysis [14, 59, 64]. Long dialysis, short daily dialysis and high-flux haemodialysis have been investigated as potential methods of improving clearance of protein-bound molecules, but have failed to show clear benefit [59, 65, 66].

In contrast to conventional haemodialysis, which mainly depends on diffusion to clear solutes, haemodiafiltration combines convection and diffusion, which is potentially very useful in facilitating removal of larger molecules, such as protein-bound solutes. Haemodiafiltration has been shown in prospective cross-over studies to be superior to high-flux haemodialysis in removing IS and PCS [67, 68]. In this respect, the effectiveness of pre- and post-dilution haemodiafiltration was comparable [67, 68]. The mechanism for the improved clearance of protein-bound solutes is not well understood but seemed to be dependent on a combination of both diffusion and convection since haemofiltration (which does not involve diffusion) reduced the serum levels of protein-bound solutes but not to the same extent as haemodiafiltration [67].

The use of super-flux cellulose triacetate membranes has also been evaluated and found to be superior to low-flux haemodialysis with respect to removing IS and most protein-bound compounds, although this might be at least partly explained by an increase in removal of albumin [69]. Similarly, dialysis with the use of a nanoporous carbon monolith (pores 2–100 nm) was able to almost completely remove IS and PCS, whereas the use of a microporous monolith (<2 mm) resulted in only partial removal, and standard high-flux haemodialysis resulted in insignificant removal [70]. A potential issue with enhanced dialysis of toxins is the rebound release of further toxins from tissues, which is observed with water-based solutes. However, Martinez and colleagues demonstrated that the rebound movement of PCS and protein solutes in the first 30 minutes post-dialysis appeared to be negligible [71].

Eloot and colleagues utilised kinetic modelling to try to determine optimal dialysis parameters to facilitate protein-bound solute removal, and found that regardless of longer or more frequent dialysis, increased volume of blood processing per week was required to increase clearance [72].

In a cross-over study of 14 patients, high-clearance dialysis (high dialysate flow rate and large dialyzer) resulted in significantly greater PCS and IS clearance compared with low-clearance dialysis (PCS 23 ± 4 ml/min vs. 12 ± 3 ml/min, $p < 0.001$; IS 30 ± 5 ml/min vs. 17 ± 4 ml/min, $p < 0.001$). However, there was no significant change in serum PCS levels with high-clearance dialysis although there was a significant decrease in IS levels [73]. The authors suggested that this lack of reduction in serum PCS levels may be due to concurrent PCS generation, and thus treatment to suppress PCS production would be required in order to achieve significant reductions in serum PCS.

5. Summary and future directions

In summary, IS and PCS are products of bacterial metabolism within the gut. Serum IS and PCS levels are increased in patients with CKD and have been associated with CKD progression, vascular disease acceleration, adverse metabolic profile and poorer cardiovascular and overall mortality. There are several methods of lowering serum IS and PCS levels, including reduced intestinal bacterial production through dietary modification of protein and/or fibre intake or pre-, pro- and synbiotic use, gastrointestinal sequestration through oral adsorbent use, reduced cellular uptake of IS through OAT inhibition, and increased clearance through enhanced dialysis. Though these treatments have been shown in some studies to successfully reduce IS and PCS levels in sera and/or cells, it is less clear whether this translates into meaningful and sustained improvements in clinical outcomes. The studies conducted to date have been limited by small patient numbers, relatively short follow-up duration and poor methodologic quality. Given the biological plausibility and clinical importance of the adverse health outcomes thought to be mediated by these toxins, further high-quality studies are needed to evaluate the short- and long-term effects of IS and PCS lowering treatments on patient-level clinical outcomes.

Author details

Melissa Nataatmadja[1], Yeoungjee Cho[1,2,3], Katrina Campbell[1,3] and David W. Johnson[1,2,3]*

*Address all correspondence to: david.johnson2@health.qld.gov.au

1 Department of Nephrology, Princess Alexandra Hospital, Brisbane, Queensland, Australia

2 Australasian Kidney Trials Network, School of Medicine, University of Queensland, Brisbane, Queensland, Australia

3 Translational Research Institute, Brisbane, Queensland, Australia

References

[1] Mafra D, Barros AF, Fouque D. Dietary protein metabolism by gut microbiota and its consequences for chronic kidney disease patients. Future Microbiology. 2013;**8**(10):1317-1323

[2] Vaziri ND. Effect of synbiotic therapy on Gut-Derived uremic toxins and the intestinal microbiome in patients with CKD. Clinical Journal of the American Society of Nephrology. 2016;**11**(2):199-201

[3] Vaziri ND, Yuan J, Rahimi A, Ni Z, Said H, Subramanian VS. Disintegration of colonic epithelial tight junction in uremia: A likely cause of CKD-associated inflammation. Nephrology Dialysis Transplantation. 2012;**27**(7):2686-2693

[4] Shimizu H, Bolati D, Adijiang A, Enomoto A, Nishijima F, Dateki M, Niwa T. Senescence and dysfunction of proximal tubular cells are associated with activated p53 expression by indoxyl sulfate. American Journal of Physiology Cell Physiology. 2010;**299**(5): C1110-C1117

[5] Shimizu H, Bolati D, Adijiang A, Muteliefu G, Enomoto A, Nishijima F, Dateki M, Niwa T. NF-kappaB plays an important role in indoxyl sulfate-induced cellular senescence, fibrotic gene expression, and inhibition of proliferation in proximal tubular cells. American journal of physiology Cell Physiology. 2011;**301**(5):C1201-C1212

[6] Adijiang A, Goto S, Uramoto S, Nishijima F, Niwa T. Indoxyl sulphate promotes aortic calcification with expression of osteoblast-specific proteins in hypertensive rats. Nephrology Dialysis Transplantation. 2008;**23**(6):1892-1901

[7] Evenepoel P, Meijers BK, Bammens BR, Verbeke K. Uremic toxins originating from colonic microbial metabolism. Kidney International Supplements. 2009;**76**(114):S12-S19

[8] Briskey D, Tucker P, Johnson DW, Coombes JS. The role of the gastrointestinal tract and microbiota on uremic toxins and chronic kidney disease development. Clin Exp Nephrol. 2017 Feb;**21**(1):7-15. DOI: 10.1007/s10157-016-1255-y. pub 2016 Mar 10. Review. PMID: 26965149

[9] Meijers BK Evenepoel P. The gut-kidney axis: Indoxyl sulfate, p-cresyl sulfate and CKD progression. Nephrology Dialysis Transplantation. 2011;**26**(3):759-761

[10] Rossi M, Johnson DW, Xu H, Carrero JJ, Pascoe E, French C, Campbell KL. Dietary protein-fiber ratio associates with circulating levels of indoxyl sulfate and p-cresyl sulfate in chronic kidney disease patients. Nutrition, Metabolism & Cardiovascular Diseases. 2015;**25**(9):860-865

[11] Toyohara T, Suzuki T, Morimoto R, Akiyama Y, Souma T, Shiwaku HO, Takeuchi Y, Mishima E, Abe M, Tanemoto M, Masuda S, Kawano H, Maemura K, Nakayama M, Sato H, Mikkaichi T, Yamaguchi H, Fukui S, Fukumoto Y, Shimokawa H, Inui K, Terasaki T, Goto J, Ito S, Hishinuma T, Rubera I, Tauc M, Fujii-Kuriyama Y, Yabuuchi H, Moriyama Y, Soga T, Abe T. SLCO4C1 transporter eliminates uremic toxins and attenuates hypertension and renal inflammation. Journal of the American Society of Nephrology. 2009;**20**(12):2546-2555

[12] Vanholder R, De Smet R, Glorieux G, Argiles A, Baurmeister U, Brunet P, Clark W, Cohen G, De Deyn PP, Deppisch R, Descamps-Latscha B, Henle T, Jorres A, Lemke HD, Massy ZA, Passlick-Deetjen J, Rodriguez M, Stegmayr B, Stenvinkel P, Tetta C, Wanner C, Zidek W. Review on uremic toxins: Classification, concentration, and interindividual variability. Kidney International. 2003;**63**(5):1934-1943

[13] Rossi M, Campbell K, Johnson D, Stanton T, Pascoe E, Hawley C, Dimeski G, McWhinney B, Ungerer J, Isbel N. Uraemic toxins and cardiovascular disease across the chronic kidney disease spectrum: An observational study. Nutrition, Metabolism & Cardiovascular Diseases. 2014;**24**(9):1035-1042

[14] Itoh Y, Ezawa A, Kikuchi K, Tsuruta Y, Niwa T. Protein-bound uremic toxins in hemodialysis patients measured by liquid chromatography/tandem mass spectrometry and their effects on endothelial ROS production. Analytical and Bioanalytical Chemistry. 2012;**403**(7):1841-1850

[15] Lin CJ, Wu V, Wu PC, Wu CJ. Meta-Analysis of the associations of p-Cresyl Sulfate (PCS) and indoxyl sulfate (IS) with cardiovascular events and All-Cause mortality in patients with chronic renal failure. PLoS One. 2015;**10**(7):e0132589

[16] Rossi M, Campbell KL, Johnson DW, Stanton T, Haluska BA, Hawley CM, Dimeski G, McWhinney BC, Ungerer JP, Kaisar OM, Isbel NM. Uremic toxin development in living kidney donors: A longitudinal study. Transplantation. 2014;**97**(5):548-554

[17] Wu IW, Hsu KH, Lee CC, Sun CY, Hsu HJ, Tsai CJ, Tzen CY, Wang YC, Lin CY, Wu MS. p-Cresyl sulphate and indoxyl sulphate predict progression of chronic kidney disease. Nephrology Dialysis Transplantation. 2011;**26**(3):938-947

[18] Motojima M, Hosokawa A, Yamato H, Muraki T, Yoshioka T. Uremic toxins of organic anions up-regulate PAI-1 expression by induction of NF-kappaB and free radical in proximal tubular cells. Kidney International. 2003;**63**(5):1671-1680

[19] Niwa T, Ise M. Indoxyl sulfate, a circulating uremic toxin, stimulates the progression of glomerular sclerosis. Journal of Laboratory and Clinical Medicine 1994;**124**(1):96-104

[20] Watanabe H, Miyamoto Y, Honda D, Tanaka H, Wu Q, Endo M, Noguchi T, Kadowaki D, Ishima Y, Kotani S, Nakajima M, Kataoka K, Kim-Mitsuyama S, Tanaka M, Fukagawa M, Otagiri M, Maruyama T. p-Cresyl sulfate causes renal tubular cell damage by inducing oxidative stress by activation of NADPH oxidase. Kidney International. 2013;**83**(4):582-592

[21] Sun CY, Chang SC, Wu MS. Uremic toxins induce kidney fibrosis by activating intrarenal renin-angiotensin-aldosterone system associated epithelial-to-mesenchymal transition. PLoS One. 2012;**7**(3):e34026

[22] Koppe L, Pillon NJ, Vella RE, Croze ML, Pelletier CC, Chambert S, Massy Z, Glorieux G, Vanholder R, Dugenet Y, Soula HA, Fouque D, Soulage CO. p-Cresyl sulfate promotes insulin resistance associated with CKD. Journal of the American Society of Nephrology. 2013;**24**(1):88-99

[23] Yamamoto H, Tsuruoka S, Ioka T, Ando H, Ito C, Akimoto T, Fujimura A, Asano Y, Kusano E. Indoxyl sulfate stimulates proliferation of rat vascular smooth muscle cells. Kidney International. 2006;**69**(10):1780-1785

[24] Barreto FC, Barreto DV, Liabeuf S, Meert N, Glorieux G, Temmar M, Choukroun G, Vanholder R, Massy ZA. Serum indoxyl sulfate is associated with vascular disease and mortality in chronic kidney disease patients. Clinical Journal of the American Society of Nephrology. 2009;**4**(10):1551-1558

[25] Liabeuf S, Barreto DV, Barreto FC, Meert N, Glorieux G, Schepers E, Temmar M, Choukroun G, Vanholder R, Massy ZA. Free p-cresylsulphate is a predictor of mortality in patients at different stages of chronic kidney disease. Nephrology Dialysis Transplantation. 2010;**25**(4):1183-1191

[26] Melamed ML, Plantinga L, Shafi T, Parekh R, Meyer TW, Hostetter TH, Coresh J, Powe NR. Retained organic solutes, patient characteristics and all-cause and cardiovascular mortality in hemodialysis: Results from the retained organic solutes and clinical outcomes (ROSCO) investigators. BMC Nephrology. 2013;**14**:134

[27] Meijers BK, Claes K, Bammens B, de Loor H, Viaene L, Verbeke K, Kuypers D, Vanrenterghem Y, Evenepoel P. p-Cresol and cardiovascular risk in mild-to-moderate kidney disease. Clinical Journal of the American Society of Nephrology. 2010;**5**(7):1182-1189

[28] Bammens B, Evenepoel P, Keuleers H, Verbeke K, Vanrenterghem Y. Free serum concentrations of the protein-bound retention solute p-cresol predict mortality in hemodialysis patients. Kidney International. 2006;**69**(6):1081-1087

[29] Marzocco S, Dal Piaz F, Di Micco L, Torraca S, Sirico ML, Tartaglia D, Autore G, Di Iorio B. Very low protein diet reduces indoxyl sulfate levels in chronic kidney disease. Blood Purification. 2013;**35**(1-3):196-201

[30] Fouque D, Laville M. Low protein diets for chronic kidney disease in non diabetic adults. Cochrane Database Syst Rev. 2009 Jul 8;(3):CD001892. DOI: 10.1002/14651858.CD001892.pub3. Review. PMID: 19588328

[31] Johnson DW. Dietary protein restriction as a treatment for slowing chronic kidney disease progression: The case against. Nephrology (Carlton). 2006;**11**(1):58-62

[32] Johnson DW, Atai E, Chan M, Phoon RK, Scott C, Toussaint ND, Turner GL, Usherwood T, Wiggins KJ. KHA-CARI guideline: Early chronic kidney disease: Detection, prevention and management. Nephrology (Carlton). 2013;**18**(5):340-350

[33] Sirich TL, Plummer NS, Gardner CD, Hostetter TH, Meyer TW. Effect of increasing dietary fiber on plasma levels of colon-derived solutes in hemodialysis patients. Clinical Journal of the American Society of Nephrology. 2014;**9**(9):1603-1610

[34] Xu H, Rossi M, Campbell KL, Sencion GL, Arnlov J, Cederholm T, Sjogren P, Riserus U, Lindholm B, Carrero JJ. Excess protein intake relative to fiber and cardiovascular events in elderly men with chronic kidney disease. Nutrition, Metabolism & Cardiovascular Diseases. 2016;**26**(7):597-602

[35] Hida M, Aiba Y, Sawamura S, Suzuki N, Satoh T, Koga Y. Inhibition of the accumulation of uremic toxins in the blood and their precursors in the feces after oral administration of Lebenin, a lactic acid bacteria preparation, to uremic patients undergoing hemodialysis. Nephron. 1996;**74**(2):349-355

[36] Francois IE, Lescroart O, Veraverbeke WS, Marzorati M, Possemiers S, Evenepoel P, Hamer H, Houben E, Windey K, Welling GW, Delcour JA, Courtin CM, Verbeke K, Broekaert WF. Effects of a wheat bran extract containing arabinoxylan oligosaccharides on gastrointestinal health parameters in healthy adult human volunteers: A double-blind, randomised, placebo-controlled, cross-over trial. British Journal of Nutrition. 2012;**108**(12):2229-2242

[37] Nakabayashi I, Nakamura M, Kawakami K, Ohta T, Kato I, Uchida K, Yoshida M. Effects of synbiotic treatment on serum level of p-cresol in haemodialysis patients: A preliminary study. Nephrology, Dialysis, Transplantation. 2011;**26**(3):1094-1048

[38] Guida B, Germano R, Trio R, Russo D, Memoli B, Grumetto L, Barbato F, Cataldi M. Effect of short-term synbiotic treatment on plasma p-cresol levels in patients with chronic renal failure: A randomized clinical trial. Nutrition, Metabolism & Cardiovascular Diseases. 2014;**24**(9):1043-1049

[39] Rossi M, Klein K, Johnson DW, Campbell KL. Pre-, pro-, and synbiotics: Do they have a role in reducing uremic toxins? A systematic review and meta-analysis. International Journal of Nephrology. 2012;**2012**:673631

[40] Rossi M, Johnson DW, Morrison M, Pascoe E, Coombes JS, Forbes JM, McWhinney BC, Ungerer JP, Dimeski G, Campbell KL. SYNbiotics easing renal failure by improving gut microbiologY (SYNERGY): A protocol of placebo-controlled randomised cross-over trial. BMC Nephrology. 2014;**15**:106

[41] Rossi M, Johnson DW, Morrison M, Pascoe EM, Coombes JS, Forbes JM, Szeto CC, McWhinney BC, Ungerer JP, Campbell KL. Synbiotics easing renal failure by improving gut microbiology (SYNERGY): A randomized trial. Clinical Journal of the American Society of Nephrology. 2016;**11**(2):223-231

[42] Buffie CG, Jarchum I, Equinda M, Lipuma L, Gobourne A, Viale A, Ubeda C, Xavier J, Pamer EG. Profound alterations of intestinal microbiota following a single dose of

clindamycin results in sustained susceptibility to Clostridium difficile-induced colitis. Infection and Immunity. 2012;**80**(1):62-73

[43] Okada K, Takahashi S, Nagura Y, Hatano M, Shimamura T. Early morphological changes of tubules in rats with chronic renal failure. Nihon Jinzo Gakkai Shi. 1992;**34**(1):65-70

[44] Horike K, Usami T, Kamiya Y, Kamiya T, Yoshida A, Itoh S, Yamato H, Ise M, Kimura G. Oral carbonaceous absorbent modifies renal function of renal ablation model without affecting plasma renin-angiotensin system or protein intake. Clinical and Experimental Nephrology. 2003;**7**(2):120-124

[45] Evenepoel P, Bammens B, Verbeke K, Vanrenterghem Y. Acarbose treatment lowers generation and serum concentrations of the protein-bound solute p-cresol: A pilot study. Kidney International. 2006;**70**(1):192-198

[46] Schulman G, Agarwal R, Acharya M, Berl T, Blumenthal S, Kopyt N. A multicenter, randomized, double-blind, placebo-controlled, dose-ranging study of AST-120 (Kremezin) in patients with moderate to severe CKD. American Journal of Kidney Diseases. 2006;**47**(4):565-577

[47] Wu IW, Hsu KH, Sun CY, Tsai CJ, Wu MS, Lee CC. Oral adsorbent AST-120 potentiates the effect of erythropoietin-stimulating agents on Stage 5 chronic kidney disease patients: A randomized crossover study. Nephrology, Dialysis, Transplantation. 2014;**29**(9):1719-1727

[48] Yamamoto S, Kazama JJ, Omori K, Matsuo K, Takahashi Y, Kawamura K, Matsuto T, Watanabe H, Maruyama T, Narita I. Continuous reduction of Protein-Bound uraemic toxins with improved oxidative stress by using the oral charcoal adsorbent AST-120 in haemodialysis patients. Scientific Reports. 2015;**5**:14381

[49] Kikuchi K, Itoh Y, Tateoka R, Ezawa A, Murakami K, Niwa T. Metabolomic search for uremic toxins as indicators of the effect of an oral sorbent AST-120 by liquid chromatography/tandem mass spectrometry. Journal of Chromatography B. 2010;**878**(29):2997-3002

[50] Miyazaki T, Aoyama I, Ise M, Seo H, Niwa T. An oral sorbent reduces overload of indoxyl sulphate and gene expression of TGF-beta1 in uraemic rat kidneys. Nephrology, Dialysis, Transplantation. 2000;**15**(11):1773-1781

[51] Takahashi N, Kawaguchi T, Suzuki T. Therapeutic effects of long-term administration of an oral adsorbent in patients with chronic renal failure: Two-year study. International Journal of Urology. 2005;**12**(1):7-11

[52] Sanaka T, Akizawa T, Koide K, Koshikawa S. Protective effect of an oral adsorbent on renal function in chronic renal failure: Determinants of its efficacy in diabetic nephropathy. Therapeutic Apheresis and Dialysis. 2004;**8**(3):232-240

[53] Shoji T, Wada A, Inoue K, Hayashi D, Tomida K, Furumatsu Y, Kaneko T, Okada N, Fukuhara Y, Imai E, Tsubakihara Y. Prospective randomized study evaluating the efficacy of the spherical adsorptive carbon AST-120 in chronic kidney disease patients with moderate decrease in renal function. Nephron Clinical Practice. 2007;**105**(3):c99-c107

[54] Wu HM, Sun HJ, Wang F, Yang M, Dong BR, Liu GJ. Oral adsorbents for preventing or delaying the progression of chronic kidney disease. Cochrane Database Syst Rev. 2014 Oct 15;(10):CD007861. DOI: 10.1002/14651858.CD007861.pub2. Review. PMID: 25317905

[55] Schulman G, Berl T, Beck GJ, Remuzzi G, Ritz E, Arita K, Kato A, Shimizu M. Randomized Placebo-Controlled EPPIC trials of AST-120 in CKD. Journal of the American Society of Nephrology. 2015;**26**(7):1732-1746

[56] Cha RH, Kang SW, Park CW, Cha DR, Na KY, Kim SG, Yoon SA, Han SY, Chang JH, Park SK, Lim CS, Kim YS. A Randomized, controlled trial of oral intestinal sorbent AST-120 on renal function deterioration in patients with advanced renal dysfunction. Clinical Journal of the American Society of Nephrology. 2016;**11**(4):559-567

[57] Masereeuw R, Mutsaers HA, Toyohara T, Abe T, Jhawar S, Sweet DH, Lowenstein J. The kidney and uremic toxin removal: Glomerulus or tubule? Seminars in Nephrology. 2014;**34**(2):191-208

[58] Enomoto A, Takeda M, Tojo A, Sekine T, Cha SH, Khamdang S, Takayama F, Aoyama I, Nakamura S, Endou H, Niwa T. Role of organic anion transporters in the tubular transport of indoxyl sulfate and the induction of its nephrotoxicity. Journal of the American Society of Nephrology. 2002;**13**(7):1711-1720

[59] Neirynck N, Glorieux G, Schepers E, Pletinck A, Dhondt A, Vanholder R. Review of protein-bound toxins, possibility for blood purification therapy. Blood Purification, 2013;**35**(Suppl 1):45-50

[60] Deguchi T, Kusuhara H, Takadate A, Endou H, Otagiri M, Sugiyama Y. Characterization of uremic toxin transport by organic anion transporters in the kidney. Kidney International. 2004;**65**(1):162-174

[61] Liu S, Wang BH, Kompa AR, Lekawanvijit S, Krum H. Antagonists of organic anion transporters 1 and 3 ameliorate adverse cardiac remodelling induced by uremic toxin indoxyl sulfate. International Journal of Cardiology. 2012;**158**(3):457-458

[62] Glorieux G, Tattersall J. Uraemic toxins and new methods to control their accumulation: Game changers for the concept of dialysis adequacy. Clinical Kidney Journal. 2015;**8**(4):353-362

[63] Mutsaers HA, Caetano-Pinto P, Seegers AE, Dankers AC, van den Broek PH, Wetzels JF, van den Brand JA, van den Heuvel LP, Hoenderop JG, Wilmer MJ, Masereeuw R. Proximal tubular efflux transporters involved in renal excretion of p-cresyl sulfate and p-cresyl glucuronide: Implications for chronic kidney disease pathophysiology. Toxicology In Vitro. 2015;**29**(7):1868-1877

[64] Viaene L, Annaert P, de Loor H, Poesen R, Evenepoel P, Meijers B. Albumin is the main plasma binding protein for indoxyl sulfate and p-cresyl sulfate. Biopharmaceutics & Drug Disposition. 2013;**34**(3):165-175

[65] Fagugli RM, De Smet R, Buoncristiani U, Lameire N, Vanholder R. Behavior of non-protein-bound and protein-bound uremic solutes during daily hemodialysis. American Journal of Kidney Diseases. 2002;**40**(2):339-347

[66] Basile C, Libutti P, Di Turo AL, Casino FG, Vernaglione L, Tundo S, Maselli P, De Nicolo EV, Ceci E, Teutonico A, Lomonte C. Removal of uraemic retention solutes in standard bicarbonate haemodialysis and long-hour slow-flow bicarbonate haemodialysis. Nephrology, Dialysis, Transplantation. 2011;**26**(4):1296-1303

[67] Meert N, Eloot S, Schepers E, Lemke HD, Dhondt A, Glorieux G, Van Landschoot M, Waterloos MA, Vanholder R. Comparison of removal capacity of two consecutive generations of high-flux dialysers during different treatment modalities. Nephrology, Dialysis, Transplantation. 2011;**26**(8):2624-2630

[68] Meert N, Eloot S, Waterloos MA, Van Landschoot M, Dhondt A, Glorieux G, Ledebo I, Vanholder R. Effective removal of protein-bound uraemic solutes by different convective strategies: A prospective trial. Nephrology, Dialysis, Transplantation. 2009;**24**(2):562-570

[69] De Smet R, Dhondt A, Eloot S, Galli F, Waterloos MA, Vanholder R. Effect of the super-flux cellulose triacetate dialyser membrane on the removal of non-protein-bound and protein-bound uraemic solutes. Nephrology, Dialysis, Transplantation. 2007;**22**(7):2006-2012

[70] Sandeman SR, Howell CA, Phillips GJ, Zheng Y, Standen G, Pletzenauer R, Davenport A, Basnayake K, Boyd O, Holt S, Mikhalovsky SV. An adsorbent monolith device to augment the removal of uraemic toxins during haemodialysis. Journal of Materials Science: Materials in Medicine. 2014;**25**(6):1589-1597

[71] Martinez AW, Recht NS, Hostetter TH, Meyer TW. Removal of P-cresol sulfate by hemodialysis. Journal of the American Society of Nephrology. 2005;**16**(11):3430-3436

[72] Eloot S, Schneditz D, Cornelis T, Van Biesen W, Glorieux G, Dhondt A, Kooman J, Vanholder R. Protein-Bound uremic toxin profiling as a tool to optimize hemodialysis. PLoS One. 2016;**11**(1):e0147159

[73] Camacho O, Rosales MC, Shafi T, Fullman J, Plummer NS, Meyer TW, Sirich TL. Effect of a sustained difference in hemodialytic clearance on the plasma levels of p-cresol sulfate and indoxyl sulfate. Nephrology, Dialysis, Transplantation. 2016;**31**(8):1335-1341

Chapter 9

Role of Organochlorine Pesticides in Chronic Kidney Diseases of Unknown Etiology

Rishila Ghosh, Manushi Siddharth,
Pawan Kuman Kare, Om Prakash Kalra and
Ashok Kumar Tripathi

Additional information is available at the end of the chapter

http://dx.doi.org/10.5772/intechopen.71196

Abstract

Chronic kidney disease (CKD) contributes to a significant burden on the healthcare system and economy worldwide. In the last two decades, a new form of CKD: chronic kidney disease of unknown etiology (CKDu) in which the disease is not attributed to known causes has emerged as a major health issue in different geographical areas over the world mainly from farming community and has become a global concern today. Despite intense and numerous research works dedicated to CKDu, very little is known with certainty regarding its etiology and the pathophysiology behind its development. Recent evidences are emerging in favor of possible role of agrochemicals and pesticides in the pathogenesis of CKDu. Organochlorine pesticides (OCPs) due to their longer half-life and lipophilic nature persist long in the environment and are known to be biomagnified through food chain. Some study reports by the authors and a few others constitute the important body of evidences depicting the association between chronic exposures to OCPs and occurrence of CKDu through environmental contamination in farming as well as non-farming communities in different geographical areas around the globe.

Keywords: chronic kidney disease, organochlorine pesticides, end stage renal disease, eGFR, CKDu

1. Chronic kidney disease (CKD)

1.1. Overview

Chronic kidney disease (CKD) refers to a gradual and progressive decline of renal function as a result of damage to renal microstructure due to various causes ultimately leading to end-stage renal disease (ESRD). Most, but not all forms of CKD are irreversible and progressive [1]. The progression of the disease is often silent to start with, but gradually over a period of time the disease reaches a stage in which due to increased renal damage and kidney dysfunction renal replacement therapy (RRT) in the form of dialysis or renal transplant becomes necessary to sustain life. Currently, 10% of the global population regardless of ethnic origin are affected by CKD and it has become a major burden on the healthcare system worldwide [2]. Globally, CKD is the 12th most common cause of death and 17th cause of disability [3]. It is estimated that nearly 1,00,000 new patients of end-stage renal disease (ESRD) enters RRT programs annually in India [4]. Worldwide, over two million people are on renal replacement therapy but this figure nearly represents 10% of those who need it [5]. With this alarming number, CKD has emerged as a global epidemic. The adverse outcomes like cardiovascular disease (CVD) and premature death are universal [6].

1.2. Definition and classification

Keeping in mind the global impact of CKD, a simple definition and classification was necessary for international development, dissemination, and implementation of clinical practice guideline. One such initiative was undertaken by KDIGO (Kidney Disease: Improving Global Outcomes) through one of the series of International Controversies Conferences in which, by the consensus of a large number of nephrologists worldwide, the definition and classification of CKD devised by KDOQI (Kidney Disease Outcomes Quality Initiative) was accepted with a minor modification (**Table 1**).

The National Kidney Foundation (NFK) of the United States of America classified the progression of CKD in five stages depending on the extent of renal dysfunction symptomatology and therapeutic guidelines (**Table 2**).

The term chronic renal failure applies to the reduction of significant number of functional nephron and typically corresponds to CKD stage 3–5. For obvious reason, the late stage 4 and stage 5 pose a large social, human, and economic burden. The term ESRD represents a stage in which the accumulation of toxic substances, fluid, and electrolytes which are excreted otherwise by normal kidneys produces significant clinical symptoms and even cause death unless removed from the body by renal replacement therapy in the form of kidney transplant or regular dialysis. In most of the cases but not all, patients of CKD with stage 3 or 4 progress to ESRD at a rate of 1.5% per year, whereas patients with stage 1 or 2 progress to more advanced stages approximately 0.5% per year [7].

Kidney damage for ≥3 months, as defined by structural or functional abnormalities of the kidney, with or without decreased glomerular filtration rate (GFR), that can lead to decreased GFR, manifested by either:
Pathologic abnormalities; or
Markers of kidney damage, including abnormalities in the composition of the blood or urine; or
Abnormalities in imaging tests
GFR < 60 mL/min/1.73m^2 for ≥3 months, with or without kidney damage
Adapted from: Levey et al. [6].

Table 1. Criteria for chronic kidney disease (CKD).

http://dx.doi.org/10.5772/intechopen.71196

Stages	GFR	Common features
1	≥90*	–
2	60–90*	↑ Parathyroid hormone, ↓ renal calcium reabsorption
3	30–59	Left ventricular hypertrophy, anemia secondary to erythropoietin deficiency
4	15–29	↑ Serum triglycerides, hyperphosphatemia, hyperkalemia, metabolic acidosis, fatigue, nausea, anorexia, and bone pain
5	<15	Renal failure: severe uremic symptoms

↑: increase; ↓: decrease. Adapted from: Lopez-Novoa et al. [1].*CKD is defined as either GFR < 60 mL/min/1.73m2 for 3 months or a GFR above those values in the presence of evidence of kidney damage such as abnormalities in blood or urine (e.g., proteinuria) tests or imaging studies.

Table 2. Stages of chronic kidney disease.

1.3. Etiology

Some decades ago, the leading cause of CKD was glomerulonephritis secondary to infection. Introduction of antibiotics and improved sanitary practice have changed the scenario; presently, the most common causes of CKD in adults are diabetes and hypertension in the developed world [8]. The leading causes of CKD in USA according to the 2012 US Renal Data System Annual Data Report are diabetes (49.1%), hypertension (28%), and glomerulonephritis (4.7%) [9]. As a fact, about 50% of ESRD patients in USA are diabetic and about 50–60% of all patients with CKD are hypertensive [10]. According to the CKD Registry of India, the most common cause of CKD in Indian population is diabetes (31%) followed by CKD of undetermined etiology (16%) followed by chronic glomerulonephritis (14%) and hypertensive nephrosclerosis (13%) with almost equal frequency. Other less common causes were: interstitial nephritis (7%), chronic obstructive uropathy (3.4%), miscellaneous (11.7), renovascular disease (0.8%), and graft failure (0.3%) [11] (**Figure 1**).

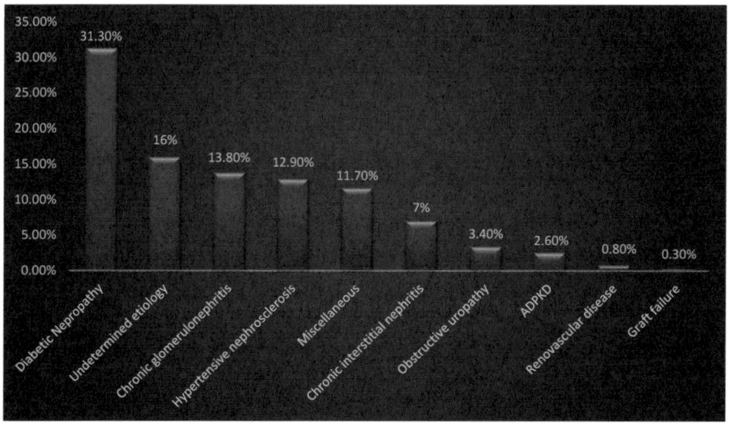

Figure 1. Etiological spectrum of Indian CKD patients of chronic kidney disease of unknown etiology (CKDu).

2. Chronic kidney disease of unknown etiology (CKDu)

2.1. Overview

In the mid of 1990s, a new form of CKD was identified among the rice paddy farmers of North Central Province (NCP) of Sri Lanka. This form of CKD is otherwise known as chronic kidney disease of unknown etiology (CKDu) [12]. Over the last two decades, similar kind of cases in significant number was reported from other farming areas of Sri Lanka and different parts of the world including Central America, among immigrants in UK from South-east Asia and India. Different terms have been used to describe CKDu in literature: chronic kidney disease of uncertain origin; chronic kidney disease of unknown origin; agrochemical nephropathy, etc. [13]. In some cases, it is named after the region or country of its origin: Central American nephropathy [14]; Salvadoran agricultural nephropathy; Mesoamerican endemic nephropathy (MeN); chronic tubulo-interstitial kidney disease of Central America; Udhanam endemic nephropathy (India); Sri Lankan agricultural nephropathy; or chronic interstitial nephritis in agricultural communities (CINAC) [15].

2.2. Global impact and epidemiological pattern

Since the first case was reported, it has become the most alarming public health issue of Sri Lanka with more than 60,000 patients and more than 20,000 deaths annually. Hospital records show a steady increase of CKDu from the year 2000 to 2015 [12]. According to the NCP (North Central Province) statistics, the cause is unknown for 2809 (70.2%) of the newly diagnosed cases of CKD and only 15.7 and 9.6% cases were diagnosed to have hypertension and diabetes, respectively. The male to female ratio was 2.6:1 showing a male preponderance. The majority of patients of CKD with undetermined etiology were in stage 4 (40%) at presentation [16].

In Central America, increasing number of CKD patients and CKD-specific mortality has been observed over the last 20 years particularly in Nicaragua and El Salvador. In the farming community of El Salvador, CKD is the fifth leading cause of death in adults. Women, men, adolescents and children, all who live in these farming communities are affected, irrespective of whether they are involved in agricultural activity or not. In Nicaragua, another endemic area for CKDu in Central America, the studies showed positive association between CKD and agricultural work, exposure to pesticides, dehydration, hypertension, drinking of *lija* (homemade liquor), and a family history of CKD [17]. Another endemic country in Central America is Costa Rica where the disease appeared in agricultural workers who work for long hours in sugarcane plantations. Clinical presentation and histopathology were consistent with chronic interstitial nephritis. The authors suspected work environment related factors to be associated with the disease [18]. A recent cross-sectional study conducted in 2009–2011 in females in agricultural communities of El Salvador, shows the prevalence of CKDu in women of these communities to be 6.7%. The key factors behind CKDu in women are probably chronic exposure to toxic agents and environmental toxins [19].

The prevalence of ESRD in Egypt's El Minia Governorate has increased from 250 to 367 per million populations from 2002 to 2007. The etiology is unknown in 27% patients [20, 21]. A case control study among ESRD patients from this area has shown association with rural residence, unsafe drinking water, family history of CKD, pesticide exposure, and medicinal plant use [21]. The authors concluded that the disease may be attributed to environmental factors.

2.3. Indian scenario

According to the report of the CKD Registry of India, of 52,273 CKD patients during 2006–2010, chronic kidney disease of unknown etiology was found in 16% of the CKD patients and was estimated to be the second leading cause only after diabetes mellitus. In this study, CKDu was more frequent in young low income patients and is clinically characterized by no or mild hypertension or proteinuria. Since there are few symptoms, disease is usually diagnosed at an advanced stage [11].

Another study from the Udhanam coastal region of Andhra Pradesh, India revealed prevalence of proteinuria to be 15.3% (54/354) in an agricultural community primarily involved in the cultivation of coconut, jackfruit, rice, and cashew with a higher prevalence in men compared to women (20% vs. 12% respectively). The prevalence of reduced GFR among males and females was 67 and 57%, respectively. The total prevalence of reduced GFR was 61% combining both males and females. Younger population showed mild to moderate proteinuria and renal histopathology studies revealed chronic tubulointerstitial nephritis. The authors suspected environmental exposure to toxic agents as the most likely cause [22]. In a recent publication by Jayasumana et al., the authors mentioned about an epidemic of CKD, not associated with the traditional risk factors from a few coastal areas of the same geographical region of Andhra Pradesh [12]. According to them, more than 4000 cases have already been diagnosed among paddy and coconut farmers of this area. The source of this information is through a personal communication with Dr. Gangadhar, Nephrologist, Nizam's Institute of Medical Sciences, Hyderabad, India [13]. No significant data of CKDu particularly among CKD patients in general population of urban or rural area are available so far.

2.4. CKDu: clinical profile and case definition

The clinical profile of CKDu patients from different geographical regions has striking similarities. Due to the slower rate of progression, majority of the affected individuals are asymptomatic for long time particularly during the early course of the disease [23]. The urine sediment shows no significant abnormalities in the markers of renal damage. Proteinuria is rare and moderate if present and can be described as "tubular" since β2 microglobulin and other tubular markers are found to be elevated in urine [24]. In the year of 2009, Ministry of Health of Sri Lanka developed the criteria for case definition of CKDu. According to these criteria, chronic kidney disease is considered to be of unknown etiology if there is: (1) no past history of, or current treatment for diabetes mellitus or chronic or severe hypertension, snake bites, urological disease of known etiology or glomerulonephritis; (2) normal glycosylated hemoglobin level ($HbA1_C < 6.5\%$); and (3) blood pressure < 160/100 mm Hg untreated or <140/90 mm Hg on up to two antihypertensive drugs [25].

2.5. CKDu: histopathological pattern

The morphological pattern of CKDu is described as chronic tubulo-interstitial nephritis, from two of the important endemic geographical areas: Sri Lanka and El Salvador [26, 27]. The prominent findings are interstitial fibrosis and tubular atrophy with or without inflammatory monocyte infiltration. In a retrospective study of 251 renal biopsies from patients in Sri Lanka, histopathological features of the first four stages of CKDu have been described [28]. The predominant feature of stage 1 disease is mild to moderate interstitial fibrosis without the evidence of interstitial inflammation in most of the cases. Glomerulosclerosis was absent in 62.3% of the specimens. Stage 2 CKD specimens show moderate interstitial fibrosis with or without mild interstitial inflammation. Features of Stage 3 CKD had moderate to severe interstitial fibrosis, moderate inflammation, tubular atrophy, and glomerulosclerosis. In a recent study from El Salvador, more severe tubular atrophy and less glomerular lesion were found among patients of CKDu involved in sugarcane farming along with more mononuclear inflammatory infiltration when compared to non-agricultural workers [29].

2.6. CKDu: probable etiological factors

Most of the available literature points toward the exposure to environmental contaminants and agrochemicals as possible etiological factors. The countries and regions where CKDu has clustered, followed age-old practice of traditional agriculture for centuries prior to the introduction of biotechnologically produced high yield seeds, chemical fertilizers, and pesticides as a part of "green revolution" in the 1960s [30]. Interestingly, it was only after the green revolution that a high prevalence of CKD cases was reported from rural agricultural communities from the endemic areas all over the world, suggesting that a factor related to the changed agricultural practice could be a trigger to this disease [31]. Recently, evidence implicating agrochemicals, particularly fertilizers emerged in Sri Lanka, where CKDu patients were found to have higher urinary excretion of cadmium having a dose-dependent association with CKDu severity [32]. Other risk factors identified for CKDu are being a farmer, handling pesticides, drinking well water, having taken herbal or Ayurvedic medicines, etc. [33]. In a recent study, Jayasumana et al. [13] proposed a well-researched theory of renal tubular damage by heavy metals which absorbed into the body as a lattice structure formed by chelation of metal ions with glyphosate, a widely used herbicides by the farmers of the endemic area. This theory, though attractive has yet to be proven by bench research and many academic chemists do not support this view. The high prevalence of CKD in the villages located downstream [34], and among consumers of water from shallow wells [16, 35] strongly indicates the possibility of entry of toxins through contaminated drinking water [13]. Genetic susceptibility is another possible risk factor according to some studies [36].

The etiology of CKDu in Central America appears to be multifactorial. Two main hypotheses have emerged. One identifies the trigger as exposure to agrochemicals and pesticides either due to exposure during agricultural activity or through contaminated physical environment, water, and food. Occurrence of extra-renal manifestations in CKDu patients suggests generalized toxicity affecting different organ systems with renal damage being a part of systemic pathology. The second hypothesis is the effect of heat stress compounded with strenuous labor and insufficient fluid intake triggering repeated episodes of subclinical acute renal injury that could lead to chronic kidney disease [37, 38].

Available literatures on CKDu mostly show prevalence of this disease from agricultural communities of low socio-economic strata. But there is increasing concern among scientists that the health hazards of agrochemicals are no longer limited to the agricultural communities. Due to extensive and widespread contamination of food, water, soil, air, flora and fauna by environmental pollutants like OCPs, general populations not involved in agriculture and populations from non-rural area are also exposed to these toxic chemicals as well.

Agrochemicals are chemicals such as inorganic fertilizers, liming agents and acidifying agents, pesticides, plant hormones or phytohormones, and plant growth agents used to improve the production of crops. The obvious benefit of using agrochemicals is the improved production of quality and quantity of vegetables, fruits, and crops, but not without a toll. Widespread and uncontrolled use of these chemicals for long time caused extensive contamination of the environment and thus caused significant adverse effect on the ecosystem and the health of the living organisms as well as humans.

3. Pesticides

A pesticide is a substance or mixture of substances used to kill a pest. It may be a chemical substance, biological agents (such as virus or bacteria), antimicrobial, disinfectant or device used against any pest [39]. The Food and Agriculture Association (FAO) of the United Nations has defined the term pesticide as "any substance or mixtures of substances intended for preventing, destroying or controlling any pest, including vectors of human or animal disease, unwanted species of plants or animals causing harm during or otherwise interfering with the production, processing, storage, transport, or marketing of food, agricultural commodities, wood and wood product or animal feedstuffs, or substances which can be administered to animals for the control of insects, arachnids or other pests in or on their bodies." Pesticides include variety of different compounds such as insecticides, ovicides, larvicides, adulticides, herbicides, fungicides, rodenticides, etc. [40]. The use of pesticides was of great help in increasing the yield of crops in agriculture and in public health programmes for controlling vector-borne diseases. On the other hand, due to their potential toxicity to human and animals, it has become a global concern for environmental pollution and health hazard. More than 98% of sprayed pesticides and 95% of herbicides reach a destination other than their targeted species including air, water, soil, food, and non-targeted living species. Some of them are persistent organic pollutants (POPs) and contribute to significant soil contamination. In this way, they have become an integral part of the ecosystem and environment, and as they are meant for destruction of some particular species, they leave a devastating effect on other non-targeted species as well as humans leading to a potential hazard to their health [39].

3.1. Organochlorine pesticides (OCPs)

Organochlorine pesticides have a long history of indiscriminate and uncontrolled use for about five decades for both agricultural and sanitary purposes. Some of the OCPs which have been banned or restricted in the last two decades in India are shown in **Table 3**.

Others which are in main use include lindane, endosulfan, dicofol, methoxychlor, and pentachlorophenol [39]. Organochlorine pesticides (OCPs), due to their chemical stability and extremely resistant nature to degradation, persist for long in the environment (**Table 4**).

These compounds are mainly found associated with organic matter in soil and in animal tissue due to their strong lipophilic property. They bioaccumulate in the adipose tissue of animals as well as humans and even get biomagnified through food chain [41]. Increased level of different OCP residues has been detected in different human samples such as placenta, blood, semen, amniotic fluid, breast milk, etc. [42–45]. Some of the notable examples are: dichlorodiphenyltrichloroethane (DDT) and its analogues (such as methoxychlor), dicofol, aldrin, endrin, heptachlor, endosulfan, chlordane, dieldrin, lindane, mirex, etc. [39].

Compounds	Status in India	Year
Aldrin	Banned	1996
Chlordane	Banned	1996
DDT	Restricted use	1980
Dieldrin	Restricted use	1990
	Complete ban	2003
Endrin	Banned	1990
HCH	Banned	1997
Heptachlor	Banned	1996

Adapted from: Free Wikipedia, the free encyclopedia.

Table 3. Current status of organochlorine pesticides in India.

Organochlorine pesticides	Half-life in soil
α-HCH	2–8 years
β-HCH	1–7 years
γ-HCH	1.2–6.5 years
Aldrin	0.3–3.0 years
Dieldrin	2.5–8.0 years
α-Endosulfan	35–67 days
β-Endosulfan	104–265 days
p,p′-DDT	2.8–10.0 years
p,p′-DDE	1–15 years

Adapted from: Agrawal and Sharma [39] and Free Wikipedia, the free encyclopedia [49].

Table 4. Environmental half-life of organochlorines.

3.2. Exposure to OCPs

Exposure to organochlorine pesticides may occur by direct exposure through handling or spraying during agricultural activity particularly by inadequately educated farmers, without proper protective gears, by using some personal care products like lice shampoo or indirectly through contaminated food and water. Organochlorine pesticides are carried long distance via atmospheric and oceanic currents from the site of its manufacture or use and build up in the fatty tissues of animals [46]. Many studies have linked OCP exposure with consumption of contaminated animal products, mostly meat, fish, and marine mammals [47, 48]. Fetuses and children may get exposed to pesticides *in utero* as well as through breast milk [49]. Even after replacement of organochlorine pesticides by organophosphate, consumer products such as edible crops, fruits, and milk show substantial levels of organochlorine pesticides residue. In a multicentric study, residues of OCPs, especially DDT and HCH have been detected in humans and in environment [50]. Before the imposition of ban, endosulfan was in extensive use in agricultural practice and this led to its occurrence in a variety of food items in India [51]. High levels of DDT and HCH have been reported in human blood, fat, and milk samples in India [52, 53]. A recent study from Punjab, India has shown p,p'-DDE as the major contaminant detected in human breast milk samples [54].

3.3. Detectable blood levels of OCPs in general population

Detectable blood levels of organochlorine pesticides (OCPs) such as DDT, DDE, HCH, endosulfan, and aldrin have been reported from different parts of the worlds like Spain, Canada, Mexico, Egypt, Pakistan and different parts of India in agro professional as well as in the non-agro professional general population. In a recent published report from Mexico, p,p'-DDE was detected in 100% of the blood samples of the participants. p,p'-DDT was detected in 41.3% of samples. β-HCH was present in 48.6% of samples and o,p'-DDT was found in only 3.3% of the samples analyzed [55]. Published data on the level of OCPs from the blood samples of general population from different parts of India have shown the presence of a number of OCPs. The OCPs levels ranged from 2.92 to 4.52 parts per billion (ppb) for α-HCH, 1.93–10.05 ppb for β-HCH, 1.69–5.33 ppb for γ-HCH, 0.03–3.32 ppb for aldrin, 1.97–2.77 ppb for dieldrin, 0.01–2.21 ppb for α-endosulfan, 1.18–1.49 ppb for β-endosulfan, 0.045–1.62 ppb for p,p'-DDT, and 2.18–4.26 ppb for p,p'-DDE [56]. High serum concentration of BHC and DDE (range: 0.006–0.130 ppm for BHC and 0.002–0.033 ppm for DDE) were detected in agro and non-agro professionals in and around Madurai, India [50]. A recent publication from Punjab, India, revealed the presence of p,p'-DDE, p,p'-DDD, o,p'-DDE, and β-endosulfan at mean levels of 15.26, 2.71, 5.62, and 4.02 ng/ml, respectively, from the blood samples of the study subjects. Though statistically non-significant ($p > 0.05$), higher levels of total DDT residues were detected in non-vegetarians [54]. Higher blood levels of DDT have also have been reported earlier [57]. High blood levels of endosulfan (with highest mean concentration of 0.30 mg/kg) was detected along with other organophosphate and p,p'-DDT from agro and non-agro professionals from Pakistan [58].

3.4. Association of blood OCPs levels and pathological conditions

Cumulative data from all over the world have linked a number of pathological conditions with detectable or high blood levels of OCPs such as metabolic syndrome, hypercholesterolemia, insulin resistance, preterm labor, urogenital and breast cancer, diabetes mellitus, etc. In a recent report from Thailand, the total amount of serum p,p'-DDE concentration was found to have significant correlation with plasma glucose levels [59]. Another study from Egypt has shown significant positive association of only heptachlor residue and blood glucose level among the OCPs studied [60]. A recent study from Northern Benin, West Africa has shown consistently higher serum levels of four OCPs namely p,p'-DDE, p,p'-DDT, β-HCH, and trans-nonachlor in diabetic subjects compared to non-diabetic controls [61]. In a recent publication, β-HCH and aldrin has been shown to be significantly and positively associated with the risk of having metabolic syndrome [62]. Another report from this Institute has shown significant positive association of higher blood levels of α-HCH, β-HCH, p,p'-DDE, and o',p'-DDD from mothers of preterm birth cases as compared to term controls [63]. A significant association of high blood levels of BHC and its isomers, dieldrin, heptachlor, DDT and its metabolites have been shown with the occurrence of reproductive tract cancer among women from Jaipur, India [64]. Another report from U.S. has shown that serum concentration of β-HCH, trans-nonachlor, and dieldrin has significant association with risk for prostate cancer [65].

4. OCPs exposure and CKDu

Literatures are scarce about the role of OCPs in CKDu. A recent study from the same laboratory has reported significant negative correlation of eGFR of patients of CKD of unknown etiology with blood levels of γ-HCH ($p < 0.05$), total HCH ($p < 0.05$), aldrin ($p < 0.05$), and total pesticides ($p < 0.05$). The authors also observed a tendency to accumulate pesticides by the CKD patients with decreasing eGFR. They also demonstrated a significant association of total pesticide load with increased oxidative stress in CKD patients [56]. In a previous study by the same authors from the same laboratory showed that the increased OCP levels in CKD patients were partially dependent on GSTM1/GSTT1 polymorphism and particularly GSTM1 (−)/GSTT1 (−) genotype was more vulnerable in this regard [66]. Earlier, Rutten et al. has shown the significant higher levels of HCB and p,p'-DDE in the serum of dialysed and non-dialysed uremic patients than in controls [67].

Epidemiological studies from the endemic areas strongly suggest the role of agrochemicals and pesticides in the development of CKDu. The detectable blood levels of these persistent organic pollutants in the general population worldwide confirms chronic exposure of humans to these toxins which are known to have significant and diverse adverse effect on different organ systems including kidney. In view of the available literatures till date, it seems to be plausible that chronic exposure to OCPs have a crucial role in the development and progression of CKDu although precise underlying mechanisms and evidence-based effective preventive and therapeutic strategies remains an unmet goal till date. Future research works with improved study design should focus on this important issue and fresh body of evidences is expected to emerge more and more in the days ahead.

http://dx.doi.org/10.5772/intechopen.71196

Acknowledgements

The author acknowledges Dr. Debashis Adhikary for his generous help in editing the draft and providing important suggestions which made this endeavor a success.

Author details

Rishila Ghosh[1], Manushi Siddharth[2], Pawan Kuman Kare[1], Om Prakash Kalra[3] and Ashok Kumar Tripathi[1]*

*Address all correspondence to: aktripathiucms@gmail.com

1 Department of Biochemistry, Environmental Biochemistry and Immunology Laboratory, University College of Medical Sciences (University of Delhi) and G.T.B. Hospital, Delhi, India

2 Multidisciplinary Research Unit, University College of Medical Sciences (University of Delhi) and G.T.B. Hospital, Delhi, India

3 Department of Medicine, University College of Medical Sciences (University of Delhi) and G.T.B. Hospital, Delhi, India

References

[1] Lopez-Novoa JM, Rodriguez-Pena AB, Ortiz A, Martinez-Salgado C, Lopez Hernandez FJ. Etiopathology of chronic tubular, glomerular and renovascular nephropathies: Clinical implications. Journal of Translational Medicine. 2011;**1479**:9-13

[2] World Kidney Day: Chronic Kidney Disease. 2015; http://www.worldkidneyday.org/faqs/chronic-kidney-disease/

[3] Prabahar MR, Chandrasekaran V, Soundararajan P. Epidemic of chronic kidney disease in India—What can be done? Saudi Journal of Kidney Diseases and Transplantation. 2008;**19**:847-853

[4] Kher V. End stage renal disease in developing countries. Kidney International. 2002; **62**:350-362

[5] Couser WG, Rrmuzzi G, Mendis S, Tonelli M. The contribution of chronic kidney disease to the global burden of major noncommunicable diseases. Kidney International. 2011;**12**:1258-1270

[6] Levey AS, Eckardt KU, Tsukamoto Y, Levin A, Coresh J, Rossert J, et al. Definition and classification of chronic kidney disease: Improving global outcomes (KDIGO). Kidney International. 2005;**67**:2089-2100

[7] Hsu CY, Vittinghoff E, Lin F, Shlipak MG. The incidence of end-stage renal disease in increasing faster than the prevalence of chronic renal insufficiency. Annals of Internal Medicine. 2004;**2**:95-101

[8] Molitch ME, DeFrozo RA, Franz MJ, Keane WF, Mogensen CE, Parving HH, et al. Nephropathy in diabetes. Diabetes Care. 2004;**7**:S79-S83

[9] Collins AJ, Foley RN, Chavers B. US Renal Data System 2013 Annual Data Report. American Journal of Kidney Diseases. 2014;**63**:A1-A7

[10] U.S. Renal Data System, USRDS. 2009 Annual Data Report: Atlas of Chronic Kidney Disease and End-Stage Renal Disease in the United States. Bethesda, MD: National Institutes of Health, National Institute of Diabetes and Digestive and Kidney Diseases; 2009

[11] Rajapurkar MM, John GT, Kirpalani AL, Abraham G, Agarwal SK, Almeida AF, et al. What do we know about chronic kidney disease in India: First report of the Indian CKD registry? BMC Nephrology. 2012;**13**:1-10

[12] Jayasumana MA, Paranagama PA, Dahanayake KS, Wijewardena KC, Amarasinghe MD, Fonseka SI. Possible link of chronic arsenic toxicity to chronic kidney disease of unknown etiology in Sri Lanka. Journal of Natural Science Research. 2013;**3**:64-73

[13] Jayasumana C, Orantes C, Herrera R, Almaguer M, Lopez L, Silva LC, et al. Chronic interstitial nephritis in agricultural communities: A worldwide epidemic with social, occupational and environmental determinants. Nephrology, Dialysis, Transplantation. 2016;**0**:1-8

[14] Ministry of Public Health and Social Assistance of El Salvador, Pan American Health Organization. Asociación de Nefrología e Hipertensión Arterial de El Salvador. Recomendaciones del Primer Taller de Salud Renal al Ministerio de Salud y Asistencia Social de El Salvador [Internet]. San Salvador: Ministry of Public Health and Social Assistance of El Salvador; 2010 [cited 2013 Oct 21]. Available from: http://nefrologiaelsalvador.com/wp-content/uploads/2013/05/DECLARACION-TALLER-SALUD-RENAL-160310.doc Spanish

[15] Almaguer M, Herrera R. Chronic kidney disease of unknown etiology in agricultural communities. MEDICC Review. 2014;**16**:9-15

[16] Jayasekara KB, Dissanayake DM, Sivakanesan R. Epidemiology of chronic kidney disease, with special emphasis on chronic kidney disease of uncertain etiology, in north central region of Sri Lanka. Journal of Epidemiology. 2015;**25**:275-280

[17] Brooks D. Final Scoping Study Report. Epidemiology of Chronic Kidney Disease in Nicaragua [Internet]. Boston: Boston University School of Public Health; 2009. Available from: http://www.cao-ombudsman.org/cases/documentlinks/documents/03H_BU_FINAL_report_scope study CRI_18.Dec.2009.pdf

[18] Cerdas. Chronic kidney disease in Costa Rica. Kidney International. Supplement. 2005;**97**: S31-S33

[19] Navarro CMO, Valdes RH, Lopez MA, Calero DJ, de Morales JF, Ascencio NPA et al. Epidemiological characteristics of chronic kidney disease of non-traditional causes in woman of agricultural communities of El Salvador. Clinical Nephrology. 2015;**83**:S24-S31

[20] Kamell EG, El-Minshawy O. Environmental factors incriminated in the development of end stage renal disease in El-Mina Governorate, Upper Egypt. International Journal of Nephrology and Urology. 2010;**3**:431-437

[21] El-Minshawy O. End stage renal disease in the El-Mina governorate, Upper Ezypt: An epidemiological study. Saudi Journal of Kidney Diseases and Transplantation. 2011;**5**: 1048-1054

[22] Machiraju RS, Yaradi K, Gowrishankar S, Edwards KL, Attaluri S, Miller F, et al. Epidemiology of Udhanam endemic nephrology. Journal of the American Society of Nephrology. 2009;**643A**:20

[23] Athuraliya NT, Abeysekera TD, Amerasinghe PH, Kumarasiri R, Bandara P, Karunaratne U, et al. Uncertain etiologies of proteinuric-chronic kidney disease in rural Sri Lanka. Kidney International. 2011;**11**:1212-1221

[24] Noiri C, Shimizu T, Takayanagi K. Clinical significance of fractional magnesium excretion (FEMg) as a predictor of interstitial nephropathy and its correlation with conventional parameters. Clinical and Experimental Nephrology. 2015;**19**:1071-1078

[25] Ministry of Health. Chronic Kidney Disease of Unknown Etiology; Circular no 01-10/2009. Colombo, Sri Lanka: Ministry of Health; 2009

[26] Nanayakkara S, Komiya T, Ratnatunga N. Tubulointerstitial damage as the major pathological lesion in endemic chronic kidney disease among farmers in North Central Province of Sri Lanka. Environmental Health and Preventive Medicine. 2012;**17**:213-221

[27] Lopez-Marin L, Chavez Y, Garcia XA, Flores WM, Garcia YM, Herrera R. Histopathology of chronic kidney disease of unknown etiology in Salvadoran agricultural communities. MEDICC Review. 2014;**16**:49-54

[28] Wijetunge S, Ratnatunga NV, Abeysekera TD. Endemic chronic kidney disease of unknown etiology in Sri Lanka: Correlation of pathology with clinical stages. Indian Journal of Nephrology. 2015;**25**:274-280

[29] Lopez-Marin L, Chavez Y, Garcia XA. Histopathology of chronic kidney disease of unknown etiology in Salvadoran agricultural communities. MEDICC Review. 2014;**16**:49-54

[30] Pimentel D. Green revolution agriculture and chemical hazards. Science of the Total Environment. 1996;**188**:S86-S98

[31] Wimalawansa SA, Wimalawansa SJ. Impact of changing agricultural practices on human health: Chronic kidney disease of multi-factorial origin in Sri Lanka. Journal of Agricultural Research. 2014;**3**:110-234

[32] Jayatilake N, Mendis S, Maheepala P, Mehta FR. CKDu National Research Project Team. Chronic kidney disease of uncertain aetiology: Prevalence and causative factors in a developing country. BMC Nephrology 2013;**14**:1-13

[33] Wanigasuriya KP, Peiris-John RJ, Wickremasinghe R. Chronic renal failure in North Central Province of Sri Lanka: An environmentally induced disease. Transactions of the Royal Society of Tropical Medicine and Hygiene. 2007;**101**:1013-1017

[34] Jayasekara JM, Dissanayake DM, Adhikari SB. Geographical distribution of chronic kidney disease of unknown origin in north central region of Sri Lanka. Ceylon Medical Journal. 2013;**58**:6-10

[35] Meharg AA, Norton G, Deacon C. Variation in rice cadmium related to human exposure. Environmental Science and Technology. 2013;**47**:5613-5618

[36] Nanayakkara S, Senevirathna S, Abeysekera T. An integrative study of the genetic, social and environmental determinants of chronic kidney disease characterized by tubulointerstitial damages in the north central region of Sri Lanka. Journal of Occupational Health. 2014;**56**:28-38

[37] Peraza S, Wesseling C, Aragon A, Leiva R, Garcia RA, Torres C, et al. Decreased kidney function among agricultural workers in El Salvador. American Journal of Kidney Diseases. 2012;**4**:531-540

[38] Herrera R, Orantes CM, Almaguer M, Alfonso P, Bayarre HD, Leiva IM, et al. Clinical characteristics of chronic kidney disease of non-traditional causes in Salvadoran farming communities. MEDICC Review. 2014;**2**:39-48

[39] Agrawal A, Sharma B. Pesticides induced oxidative stress in mammalian systems. International Journal of Biomedical Research. 2010;**3**:90-104

[40] Ellenhorn MJ, Schonwald S, Ordog G, Wasserberger J. Ellenhorn's Medical Toxicology: Diagnosis and Treatment of Human Poisoning. Maryland: Williams & Wilkins; 1997. p. 1614-1663

[41] Siddiqui MK, Srivastava S, Srivastava SP, Mehrotra PK, Mathur N. Persistent chlorinated pesticides and intra-uterine foetal growth retardation: A possible association. International Archives of Occupational and Environmental Health. 2003;**76**:75-80

[42] Pant N, Mathur N, Banerjee AK, Srivastava SP, Saxena DK. Correlation of chlorinated pesticides concentration in semen with seminal vesicle and prostatic markers. Reproductive Toxicology. 2004;**19**:209-214

[43] Devanathan G, Subramanian A, Someya M, Sudaryanto A, Isobe T. Persistent organochlorines in human breast milk from major metropolitan cities in India. Environmental Pollution. 2009;**157**:148-154

[44] Sharma E, Mustafa M, Pathak R, Guleria K, Ahmed RS. A case control study of gene environmental interaction in fetal growth restriction with special reference to organochlorine pesticides. European Journal of Obstetrics & Gynaecology and Reproductive Biology. 2012;**161**:163-169

[45] Dewan P, Jain V, Gupta P, Banerjee BD. Organochlorine pesticide residues in maternal blood, cord blood, placenta and breast milk and their relation to birth size. Chemosphere. 2013;**90**:1704-1710

[46] Bentzen TW, Follman EH, Amstrup SC, York GS, Woller MJ, Muir DCG, et al. Dietary biomagnification of organochlorine contaminants in Alaskan polar bears. Canadian Journal of Zoology. 2008;**3**:177-191

[47] Mwevura H, Othman OC, Mehe GL. Organochlorine pesticide residues in edible biota from the coastal area of Dares Salaam city. Journal of Marine Science. 2002;**1**:91-96

[48] Fitzgerald E, Hwang SA, Deres DA, Bush B, Cook K, Worswick P. The association between local fish consumption and DDE, mirex, and HCB concentrations in the breast milk of Mohawk women at Akwesanse. Journal of Exposure Analysis and Environmental Epidemiology. 2001;**11**:381-388

[49] Jurewicz J, Hanke W. Prenatal and childhood exposure to pesticides and neurobehavioral development: Review of epidemiological studies. International Journal of Occupational Medicine and Environmental Health. 2008;**2**:121-132

[50] Subhramanium K, Solomon J. Organochlorine pesticides BHC and DDE in human blood in and around Madurai, India. Indian Journal of Clinical Biochemistry. 2006;**2**:169-172

[51] Thakur JS, Rao BT, Rajwanshi A, Parwana HK, Kumar R. Epidemiological study of high cancer among rural agricultural community of Punjab in northern India. Environmental Research and Public Health. 2008;**5**:399-407

[52] Chatterjee SK, Kashyap SK, Gupta SK. Pesticide Pollution Due to Chlorinated Insecticides Especially DDT in the Environment of Man and Other Livestock in the Country. Report of a DST Project. Ahmedabad: National Institute of Occupational Health; 1980

[53] Raha P, Agarwal NR, Samanta S. Organochlorine pesticide residues in mother milk. In: Agnihotri NP, Walia S, Gajbhiya VT, editors. Green Pesticides, Crop Protection and Safety Evaluation. Society of Pesticide Science; 1999. p. 231-234

[54] Bedi JS, Gill JPS, Kaur P, Sharma A, Aulakh RS. Evaluation of pesticide residues in human blood samples from Punjab (India). Veterinary World. 2015;**8**:66-71

[55] Waliszewski SM, Caba M, Herrero-Mercado M, Saldariaga-Norena H, Meza E, et al. Organochlorine pesticide residue levels in blood serum of inhabitants from Veracruz, Mexico. Environmental Health and Monitoring. 2012;**184**:5613-5621

[56] Siddharth M, Datta SK, Bansal S, Mustafa M, Banerjee BD, Kalra OP, et al. Study on organochlorine pesticide levels in chronic kidney disease patients: Association with estimated glomerular filtration rate and oxidative stress. Journal of Biochemical and Molecular Toxicology. 2012;**26**:241-247

[57] Kumar A, Baroth A, Soni I, Bhatnagar P, John PJ. Organochlorine pesticide residues in milk and blood of women from Anupgarh, Rajasthan, India. Environmental Monitoring and Assessment. 2006;**116**:1-7

[58] Latif Y, Sherazi STH, Bhanger MI, Nizamani S. Evaluation of pesticide residues in human blood samples of agro professionals and non-agro professionals. American Journal of Analytical Chemistry. 2012;**3**:587-595

[59] Teeyapant P, Ramchiun S, Polputpisatkul D, Uttawichai C, Parnmen S. Serum concentrations of organochlorine pesticides p,p′-DDE in adult Thai residents with background levels of exposure. The Journal of Toxicological Sciences. 2014;**39**:121-127

[60] Sharaf NE, Amer NM, Ibrahim KS, El-Tahlawy EM, Abdelgelil KS. Pesticides usage in agriculture among rural women in Egypt: Association between serum organo-chlorine pesticide residues and occurrence of diabetes. World Journal of Medical Sciences. 2013;**1**:8-15

[61] Azandjeme CS, Bouchard M, Francois D, Houinato D, Delisle H. Serum concentrations of organochlorine pesticides associated with diabetes and obesity in northern Benin (West Africa). Journal of Environmental and Occupational Sciences. 2014;**3**:121-129

[62] Tomar LR, Agarwal MP, Avasthi R, Tyagi V, Mustafa MD, Banerjee BD. Serum organochlorine pesticide levels in patients with metabolic syndrome. Indian Journal of Endocrinology and Metabolism. 2013;**17**:S342-S344

[63] Md M, Garg N, Banerjee BD, Sharma T, Tyagi V, Dar SA, et al. Inflammatory-mediated pathway in association with organochlorine pesticides levels in the etiology of idiopathic preterm birth. Reproductive Toxicology. 2015;**57**:111-120

[64] Mathur V, John PJ, Soni I, Bhatnagar P. Blood levels of organochlorine pesticide residues and risk of reproductive tract cancer among women from Jaipur, India. Advances in Experimental Medicine and Biology. 2008;**617**:387-394

[65] Xu X, Dailey AB, Talbott EO, Iiacqua VA, Kearney G, Asal NR. Associations of serum concentrations of organochlorine pesticides with breast cancer and prostate cancer in U.S. adults. Environmental Health Perspectives. 2010;**118**:60-66

[66] Siddarth M, Datta SK, Mustafa MD, Ahmed RS, Banerjee BD, Kalra OP, Tripathi AK. Increased level of organochlorine pesticides in chronic kidney disease patients of unknown etiology: Role of GSTM1/GSTT1 polymorphism. Chemosphere. 2014;**96**(1-7)

[67] Rutten GA, Schoots AC, Vanholder R, Desmet R, Ringoir SM, Cramers CA. Hexachlorobenzene and 1,1-di(4-chlorophenyl)-2,2-dichloroethene in serum of uremic patients and healthy persons: Determination by capillary gas chromatography an electron capture detection. Nephron. 1988;**48**:217-221

Chapter 10

Nutritional Status Disorders in Chronic Kidney Disease: Practical Aspects (Systematic Review)

Ludmila Y. Milovanova, Victor V. Fomin,
Lidia V. Lysenko (Kozlovskaya), Yuriy S. Milovanov,
Nikolay A. Mukhin, Vasiliy V. Kozlov,
Marina V. Taranova, Svetlana Y. Milovanova,
Marina V. Lebedeva and Aigul Zh. Usubalieva

Additional information is available at the end of the chapter

http://dx.doi.org/10.5772/intechopen.69297

Abstract

Despite the significant achievements in the management of chronic kidney disease (CKD) patients, the mortality rate of these patients still remains high. Nutritional status disorders (NSD) are considered now as one of the prognostic risk factors not only for dialysis but also for predialysis CKD stages. Since the publication of KDIGO 2012 guidelines for CKD patient's management, there has been some significant advancement in our understanding of main NSD mechanisms in CKD, including different nosological group patients (first, in diabetic and systemic diseases patients). At the same time, there is still an urgent need for randomized trials for better-informed decisions and future optimization of CKD patients' care. This chapter provides the current data on all aspects of NSD in CKD: etiology, diagnosis, prevention, and treatment approaches, as well as on risk factors of NSD at predialysis stages and in chronic hemodialysis patients. Considerable attention was devoted to the diagnosis and differential diagnosis of NSD in CKD patients. It was determined that the overall strategy for dietary treatment contributed to improving the life quality of patients and slowing down of CKD progression. The review is written based on the published results of clinical studies performed on the position of evidence-based medicine.

Keywords: chronic kidney disease, nutrition status disorders, protein energy wasting, Klotho

1. Introduction

One of the actual problems of nephrology is to improve quality of life and overall survival of patients with chronic kidney disease (CKD), the prevalence of which is steadily growing throughout the world. Therefore, the retardation of CKD progression and prevention of its complications, as well as the delay of renal replacement therapy (RRT) onset, are the primary medical and social-economical goal [1–3].

The rate of renal failure progression depends on a range of factors, and among them, nutritional status disorders (NSD) have the important prognostic value [2, 3]. Early detection of NSD requires a further in-depth examination of a patient to identify the potential cause (or causes) of NSD. NSD develops 2.5 times more often in patients with systemic disease that is caused by both the underlying disease activity (increased levels of inflammatory cytokines) and duration of corticosteroid therapy in addition to the general CKD risk factors [4]. NSD at predialysis CKD stages is found mainly to occur in diabetes mellitus, in patients with severe anemia (hemoglobin <100 g/l) or with high proteinuria (more than 2.5 g/day), as well as in patients who eat low-calorie nutrition (less than 30 kcal/kg/day) [1, 2, 5].

Low-protein diet (LPD) is considered now as more optimal for CKD patients. LPD, reducing glomerular hypertension, favors decreasing proteinuria as well as hemodynamic damage of renal glomeruli and thus contributing to a slowdown of CKD progression [2, 6, 7]. The influence of LPD on CKD progression is more expressed in case of diabetic nephropathy (DN). The annual rate of glomerular filtration rate (GFR) decline in patients who follow LPD and slow down by 1.5–2 times compared with standard diet, and outcome to the end-stage of CKD is observed less often almost by three times [5, 7]. Renal protective effects of LPD are connected with its hemodynamic and metabolic abilities. The adjustment of protein and phosphorus contents in the diet in accordance with patient's residual renal function contributes to reducing hemodynamic load to the residual nephrons, in addition to the decreasing of uremic intoxication. As a result, the glomerular hypertrophy process as well as the renin-angiotensin-aldosterone system (RAAS) activation decreases, intraglomerular autoregulation normalizes, and intraglomerular and systemic hypertension reduces. LPD also partially corrects such unfavorable uremic, metabolic, and endocrine complications, such as hypoalbuminemia, dyslipidemia, anemia, hyperphosphatemia with parathyroid glands hyperplasia, and thereby it helps to reduce the risk of uremic hyperparathyroidism, vascular calcification, and atherosclerosis [2, 8, 9]. LPD in combination with ketoanalogs of essential amino acids enhances also antihypertensive and antiproteinuric effects of angiotensin receptor blockers (ARB), corrective action of erythropoietins in anemia, effects of synthetic vitamin D analogs and calcimimetics on hyperparathyroidism symptoms, and hypolipidemic effect of statins [4, 10, 11].

It was found that the mortality rate of dialysis patients is inversely related to the amount of protein intake (protein quota), body mass index, and serum albumin [1, 12].

Improvement of the approaches to the early diagnosis, treatment, and prevention of NSD in CKD patients is an important strategy to reduce cardiovascular (CV) and overall mortality, to increase quality of life, as well as to reduce the cost of hospital and RRT treatment [1, 13].

http://dx.doi.org/10.5772/intechopen.69297

The review was written based on the published results of clinical studies performed on the position of evidence-based medicine. It is intended not only for nephrologists but also for internists, cardiologists, and endocrinologists.

2. Methods

Literature searches were made of 10 major databases among which were PubMed, Medline, Embase, Cochrane Library, CINAHL, and e-library. The search was carried out to find all articles relevant to CKD and Nutrition Status Disorders. This search encompassed original articles, systematic reviews, and meta-analyses. There was no language restriction.

2.1. Agreed criteria for article inclusion in the review

Articles should be full-text. Brief publications and abstracts were not included:

- Research should include at least 20 patients in each group. The minimum mean duration of a study was 6 months.
- Analyzed literature over past 15 years.
- The article has the detailed research protocol for assessing its quality.
- Patients examination must meet KDIGO 2012 guidelines.
- Randomized controlled trials.
- Retrospective nonrandomized trials.

3. Nutritional status disorders in chronic kidney disease patients

The International Society of Renal Nutrition and Metabolism (ISRNM) [14] recommended the term "Protein-energy wasting (PEW)" to describe the state of decreased body stores of protein and energy in CKD patients and proposed a common nomenclature and diagnostic criteria for these alterations in the context of CKD.

3.1. Prevalence PEW in CKD

PEW was traditionally considered for a long time as the problem of patients who receive RRT. Meanwhile, the results of epidemiological studies conducted for recent years have convincingly demonstrated that nutritional status disorders appear to be revealed much earlier, before dialysis treatment starting, from stages 3B–4 CKD, and impact on prognosis of patients on dialysis [1, 2, 12, 13, 15]. The incidence of PEW depends on the stage of CKD (**Table 1**): among CKD patients with a glomerular filtration rate (GFR) of 44–30 ml/min/1.73m^2, PEW is detected in 4.2% of cases in average, whereas in CKD patients with GFR of 29-15 ml/min/1.73m^2 in 21.3%, and almost all patients with end-stage of CKD have PEW [1, 2, 7, 13, 15, 16].

CKD stage	Description	GFR, ml/min/1.73 m²	Incidence of PEW
1	Kidney damage with normal or increased GFR	≥90	No
2	Kidney damage with mildly decreased GFR	89–60	No
3		59–30	
3a	Mild-to-moderate decrease in GFR	59–45	No
3b	Moderate-to-severe decrease in GFR	44–30	4.2%
4	Severely decreased GFR	29–15	21.3%
5	End-stage of renal failure	<15 or RRT onset	74.5%

GFR: glomerular filtration rate, is calculated by CKD-EPI creatinine equation (2009); PEW: protein-energy wasting; and RRT: renal replacement therapy.

Table 1. Incidence of PEW depending on CKD stage.

At the predialysis stages, PEW is typical for patients with DN because of insulin deficiency or insulin resistance, accelerating protein catabolism, as well as due to a high incidence of infectious complications, diabetic neuropathy of gastrointestinal tract with malabsorption, [1, 5, 15, 17]; for patients with systemic diseases; high proteinuria (more than 2.5 g/day); severe anemia (hemoglobin <100 g/L); for those who receive prolonged corticosteroid therapy (more than 6 months); for patients who eat low-calorie foods (less than 30 kcal/kg/day) [1, 2, 4, 15].

3.2. Etiology and pathogenesis

In contrast to the end products of fat and carbohydrate metabolism (CO_2 and H_2O) that are excreted through the lungs and skin, the products of protein metabolism can be excreted only by kidneys [7, 16].

Qualitative protein food composition is very important because the absence or deficiency of at least one of any essential amino acid (EAA) may be a limiting factor for protein biosynthesis in the body. Even when the dietary intake provides all amino acids, the body may suffer from a protein deficiency if the absorption of any amino acid decreases in the intestine, or when it breaks up more than usual under the influence of gut microbiota. In these cases, limited protein synthesis will occur or the body will compensate for the lack of amino acid required for protein biosynthesis by breaking down its own proteins [9, 18]. Changes in protein metabolism in uremia are closely related to amino acid metabolism disturbance. Due to a decrease in the metabolically active mass of the kidneys, the deficiency of the enzymes synthesized in the kidneys, which are necessary for the formation of amino acids, develops [9, 13]. Decrease in plasma concentration of EAA can also be largely due to acidosis [15, 17].

The degree of protein and amino acids assimilation from food also depends on the quantitative and qualitative composition of carbohydrates and lipids. Experimental and clinical data indicate that a diet with insufficient fat and low-calorie diet contribute to the increased oxidation of amino acids, intensified degradation, and, partly, even protein synthesis [7, 18]. Protein metabolism, in turn, is closely integrated with the exchange of carbohydrates, lipids, and nucleic acids through amino acids or α-ketoacids (α-ketoglutarate, oxaloacetate, and pyruvate). Thus, aspartic acid or alanine through the transamination way is reversibly converted to pyruvate oxaloacetate, which are subsequently directly included in the carbohydrate metabolism. An inverse relationship was found between the leptin concentration and the nutritional status (NS) parameters and a direct relationship with the leptin of the C-reactive protein (CRP) [19].

Proteins (and consequently, amino acids as products of their hydrolysis) are directly involved in the biosynthesis of a number of hormones and other biologically active compounds that regulate metabolic processes in the body. With insufficient intake of protein from food, the protein from its own pool disintegrate into free amino acids, which ensure the synthesis of the necessary cytoplasmic fractions of protein, enzymes, hormones, and other biologically active compounds [16, 18].

PEW in CKD can also be exacerbated by eating mostly plant proteins of low biological value and low-calorie diet. This increases the insulin secretion, which inhibits lipolysis and mobilization of skeletal muscle proteins. These disturbances lead to that the levels of amino acids in the blood drop the levels of amino acids in the blood drop, the synthesis of albumin and other proteins decreases, leading to hypoalbuminemia. The adaptation mechanism includes hormonal changes. These changes help mobilize free fatty acids from adipose tissue and amino acids from the muscles. Gluconeogenesis and oxidation of amino acids provide the energy that is necessary for the organism-sustaining processes, as a result, protein synthesis is inhibited, metabolism is slowed down, and muscle mass and body fat stores decrease [1, 6, 9].

An important role in the development of PEW is assigned to cytokines and chemokines, which begin to accumulate in the blood of patients as the stage of CKD progresses. Cytokines, suppressing appetite, cause loss of body weight [13, 18]. Patients with CKD, stages 4–5, are prone to negative nitrogen balance and hypercatabolism due to anorexia, inhibition of protein and amino acid synthesis, and the deficiency of vitamins and microelements [1, 16].

In acute and chronic infections or immune inflammations, there are effects of tumor necrosis factor α (TNF α), interleukin 2 and 6 (IL-2 and IL-6), etc., which also contribute to the development of hypoalbuminemia and worsen the prognosis [1, 20].

At the same time, in chronic renal failure patients who ignore the use of protein restricted diet and consume protein in the amounts greater than recommended for their stage of CKD, progressively increased levels of glycation products are observed, which trigger a complex cascade of reactions involving the generation of active forms of oxygen. Amino acids, proteins, carbohydrates, and lipids (primarily unsaturated fatty acids both free and in the composition of phospholipids) are subjected to reactions of free radical oxidation involving reactive oxygen species [1, 16]. Acidosis, induced by uncontrolled protein intake, leads to suppression of amino acid synthesis, increases their decarboxylation in muscles, and reduces albumin synthesis [17].

3.3. Classification

In clinical practice in the predialysis patient population, PEW is divided into three degrees: mild, moderate, and severe [1, 14, 21]. The degree of PEW is established by determining the ratio of body weight/recommended body weight × 100%. A decreased ratio down to 80% means a mild degree of nutritional disorder, a decrease from 80–70%—moderate, and less than 70%—severe nutrition disorder.

3.4. Clinical presentation

Complaints depending on the underlying pathology that caused signs of PEW: a weight loss over the past 6 months, poor appetite, in case of severe PEW—refusal to eat, vomiting, nausea, bloating, diarrhea, constipation, abdominal pain, edema, cramps, cough, shortness of breath, prolonged fever, anxiety, dry skin, hair loss, deformation of the nails, and weakness.

Medical history allows to identify the *kidney disease*, which has led to the development of PEW.

3.4.1. Physical examination

Assessment of nutritional status is carried out on a four- or seven-point scale. A seven-point scale evaluation is considered more reliable [14, 21, 22].

The following basic criteria are important:

- The dynamics of the patient's weight since the last examination (usually for 6 months).
- The protein quota intake and calorie content of food calculated according to a 3-day food diary; the presence of symptoms of gastrointestinal dysfunction.
- The status of the patient's fat and muscle mass bases on a visual examination (shoulder line, the contouring of clavicles, shoulder blades, and ribs) and palpation (the thickness of the fat fold above the biceps and triceps, muscular mass of the triceps, and muscles between the thumb and index finger). To objectify the data, the caliper can be used to measure the fat fold thickness in several places (subscapular region, above the biceps, triceps, and iliac crest) and the shoulder circumference in the middle third.

Familiarity with the anamnesis and physical examination reveals the **clinical picture of PEW** [1, 13, 14, 21]:

- Decrease in the body weight by 10% over the last 6 months and shorter period; poor appetite.
- Reduced subcutaneous tissue.
- Possible apathy, fast fatigue, decreased taste, and slowing of peristalsis.
- Subjective assessment (according to seven-point scale) ≤ 5 points.
- Basal metabolic rate and body temperature are lowered due to decreased levels of triiodothyronine (T_3) below 3.5 pg/ml and loss of the heat-insulating function of the subcutaneous tissue.

3.4.1.1. Mild-to-moderate PEW

Symptoms of nutritional disorders are characterized by a decrease in the body weight (by 3–5% per month) and a progressive decrease in appetite with the development of anorexia. The thickness of the skin-fat fold (SFFT) above the triceps muscle of the shoulder as well as a muscular mass in the shoulder region is reduced. The blood levels of albumin, prealbumin, transferrin, and triiodothyronine (T3) decrease. Lymphopenia and impaired glucose tolerance may develop.

3.4.1.2. *Severe PEW*

It is accompanied by more pronounced changes in clinical and laboratory parameters. Physical examination reveals the intercostal depression, atrophy of the temporal muscles, and muscles of the extremities. Subcutaneous fat tissue is atrophied or absent. Apathy, rapid fatigue, and a feeling of cold are often symptoms of hypovitaminosis (vitamins B, C, folic acid, D_3 and B_{12}, and PP); deficiency of trace elements (iron, zinc, copper, and selenium), calcium, arginine and L-carnitine are added symptoms; and signs of oxidative stress, aggravating renal anemia, cardiomyopathy, myopathy, encephalopathy, and hypertension also accompany. There may be atrophy of intestinal villi and increased growth of microflora in the small intestine.

3.5. Diagnosis

Diagnostic challenges with PEW arise from a variety of causes and also because the body weight of patients changes a little due to sodium and water retention and decrease only at the last stage of CKD [1, 7, 21, 22].

3.5.1. *Anthropometric methods of assessment*

Anthropometric methods include determination of body mass index and evaluation of muscle and fat mass of the body [1, 14, 21]. The body mass index (BMI) (Quetelet index, kg/m^2) is calculated by the formula: BMI = $M/L2$, where M is the body weight in kilograms and L is the height of a person measured in meters and squared.

Measurement of the SFFT by a caliper at 4 points (subscapular region, above the biceps, triceps, and iliac crest) allows to calculate the proportion of fat component as a percentage of the total body weight, which is 15–16% in healthy men and 25% in women. If the SFFT is reduced by more than 10% from the normal value, it indicates a predominant *energy insufficiency* [1, 14, 22].

The amount of fat in the body (fat mass) can be calculated by the formula: $D = d \times S \times K$, where D is fat mass (kg); d is the average thickness of the subcutaneous fat layer together with the skin (sm) = $(d_1 + d_2 + d_3 + d_4)/8$, where d_1 is above the triceps; d_2 is above the biceps; d_3 is above the shoulder blade; d_4 is on the abdomen; S is the surface of the body = $M^{0.425} \times P^{0.725} \times 71.84 \times 10^{-4}$, where M is the weight (kg), P is height (sm), and K is a constant equal to 1.3.

About the muscle mass, it can be indirectly judged by the formula: SMV (sm) = SC (sm) – 0.314 × SFFT (mm), where SMV is the shoulder muscles volume; SC is shoulder circumference at mid-shoulder level; and SFFT is the skin-fat fold thickness above the triceps at the point of shoulder circumference measurement. Deficiency of SMV, exceeding 10%, is typical for *protein deficiency*.

For dialysis PEW, a combination of muscle deficiency with a decreased volume of adipose tissue is typical. Assessment of anthropometric parameters should be performed in all patients with CKD once every 3 months.

Anthropometric criteria of PEW are BMI <18.5 kg/m^2; SFFT in men <9.5 mm, in women <13 mm; SMV in men <23 cm, in women <21 cm. At the same time, SFFT is a reflection of body fat reserves, and SMV is an indicator of the peripheral protein pool.

3.5.2. Laboratory diagnostics

For the diagnose of impairments in the synthesis of visceral proteins, the determination of the content of albumin, transferrin, and lymphocytes number in the blood, as well as of the level and spectrum of essential amino acids, is used [1, 14, 21]. The serum albumin level only is insufficient for the decision about NS in CKD patients, since its level depends on the intravascular volume and the half-life period of albumin is approximately 21 days [14]. Therefore, a decrease in the albumin serum level is a relatively a late marker of PEW. It should be taken into account that the decrease in serum albumin level may be due to the other causes, in addition to PEW. Infections, injuries, and surgical interventions, associated with blood and plasma loses; a high level of proteinuria; and disturbances of the protein-synthetic function of the liver can cause a rapid and significant decrease in serum albumin level [14]. On the other hand, prolonged and persistent decrease in serum albumin level regardless of its cause always leads to PEW in CKD patients [1, 14]. Hypoalbuminemia is closely associated with an increase in concomitant diseases, hospitalizations, and the mortality rate of CKD patients [1, 3, 20, 23].

The association of hypoalbuminemia with inflammatory process may be established using the ratio of the levels of albumin and C-reactive protein in serum [1, 4, 13, 14].

An important diagnostic marker of PEW is also a low serum level of transferrin in the blood and is representative of the fraction of beta-globulin; its decrease is observed at an earlier stage of protein metabolism disturbance than changes in albumin levels (lifetime of transferrin is 7–8 days). However, the concentration of transferrin may increase the iron deficiency usually accompanying PEW, which should be taken into account in determining the severity of PEW [1, 14, 21].

More accurate markers of the visceral protein pool status are both short-lived transport proteins—prealbumin (lifespan is 2 days) and retino-binding protein (lifespan is 10–12 h). The prealbumin level below 0.3 g/l is associated with an increased risk of death and correlates with other indicators of PEW [13, 14, 16]. Their content in serum decreases earlier in the case of protein deficiency in the diet, although it can quickly decrease due to intercurrent diseases [14].

The degree of PEW correlates with the content of lymphocytes in blood [14, 15]. Therefore, the absolute number of lymphocytes in the blood can be used to judge the severity of PEW in patients with CKD: absolute number of lymphocytes = % of lymphocytes × number of white blood cells/100.

The laboratory signs of PEW are serum albumin <35 g/l; serum transferrin <180 mg/dl; and absolute number of blood lymphocytes <1800

The study of serum protein counts and the absolute number of lymphocytes should be carried out once every 3 months, and if necessary—once every 1.5 months [1, 14].

3.5.3. Instrumental diagnostics

From the instrumental methods for the main body components assessing, the method of 2-hour bioimpedanceometry is most often used in practical work in connection with the ability to quantitatively determine not only fatty tissue and muscle mass of the body but also the distribution of fluid in the body [22, 24]. Complex instrumental methods for analyzing NS of the body (neutron activation analysis, two-photon X-ray absorptiometry, etc.) are not widely available due to high cost.

Bioimpedansometry measures the volume of the total fluid and the proportion of extracellular and cellular fluids separately, allows to establish a nonfat body mass and a "dry weight," and thus contributes to the selection of an effective mode of HD and ultrafiltration as well as the value of the protein quota.

DEXA is a noninvasive method for assessing the condition of the three main body components (fatty tissue, muscle mass, bone mass, and bone mineral density). The state of hyperhydration of dialysis patients practically does not affect the accuracy of DEXA. The principle of the DEXA method is the scanning of a body in a rectilinear section with the help of two beams of photons emitted by an X-ray source. Different tissues (fat, muscle, and bone) absorb X-rays in varying degrees. The composition of the body is calculated from the ratio of the natural logarithms of the absorbed and unabsorbed beams [14, 22].

Fresenius Medical Care (Germany) company has developed a device that allows to determine the individual fluid balance and body composition of the patient—the Body Composition Monitor (BCM). The BCM can be used in patients with CKD, regardless of patient's treatment. The measurement is based on the bioimpedance spectroscopy technology, which allows to calculate the volume of body water (total, intra-, and extracellular), as well as muscle and fat mass of the body (**Table 2**). Since the total body water (TBW) index is equivalent to the urea volume distribution (V), it is not necessary to spend working time for calculating urea kinetic modeling and calculating TBW based on anthropometric parameters. Indicator V can be used to calculate the dose of dialysis [22].

In addition to the anthropometric (BMI, SFFT, and SMV) and laboratory (albumin, transferrin, and absolute number of lymphocytes) indicators of NS, the evaluation of protein

Parameter	Gender	Age	Normal range
BMI, kg/m^2			19.5 ± 0.33 (23–18.4)
Body fat mass, %	M	20–39	12.9 ± 0.65 (19.9–8.0)
		40–59	18.1 ± 0.41(21.9–11.0)
		60–79	20.7 ± 0.66 (24.9–13.0)
	F	20–39	29.1 ± 0.44 (32.9–21.0)
		40–59	26.4 ± 0.51 (33.9–2.30)
		60–79	27.8 ± 0.35 (35.9–24.0)
Body muscles mass, %	M	18–39	35.4 ± 0.75 (39.3–33.3)
		40–59	37.1 ± 0.85 (39.1–31.1)
		60–80	34.6 ± 0.31 (38.9–32.9)
	F	18–39	26.2 ± 0.45 (30.3–24.3)
		40–59	27.1 ± 0.65 (30.1–24.1)
		60–80	27.3 ± 0.55 (29.9–23.9)

BMI: body mass index; M: male; F: female; and BIA: bioimpedance analysis.

Table 2. Normal range of nutritional status parameters according to BIA.

intake and calorie content of food assessed according to a three-day food diary is needed [22, 25].

Integrated assessment of nutritional status can be performed also using the malnutrition inflammation score (MIS) scale. It allows to analyze anthropometric data (BMI, dry weight dynamics, body fat, and muscle mass), gastrointestinal symptoms, dialysis time, laboratory data (albumin and blood transferrin), hospitalization rates, and the risk of lethality on dialysis [14, 22].

All patients with an identified PEW should be given anthropometric measurements (or bioelectrical impedance analysis), a clinical and biochemical blood test, and a general urinalysis at least one time per 1.5 months, an analysis of protein intake and calorie content on a 3-day food diary for at least one time in 3 months [1, 15, 21].

3.6. Differential diagnosis

PEW should be differentiated with a malabsorption syndrome, given a number of common manifestations (progressive decrease in BMI and blood albumin). In contrast to malabsorption, chronic diarrhea with steatorrhea and creatoria is not typical for PEW; while there is pronounced increase in serum CRP and TNF-α, calcification of the arteries [1, 14, 20] is found [1, 14, 20].

According to the WHO, the diagnostic sign of PEW is a decrease in the mental and physical performance of patients, identified as a decrease in the quality of life when determining the psychosomatic status according to the standard questionnaires of Kidney Disease Quality of life short form (KDQOL-SF) [1].

3.7. Prognosis

Disorders of nutritional status are of great prognostic importance, since they significantly impact on the survival and level of rehabilitation of these patients. According to a single-site study [23], the mortality rate during the first year on dialysis therapy was 1% in patients with a serum albumin level > 38 g/l at the moment of admission to HD treatment, and 30% for patients in whom the serum albumin did not exceed 30 g/l.

3.8. Possibilities for PEW correction in CKD: goals and approaches

In CKD patients at the predialysis stage with PEW, the main goal of the treatment is to eliminate the factors contributing to the progression of nutritional disorders and to achieve the stabilization of renal failure [1, 14, 21]. The main aim of the diet is to inhibit glomerular hypertrophy and intraglomerular hypertension, to reduce the traffic load to tubules, to decrease cytokines and uremic toxins production: (TGF-β, ATII, oxygen radicals, TIMP (tissue inhibitor matrix metalloproteinases), indoxyl sulfate, guanidine, phosphates, oxalic acid, NO, etc.)

In most patients with CKD and systemic disease (systemic lupus erythematosus, and systemic vasculitis) with persistent disease activity, therapy (correction of the diet and hypertension, suppression of disease activity by glucocorticosteroids (GS) and/or cytostatics) can allow to slow the progression of renal failure and eliminates PEW [1, 4]. However, it should be borne in mind that the long-term (more than 6 months) use of CS in CKD patients in predialysis stages can enhance hypercatabolism, promote the development or aggravation of an existing PEW, and therefore careful and regular monitoring of anthropometric indices and serum albumin level is required for these patients [1, 13, 14].

LPD with a protein content of 0.6 g/kg body weight/day should be carefully balanced both in essential amino acid contents and in calories (at least 34 kcal/kg of ideal body weight/day). This requirement must be strictly observed in patients with 4–5 stages of CKD with digestive disorders due to uremia and also in patients with stages 3–4 of CKD in systemic diseases with persistent disease activity, long-term treatment with GS [1]. When making a 7-day menu, it is allowed to substitute products for their protein and carbohydrate equivalents, and to replace a portion of the animal protein (0.1 g/kg body weight/day or more) with a high-purity soybean protein (equivalent amount) in the LPD [1, 14, 21, 26].

It is promising to use highly purified soy protein SUPRO-760 (DuPont Protein Technologies USA) [1, 13, 14]. Protein "SUPRO" is a protein of high quality, fully digested by the body (adjusted amino acid coefficient of protein digestion—1.0). It is prescribed as an additive to food at the rate of 0.2–0.3 g soy protein per kg body weight per day [1, 14]. When compiling a diet that includes the soy protein SUPRO-760, the total amount of protein in the diet should not exceed 0.7 g/kg of body weight/day, whereas the total caloric value should not be less than 30 kcal/kg body weight/day for patients with 3B-5 stages of CKD [1, 14]. In patients who are committed to the use of predominantly vegetable protein, as well as in patients with anorexia (usually with eGFR <25 ml/min, 1.73 m^2), half the daily amount of animal origin protein in a traditional LPD (0.6 g/kg body weight/day) may be replaced with highly purified soy protein [1, 13, 14]. In most of CKD 4–5 stages, patients with anorexia, when using such diet, dyspeptic phenomena decreased, blood urea nitrogen level decreased, acidosis corrected, and the general condition improved [19].

In the clinical practice of recent years, high-energy nutrient mixtures that are balanced by the essential amino acids content such as Fresubin Renal, manufactured by Fresenius Kabi, Germany, etc., is introduced in the diet of CKD patients to treat the NSD. These specialized mixtures are made on the basis of CKD patients' requirements in protein, fat, carbohydrate, and energy and also enriched with vitamins and minerals.

In the predialysis period of CKD, the use of a low-protein mixture (3 g protein/100 ml) Suplena (Abbott Nutrition, USA), with a minimum amount of potassium, sodium, and phosphorus balanced with a vitamin-mineral complex, is also promising for prevention and treatment of PEW. The energy value of one package of a liquid mixture (237 ml) is 474 kcal [14].

The using of EAA and their α-KA (Ketosteril, Fresenius Kabi) in the LPD allows to maintain the protein balance [1, 6, 10]. EAA and KA are important components of LPD, which prevents the development of PEW, and enhance the beneficial effects of LPD [7, 13]. Ketoanalogues, in contrast to the matched their amino acids, do not contain a nitrogen group; by capturing endogenous nitrogen they are converted into amino acids in the body, and they contribute to the disintegration of urea. The ready-pharmaceutical complex of all EAA and KA in the optimal ratio (ketosteril) provides the need of CKD patients in essential amino acids with minimal nitrogen administration, correcting amino acid metabolism, and accelerating urea metabolism, reduces the risk of protein hypercatabolism, and negative nitrogen balance when applied diet with protein restriction. This reduces the insulin resistance, uremic dyslipidemia (hypertriglyceridemia), oxidative stress (formation of an active form of oxygen, RO—reactive oxygen). The need of EAA and KA addition to LPD is determined by the CKD stage (**Table 3**) [1, 14].

The use of EAA and KA allows to limit protein intake to the required minimum amount to enhance the positive effects of LPD and at the same time to prevent the development of PEW [6, 11]. With the use of ketoacids, even very low protein intake (up to 0.3 g/kg/day) can be achieved without increasing the risk of PEW developing [1]. In patients who were observed in predialysis stages of CKD who used LPD and received EAA and KA for at least 12 months, there was a significantly lower incidence of NSD and a slower decline in GFR per year than in patients who did not limit the protein content in the diet [4].

In patients with 3B-5 stages of CKD, attachment of PEW can contribute to the development or aggravation of existing arterial hypertension because of decreased synthesis of nitric oxide (NO) due to arginine deficiency. Arginine deficiency in uremia is due to insufficient intake of amino acids with food, as well as a decrease in the formation of arginine from citrulline [16, 18]. CKD patients with PEW need antihypertensive therapy more than other patients. In CKD, ACE inhibitors and ARB have an antihypertensive effect comparable to the effect of calcium channel blockers (CCB), but ACE inhibitors and ARB are more likely, than CCB, have a nephroprotective effect, slowing the progression of renal failure, especially with persistent proteinuria [27]. A "strict" LPD in combination with ACE inhibitors (with predominantly hepatic way of elimination) or ARB in patients with stage 3B-4 CKD and persistent proteinuria more than 1 g/day have a joint effect on proteinuria reduction. The antiproteinuric effect is provided by two components: a

CKD stage	GFR (ml/min/1.73 m^2)	Daily protein intake (g protein/kg body weight/day)	EAA и KA
1	≥90	0.8	Not required
2	60–89	0.8	Not required
3A	30–59	0.8	Not required
3B	30–44	0.6/0.7	1 tablet/5 kg of body weight/day
4	15–29	**1.** 0.6 2. 0.3–0.4	1 tablet/5 kg of body weight/day 1 tablet/5 kg of body weight/day
5	>10 to <15 (predialysis)	**1.** 0.6 2. 0.3–0.4	1 tablet/5 kg of body weight/day 1 tablet/5 kg of body weight/day

GFR: glomerular filtration rate is calculated by CKD-EPI creatinine equation; EAA: essential amino acids; and KA: ketoanalogs of amino acids.

Table 3. Essential ketoanalogs and amino acids requirement depending on the diet protein restriction and CKD stage (KDIGO guidelines, 2012).

decrease in the preglomerular vasodilation (due to the restriction of protein intake) and postglomerular vasoconstriction (caused by RAAS inhibition), leading to a decrease in intraglomerular hyperfiltration, the main determinant of the tubulointerstitial fibrosis progression [1]. In addition, RAAS blockers in combination with a LPD may affect the maintenance of Klotho products as a cardionephroprotective factor [27, 28]

The cardionephroprotective role of ketoacids and LPD was demonstrated in the experiment after subtotal nephrectomy. There was a decrease in proteinuria, arterial hypertension, and slowing down of left ventricular hypertrophy formation [14]. The retardation of CKD progression is associated with a lesser effect of EAA and KA on intra-glomerular hypertension, as well as with its ability as an additional source of calcium to correct hyperphosphatemia and slow the formation of uremic hyperparathyroidism. LPD in combination with EAA and KA enhances the following positive effects: antihypertensive and antiproteinuric effects of RAAS blockers, the corrective effect of erythropoietin preparations on anemia and of synthetic analogs of vitamin D, calcimimetics on hyperparathyroidism, and also the hypolipidemic effect of statins [1, 13, 14]

At the same time, CKD patients, with combined administration of EAA and active metabolites of vitamin D, due to a possible risk of hypercalcemia should stop taking vitamin D. If hypercalcemia persists, then it is necessary to reduce the dose of EAA to normalize the plasma concentration of calcium [1]. In recent years, the effect of ketosteril on the risk of vascular calcification has not been confirmed [29].

The addition of soy protein in the diet of patients with 3B-5 stages of CKD may also contribute to an antihypertensive effect. According to our data, patients with CKD 3B-5 stages who added soy protein to food achieved more effective correction of hypertension than patients who used milk protein as a food additive [4]. The antihypertensive effect of soy protein is due to the isoflavone in it, genistein (an estrogen of plant origin) that has an anti-inflammatory effect and a protective effect on the vascular endothelium (8 mg of isoflavone is contained in 1 g of soy protein). Soy protein contains more than animal protein, arginine (7.6% vs. 3.7%)—the precursor of NO and glycine (4.2% vs. 1.8%), which inhibit the stress hormone adrenalin and contribute to vasodilation [19, 30].

All patients with PEW to reduce the rate of protein catabolism (PCR) should consume at least 35 kcal/kg of body weight/day [1, 25].

At the same time, in prescribing the caloric content of the diet, in addition to taking into account the age, sex, general condition of the patient, and pathogenetic features of the disease, it is necessary to take into consideration the general regimen of the patient. In persons who comply with bed rest, energy expenditure will be significantly less than that of patients on a general regime. Therefore, the total calorie content of food cannot be the same for all patients [25].

The use of new drug groups, in particular, endothelin-1 receptor agonists, which have an antiproteinuric effect, agents that inhibit fibrogenesis and inflammation such as pyrophenidone and bardoxolone, as well as an inhibitor of aminoguanidine proteins glycation, are discussed [22].

Based on the available literature data, the correction of NSD, especially early, even at the predialysis stage not only improves the quality of life of patients but also contributes to slowing the progression of CKD and CVE, to prevent PEW at the stage of regular HD [12]. Thus, the correction of NSD becomes an important and obligatory part in the treatment of patients with CKD [1, 14]

3.9. Prophylaxis and dispensary observation

All patients with CKD are advised to consult a dietician, as well as to train in educational programs concerning the need to restrict protein, phosphorus, potassium, and salt in the diet. Primary prevention of NSD in patients with CKD traditionally is the restriction of protein in the diet adequately to the reducing degree of GFR. So if at 2–3A stages of CKD with GFR >45 ml/min/1.73m^2, the recommended daily protein intake is 0.8 g protein/kg/day, then with GFR 44-30 ml/min/1.73m^2, its intake is limited to 0.7–0.6 g/kg body weight/day and 0.6–0.3 g/kg body weight/day when GFR 29-15 ml/min/1.73m^2 [1, 14]. In CKD patients with proteinuria > 3 g/day, the total amount of protein in the daily ration is increased by 1 g protein/g of proteinuria [1, 14, 21, 22].

In a diet with a protein restriction of 0.6 g/ kg body weight, at least 60% should be a protein of animal origin as the most valuable in the content of EAA. Plant protein has a lower biological value, since it does not contain the whole composition of EAA. The exception is the soy protein, which is close to the protein of animal origin in the spectrum of EAA [1, 18, 19, 30].

In a "strict" LPD—0.3 g protein/kg/day—the whole protein could be of plant origin but it is a mandatory requirement to combine this diet with EAA and their α- keto-analogues [6, 11]. However, a strict LPD (but not lower than 0.3 g/kg/day) is permissible only if there are technical and organizational facilities for regular monitoring of nutritional status, and it should be combined with the mandatory intake of EAA and KA.

To ensure that the LPD (0.6–0.3 g protein/kg/day) did not lead to catabolism of the body's own proteins, patients, along with the addition of EAA, should consume at least 35 kcal/kg/day, and only in a background of large amounts of protein (0.8–0.7 g/kg/day) the consumption of 30 kcal/kg/day is sufficient. [25]. High energy value of food should be provided by carbohydrates and fats. [14, 25].

Nutritional value of fats is determined by the presence of fatty unsaturated acids (linoleic and linolenic) in their composition, which are not synthesized by the body, but come from food. The ratio of vegetable oils and animal fats in the diet should be 1:3. Vegetable oil (e.g., sunflower, soybean, corn, and cotton) should be present in the daily diet of the patient [14, 22].

The energy value of food is calculated on the basis of the percentage content of carbohydrates, fats, and proteins in it, and the coefficient of their biological value. The coefficient of biological energy value for carbohydrates is 4 kcal/g, for fats is 9 kcal/g, and for protein is 4 kcal/g. Combining the energy value of the protein, fat, and carbohydrates contained in the products, the caloric value of the entire diet may be calculated [14, 25].

Patients with a purine metabolism disorders (hyperuricemia and hyperuricosuria) should exclude rich broths, by-products—liver, kidneys, heart, tongues, as well as pates, sausages, veal, pork, smoked products, meat and fish canned food, beans (green peas, beans, French beans, and lentils), cocoa, chocolate, nuts, strong tea and coffee, grapes, raisins, and grape wines [1, 14].

If oxalic acid is impaired (oxaluria, oxalate kidney stones, and oxalosis), in addition to restrictions for patients with elevated uric acid, the consumption of sorrel, spinach, rhubarb, and peppers should also be limited [1, 14, 16].

Contraindications to the administration of LPD in CKD are mainly related to patients with late 5 stage of CKD (**Table 4**).

3.10. Pharmacological support for tolerance to a LPD

Long-term compliance with LPD is difficult due to anorexia as well as the tendency of CKD patients to protein hypercatabolism. The methods that affect anorexia and hypercatabolism in CKD include correction of metabolic acidosis (calcium carbonate, and α-ketoanalogs of EAA), deficiency of iron and erythropoietin, elimination of hyperleptinemia (eicosapentaenoic acid), and hyperparathyroidism (calcitriol, paricalcitol, and cinacalcet) [1, 13, 14, 21].

Treatment with calcium carbonate in the background of protein-intake restriction increases the level of plasma bicarbonate and reduces the protein catabolic rate (PCR) from 1.2 to 1.0 g/day. As a result, protein's catabolism and anorexia that are typical for acidosis are reduced, neutral or positive nitrogen balance is maintained, and parathyroid gland activation is partially inhibited [14].

EAA and KA are important components of LPD, which help to prevent the development of PEW, correct acidosis, and enhance the beneficial effects of LPD [7, 13]. The need of EAA and KA supplementation to LPD is determined by the CKD stage.

The absorption of α-keto acids in the gastrointestinal tract is quick, and their conversion to essential amino acids averages from 30% for valine and up to 70% for phenylalanine. The number of α-keto acids involved in conversion to essential amino acids is inversely proportional

Absolute contradiction	Relative contradiction
• 5 CKD stage with GFR < 10 ml/min and decompensate metabolic acidosis, uremic polyneuropathy, or uncontrolled hypertension • Cachexia (BMI < 18 kg/m^2) • Rapidly progressive glomerulonephritis • Severe nephrotic syndrome • Intolerance to dietary restrictions	• Decompensate diabetes mellitus • Severe hypercatabolism • Bacterial infection (acute, exacerbation of chronic form) • Severe anemia • Noncompliance • Anorexia • Psychopathy, mental disorders, encephalopathy

LPD: low-protein diet; GFR: glomerular filtration rate; BMI: body mass index; CKD: chronic kidney disease.

Table 4. Contraindication to LPD in CKD.

to the daily protein quota in food and directly depends on the caloric content of the diet. Some α-keto acids, e.g., ketoisoleucine, in uremia suppress protein degradation in muscles, allowing to maintain a neutral nitrogen balance in conditions of renal failure in the background of protein restriction [25].

3.11. Consumption of potassium, sodium, and phosphorus in CKD: water regime

At 3B stage CKD daily intake of potassium, phosphorus in the diet should not exceed 3000 mg and 700 mg, respectively, at the 4th stage CKD—potassium intake should be reduced by half. LPD allows to reduce the consumption of phosphorus—when consuming 0.6 g/kg protein, patients receive 500–800 mg of phosphorus a day, and when the protein quota is limited to 0.3 g/kg—250 mg of phosphorus. In case of hyperphosphatemia, it should be limited to a fish (no more than 1 time per week), as well as cereals (except rice) and other foods rich in phosphorus. As an alternative to cereals, artificial sago can be used [1, 14, 26].

In order to correct hyperkalemia, it is recommended to limit the use of dried apricots, figs, bananas, apricots, peaches, and nectarines [1, 14].

Restriction of salt intake (no more than 5 g/day) increases the antiproteinuric effectiveness of RAAS inhibitors. Exceptions include patients with increased sodium excretion in tubular lesions [26].

Most patients with CKD should be recommended a consumption of at least 2 liters of fluid/day and up to 3 liters of fluid/day in hot weather, especially when purine metabolism is disordered, oxalic acid turnover disturbances, urolithiasis, and a tendency to urinary infection [1, 14, 26]

With nephrotic syndrome, as well as in the terminal stage of CKD with a GFR value of less than 15 ml/min, when the patient cannot form more than 1 l urine/day, the fluid intake is corrected by diuresis (300–500 ml to be added to the amount of excreted urine from the previous day) [1].

3.12. Nephroprotective effect of LPD

The nephroprotective effect of LPD is associated with its hemodynamic and metabolic effects. The dietary load of protein and phosphorus, according to the possibilities of the residual function of the kidneys of the patient, in addition to reducing uremic intoxication and lowering the level of urea, creatinine, and uric acid in the blood, reduces the hemodynamic load on the residual nephrons, which slows the progress of glomerular hypertrophy, as well as activation of RAAS, normalizes intraglomerular autoregulation, and reduces intra-glomerular and systemic arterial hypertension [1, 14]. The LPD partially corrects such unfavorable uremic metabolic and endocrine disorders, as hypoalbuminemia, dyslipidemia, insulinoresistance, hyperphosphatemia with parathyroid gland hyperplasia, and anemia, and thereby reduces the risk of uremic hyperparathyroidism, vascular calcification, and atherosclerosis (**Table 5**) [7, 20, 26].

The effect of LPD on CKD advancing is more pronounced in cases of DN. In the background of LPD, the annual incidence of GFR declines by 1.5–2 times, and the outcome in the terminal stage of CKD is observed almost three times less frequently than in the standard diet [5, 7].

Mechanisms of action	Clinical effect
Protein restriction to the level, adapted to residual renal function	Decrease in level of uremic toxins, azotemia, hyperuricemia
Correction of metabolic acidosis	Correction of nutrition status: protein catabolism; hypoalbuminemia; amino acids metabolism
Inhibition of glomerular hypertrophy and intraglomerular hypertension, decrease in tubular transport overload, suppression of cytokines and uremic toxins synthesis: TGF-β, AII and RO, TIMP, indoxyl sulfate, guanidine, phosphate, oxalic acid, NO	Decrease in proteinuria, correction of hypertension, slowing down of glomerulosclerosis and tubulointerstitial fibrosis, and GRF stabilization
Partial correction of dyslipidemia: • of hypercholesteremia; • of hypertriglyceridemia; • decrease in insulin resistance	Slowing down of atherosclerosis progression, decrease in risk of cardiovascular complications and mortality
Decrease in serum phosphate and PTH levels, increase in calcitriol	Suppression of hyperparathyroidism, vascular calcification, improvement of anemia, and decrease in erythropoietin doses

TGF-β: transforming growth factor β; AII: angiotensin II; RO: reactive oxygen; TIMP: tissue inhibitor matrix metalloproteinases; NO: nitrogen oxygen; PTH: parathyroid hormone; and GFR: glomerular filtration rate is calculated by CKD EPI creatinine equation.

Table 5. Mechanisms of action and clinical effects of low-protein diet (LPD).

The effect of LPD directly depends on the correct compliance by patients with the prescribed restriction of the amount of protein in the diet (0.8–0, 6–0.3 g/kg body weight/day), depending on the stage of CKD, the ratio of animal and vegetable proteins in it, and also on high caloric intake (30–35 kcal/kg body weight/day) [1, 14, 21].

According to the re-analysis of the MDRD multicentre study (Modification of diet in renal disease), in the background of LPD in patients with GFR more than 25 ml/min, the rate of CKD progression decreased by approximately 10%, and with GFR less than 25 ml/min, it was an average of 30% for every 0.2 g/kg of protein excluded from the diet [1].

The results of the research indicate that "strict" LPD (0.3 g/kg/day of vegetable protein) and the use of a complex of EAA and KA (ketosteril 1 table/5 kg of body weight per day) in patients with stage 4 CKD provide a more effective reduction of uremia symptoms and provide an extension of the predialysis period than conventional LPD (0.6 g protein/kg/day) [6, 11]. Strengthening of the nephroprotective role of LPD by combining it with α-ketoanalogs of amino acids is associated with a lesser effect it has on intra-glomerular hypertension, as well as with their ability as an additional source of calcium to inhibit hyperphosphatemia and slow the formation of uremic hyperparathyroidism [1, 11]. LPD in combination with EAA and KA enhances the antihypertensive and antiproteinuric effects of RAAS blockers, the corrective effect of erythropoietin preparations on the anemia, the effects of synthetic analogs of vitamin D and calcimimetics on manifestations of hyperparathyroidism, and the hypolipidemic effect of statins [10].

The replacing of a portion of the animal protein (0.1–0.2 g/kg/day) in the LPD (0.6 g protein/kg body weight/day) with a highly purified soy protein (an equivalent amount) contributed to retardation of CKD progression [4]. Soy protein is less able than animal protein (meat, fish, milk, etc.) to increase hyperperfusion and hyperfiltration in remnant nephrons [30]. The results of studies on the model of unilateral ureteral obstruction in rats receiving LPD demonstrated a decrease in the expression of the nuclear factor of Kappa B transcription (NFkB), the most important mediator of activation of many proinflammatory and profibrotic cytokines and TGF-β-key as a profibrotic factor in the renal tissue [28, 30]. LPD with an addition of soy protein to the diet reduces tubulointerstitial fibrosis also due to suppression of tyrosine protein kinase as a powerful sclerosis stimulant [30]. Currently, the possibility of LPD influence to maintain the serum level of klotho protein, as an established strong early cardio and nephroprotective factor, is being actively studied [29].

4. Conclusion

Thus, the restriction of daily food protein intake to 0.3–0.6 g/kg/day prevents accumulation of toxic products, retards, and delays terminal renal failure. Replacing a portion of the animal protein in a LPD by an equivalent amount of highly purified soy protein enhances the nephroprotective effect of a LPD and favors more pronounced slowdown of CKD progression. The use of keto-analogues of essential amino acids with LPD at predialysis stage of CKD allows preserving CKD patients from nutrition status disorders and contributes to slow down of CKD complications. Control of nutrition status in CKD should be carried out regularly. A comprehensive assessment of NS in CKD patients can be quickly performed using bioimpedance analysis.

Acknowledgements

This work was supported by Russian Science Foundation (grant No. 14-15-00947 2014).

Abbreviations

ACE	Angiotensin converting enzyme
ARB	Angiotensin receptor blockers
BCM	Body Composition Monitor
BMI	Body mass index
CKD	Chronic Kidney Disease
CRP	C-reactive protein
CRF	Chronic Renal Failure
CV	cardiovascular

CVC	Cardiovascular complications
CVE	cardiovascular events
DN	diabetic nephropathy
EAA	essential amino acids
EPO	erythropoietins
FGF-23	fibroblast growth factor
GFR	Glomerular Filtration Rate
GS	glucocorticosteroids
HD	Regular Hemodialysis
KA	Keto-analogues
LVH	left ventricular hypertrophy
LPD	low protein diet
NS	nutritional status
NSD	nutritional status disorders
PTH	parathyroid hormone
PCR	protein catabolism rate
RAAS	renin angiotensin aldosterone system
PEW	protein-energy wasting
RRT	renal replacement therapy
SFFT	thickness of the skin-fal fold
SMV	Shoulder muscles volume
TBW	total body water

Author details

Ludmila Y. Milovanova*, Victor V. Fomin, Lidia V. Lysenko (Kozlovskaya), Yuriy S. Milovanov, Nikolay A. Mukhin, Vasiliy V. Kozlov, Marina V. Taranova, Svetlana Y. Milovanova, Marina V. Lebedeva and Aigul Zh. Usubalieva

*Address all correspondence to: ludm.milovanova@gmail.com

I.M. Sechenov First Moscow State Medical University, Moscow, Russian Federation

References

[1] KDIGO. Clinical Practice Guideline for the evaluation and management of chronic kidney disease. Journal of the International Society of Nephrology. 2013;**3**(Suppl. 1):1-136

[2] Bellizzi V, Cupisti A, Locatelli F, et al., on behalf of the "Conservative Treatment of CKD" study group of the Italian Society of Nephrology. Low-protein diets for chronic kidney disease patients: The Italian experience. BMC Nephrology. 2016;**17**:77. DOI: 10.1186/s12882-016-0280-0

[3] Bonanni A, Mannucci I, Verzola D, et al. Protein-energy wasting and mortality in chronic kidney disease. International Journal of Environmental Research and Public Health. 2011;**8**(5):1631-1654. DOI: 10.3390/ijerph8051631

[4] Milovanov YS, Milovanova LY, Mikhailov AA, et al. Influence of diet balanced with essential amino acids and keto acids analogs and high-nutrient blend on the progression of renal failure in patients in the pre-dialysis stage of chronic kidney disease caused by systemic autoimmune diseases. International Journal of BioMedicine. 2013;**3**(3):184-187. DOI: http://www.ijbm.org/articles/Article3_3_CR7.pdf

[5] Firouzi S, Barakatun-Nisak MY, Nor Azmi K. Nutritional status, glycemic control and its associated risk factors among a sample of type 2 diabetic individuals, a pilot study. Journal of Research in Medical Sciences. 2015;**20**(1):40-46. DOI: https://www.ncbi.nlm.nih.gov/pmc/articles/PMC4354064/

[6] Bellizzi V. Long-term outcome of patients following a very low protein diet supplemented with keto/amino acids during the pre-dialysis period. Journal of Renal Nutrition. 2012;**22**(2):7-8. DOI: 10.1093/ndt/gfu251

[7] Chauvean P, Aparicio MR. Benefits in nutritional interventions in patients with CKD stage 3-4. Journal of Renal Nutrition. 2011;**21**(1):20-22. DOI: 10.1053/j.jrn.2010.11.005

[8] Mitch WE, Remuzzi G. Diets for patients with chronic kidney disease, should we reconsider? BMC Nephrology. 2016;**17**:80-86. DOI: 10.1186/s12882-016-0283-x

[9] D'Alessandro C, Piccoli GB, Calella P, et al. "Dietaly": Practical issues for the nutritional management of CKD patients in Italy. BMC Nephrology. 2016;**17**:102-104. DOI: 10.1186/s12882-016-0296-5

[10] Aparicio M, Bellizzi V, Chauveau X, et al. Protein-restricted diets plus keto|amino acids – A valid therapeutic approach for chronic kidney disease patients. Journal of Renal Nutrition. 2012;**22**(25):1-21. DOI: 10.1053/j:jrn.2011.09.005

[11] Garneata L. Ketoanalog-supplementted very low protein diet in pre-dialysis chronic kidney disease it really work? The Romanian experience. Journal of Renal Nutrition. 2012;**22**(2):9-10 DOI: 10.1053/j.jrn.2013.01.030

[12] Caria S, Cupisti A, Sau G, et al. The incremental treatment of ESRD: A low-protein diet combined with weekly hemodialysis may be beneficial for selected patients. BMC Nephrology. 2014;**15**:172. DOI: 10.1186/1471-2369-15-172

[13] Yoshitsugu Obi, Hemn Qader, Csaba P. Latest consensus and update on protein energy-wasting in chronic kidney disease. Current Opinion in Clinical Nutrition and Metabolic Care. 2015;**18**(3):254-262. DOI: 10.1097/MCO.0000000000000171

[14] Fouque D, Kalantar-Zadeh K, Kopple J, et al. A proposed nomenclature and diagnostic criteria for protein-energy wasting in acute and chronic kidney disease. Kidney International. 2008;**73**:391-398. DOI: 10.1038/sj.ki.5002585

[15] Hyun YY, Lee KB, Han SH, et al. Nutritional status in adults with predialysis chronic kidney disease: KNOW-CKD Study. Journal of Korean Medical Science. 2017;**32**(2):257-263. DOI: 10.3346/jkms.2017.32.2.257

[16] Fouque D, Pelletier S, Mafra D, et al. Nutrition and chronic kidney disease. Kidney International. 2011;**80**:348-357. DOI: 10.3346/jkms.2017.32.2.257

[17] Franch HA, Raissi S, Wang X, et al. Acidosis impairs insulin receptor substrate-1-associated phosphoinositide 3-kinase signaling in muscle cells: Consequences on proteolysis. American Journal of Physiology. Renal Physiology. 2004;**287**:700-706. DOI: 10.1152/ajprenal.00440.2003

[18] Carrero JJ, Stenvinkel P, Cuppari L, et al. Etiology of the protein-energy wasting syndrome in chronic kidney disease: A consensus statement from the International Society of Renal Nutrition and Metabolism (ISRNM). Journal of Renal Nutrition. 2013;**23**:77-90. DOI: 10.1053/j.jrn.2013.01.001

[19] Zoccali C, Malamaci F. Adiponectin and leptin in chronic kidney disease: Causal factors or mere risk markers? Journal of Renal Nutrition. 2011;**21**(1):87-91. DOI: 10.1053/j.jrn.2010.10.014

[20] Mutsert R, Grootendorst DC, Axelsson J, et al, NECOSAD Study Group. Excess mortality due to interaction between protein-energy wasting, inflammation and cardiovascular disease in chronic dialysis patients. Nephrology, Dialysis, Transplantation. 2008;**23**:2957-2964. DOI: 10.1093/ndt/gfn167

[21] Kovesdy CP, Kopple JD, Kalantar-Zadeh K. Management of protein-energy wasting in non-dialysis-dependent chronic kidney disease: Reconciling low protein intake with nutritional therapy. American Journal of Clinical Nutrition. 2013;**97**:1163-1177. DOI: 10.3945/ajcn.112.036418

[22] Dumler F. Body composition modifications in patients under low protein diets. Journal of Renal Nutrition. 2011;**21**(1):76-81. DOI: 10.1053/j.jrn.2010.10.005

[23] Pupim LB, Caglar K, Hakim RM, et al. Uremic malnutrition is a predictor of death independent of inflammatory status. Kidney International. 2004;**66**:2054-2060. DOI: 10.1111/j.1523-1755.2004.00978.x

[24] Wilson FP, Xie D, Anderson AH, et al. Urinary creatinine excretion, bioelectrical impedance analysis, and clinical outcomes in patients with CKD: The CRIC study. Clinical

Journal of the American Society of Nephrology. 2014;**9**:2095-2103. DOI: 10.2215/CJN.03790414

[25] Avesani CM, Kamimura MA, Cupari L. Energy expenditure in chronic kidney disease patients. Journal of Renal Nutrition. 2011;**21**(1):27-30. DOI: 10.1053/j.jrn.2010.10.013

[26] Turner JM, et al. Treatment of chronic kidney disease. Kidney International - International Society of Nephrology. 2012;**81**(4):351-362. DOI:10.1038/ki.2011.380

[27] Karalliedde J, Maltese G, Hill B, et al. Effect of renin-angiotensin system blockade on soluble Klotho in patients with type 2 diabetes, systolic hypertension, and albuminuria. Clinical Journal of the American Society of Nephrology. 2013;**8**(11):1899-1905. DOI: 10.2215/CJN.02700313

[28] Adijiang A, Shimizu H, Higuchi Y, et al. Indoxil sulfate reduces klotho expression and promotes senescence in the kidneys of hypertensive rats. Journal of Renal Nutrition. 2011;**21**(1):105-109. DOI: 10.1053/j.jrn.2010.10.020

[29] Milovanova L, Kozevnikova E, Milovanov Y, et al. Influence of essential amino acids ketoanalogs and protein restriction diet on morphogenetic proteins (FGF-23 and Klotho) in CKD patients". Materials of 53rd ERA-EDTA Congress, 21-24 May 2016 Vienna DOI: 10.3252/pso.eu.53era.2016 341_SP https://www.postersessiononline.eu/173580348_eu/congresos/53era/aula/-SP_341_53era.pdf

[30] McGraw NJ, Krul ES, Grunz-Borgmann E, et al. Soy-based renoprotection. World Journal of Nephrology. 2016;**5**(3):233-257. DOI: 10.5527/wjn.v5.i3.233

Section 4

Genetic Aspects in CKD

Discovery of Single Nucleotide Polymorphism in Polycystic Kidney Disease among South Indian (Madurai) Population

Pandiaraj Veeramuthumari and William Isabel

Additional information is available at the end of the chapter

http://dx.doi.org/10.5772/intechopen.71201

Abstract

The kidneys serve an essential regulatory role in most of the animals, including vertebrates and some invertebrates. They are important in the urinary system and also serve homeostatic functions like regulation of electrolytes, maintenance of acid-base balance and regulation of blood pressure (via maintaining salt and water balance). They also serve as natural filter of the blood and remove wastes that are diverted to the urinary bladder. By producing urine, the kidneys excrete wastes such as urea and ammonia. The kidneys are responsible for reabsorption of water, glucose, amino acids and trace elements. They also produce hormones including calcitriol, renin and erythropoietin. The kidney is approximately 11–14 cm long, 6 cm wide and 4 cm thick. Each adult kidney weighs between 125 and 170 g in males and between 115 and 155 g in females. The left kidney is typically slightly larger than the right kidney. Each kidney is made up of about 1 million microprocessor units called nephrons.

Keywords: polycystic kidney disease, renal failure, single nucleotide polymorphism, polymerase chain reaction, disease complications

1. Introduction

The kidneys play an essential regulatory role in animals and are responsible for reabsorption of water, glucose, amino acids and trace elements. They also produce hormones including calcitriol, renin and erythropoietin. The kidney is approximately 11–14 cm long, 6 cm wide and 4 cm thick. Each adult kidney weighs between 125 and 170 g in males and between 115 and 155 g in females. The left kidney is typically slightly larger than the right kidney [1] **(Figure 1).** Each kidney is made up of about 1 million microprocessor units called nephrons.

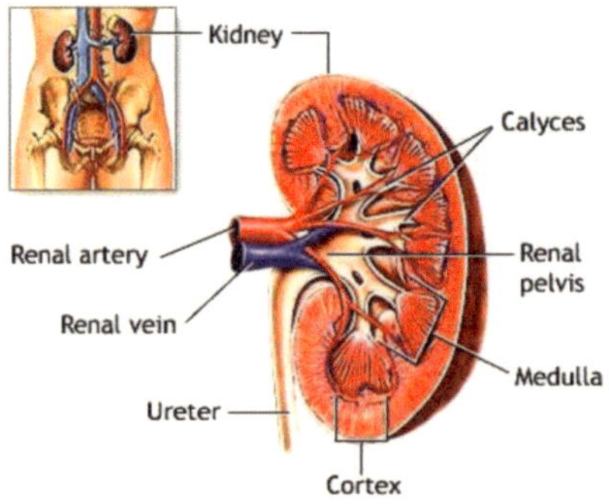

Figure 1. Structure and location of kidney. Source: [2] (http://www.sugarbp.org/kidneystucture_diabetes.htm).

The nephron is the basic structural and functional unit of a kidney [3]. Each nephron has an initial filtering component composed of a glomerulus and Bowman's capsule, which is connected to a long convoluted tubule lined by transporting epithelia.

Sodium chloride, potassium and glucose are filtered and reabsorbed along with water in the nephron back into the bloodstream. This maintains a correct balance of trace element within the blood, which assists in blood pressure regulation and normal levels of blood sugars. Hence, the kidneys are found to play a crucial role in regulating the amount of water and chemicals (electrolytes) in the body such as sodium, potassium and phosphorus [4].

1.1. Different types of kidney diseases

Usually both the kidneys are affected by various forms of diseases and then the waste products and excess fluid build up, causing severe swelling and symptoms of uremia (kidney failure). They are congenital kidney disease, hereditary kidney disorders and acquired kidney diseases.

1.1.1. Congenital disease

It involves malformation of the genitourinary tract, usually leading to some type of obstruction that subsequently produces infection and/or destruction of kidney tissue, which may eventually progress to chronic kidney failure. For example, horseshoe kidney, also known as *ren arcuatus* (in Latin), renal fusion or super kidney, is a congenital disorder affecting about 1 in 500 people [5, 6].

1.1.2. Hereditary disorders

Hereditary diseases are Alport's syndrome or hereditary nephritis, primary hyperoxaluria, cystinuria and polycystic kidney disease (PKD). The chapter found that polycystic kidney disease is more common among the population.

1.1.2.1. Polycystic kidney disease (PKD)

Epithelial cell polarity is vitally important for correct function of different tubule segments [3]. Cell polarity defects have been linked to a number of hereditary kidney diseases including polycystic kidney diseases (PKDs) characterized by the accumulation of fluid-filled cysts in the cortex and medulla [7–10]. There are two types of PKDs. They are autosomal dominant polycystic kidney disease (ADPKD) and autosomal recessive polycystic kidney disease (ARPKD) [10].

1.1.3. Acquired kidney diseases

These diseases are numerous and are generally known as nephritis (inflammation of the kidney). The most common type of nephritis is glomerulonephritis and has many causes. The acquired kidney diseases are renal agenesis, multicystic dysplastic kidney, renal dysplasia, diabetic nephropathy, glomerulonephritis, hydronephrosis, interstitial nephritis, kidney stones, kidney tumors: Wilms tumor and renal cell carcinoma, lupus nephritis, minimal change disease (MCD), nephrotic syndrome, pyelonephritis and renal failure.

2. Renal failure

In renal failure, the kidneys lose their normal function due to various factors including infections, autoimmune diseases, diabetes and other endocrine disorders, cancer, and toxic chemicals [11]. Genetic variability on the development of renal failure is becoming clearer and emphasizes the need to elucidate the genetic basis for renal diseases and associated complications. Studies on genetic variability in renal failure would lead to better understanding of different phenotypes observed in polycystic kidney disease and would enable us to determine whether a patient is genetically predisposed to such complications.

2.1. Acute renal failure

Acute kidney injury (AKI), previously called acute renal failure (ARF), is a rapid loss of kidney function due to low blood volume from any cause, exposure to substances harmful to the kidney and obstruction of the urinary tract [12, 13]. Elevated blood urea nitrogen and creatinine or inability of the kidneys to produce sufficient amounts of urine is noted in these patients.

2.2. Stage 5 chronic kidney diseases

Stage 5 CKD is often called **end stage renal disease (ESRD).** The symptoms of Stage 5 CKD are:

- Increase in serum creatinine or protein in the urine are observed.
- The patients develop hypertension or congestive heart failure due to fluid overload and production of vasoactive hormones created by the kidney via the RAS (renin-angiotensin system).

- Urea accumulates, leading to azotemia and ultimately uremia. Urea is excreted by sweating and crystallizes on skin ("uremic frost") (http://en.wikipedia.org/wiki/Chronic_kidney_disease; "Chronic Kidney Disease". medscape.) [14].
- Later this progresses to secondary hyperparathyroidism, renal osteodystrophy and vascular calcification that further impair cardiac function.
- Metabolic acidosis, due to accumulation of sulfates, phosphates, uric acid, etc., leads to excitability of cardiac and neuronal membranes by promoting hyperkalemia [15].

People with chronic kidney disease (hyperlipidemia) suffer from accelerated atherosclerosis and are likely to develop cardiovascular disease than the general population [16].

3. Polycystic kidney disease (PKD)

There are two forms of **PKD:**

(i) Autosomal dominant polycystic kidney disease (ADPKD)

(ii) Autosomal recessive polycystic kidney disease (ARPKD)

3.1. Autosomal dominant polycystic kidney disease (ADPKD)

Autosomal dominant polycystic kidney disease occurs worldwide and in all races. ADPKD is one of the most commonly inherited conditions in humans with an incidence of 1:500 to 1:1000 [17, 18]. It is genetically heterogeneous with two genes identified: PKD1 (16p13.3) and PKD2 (4q21) [9, 19, 20].

3.2. Autosomal recessive polycystic kidney disease (ARPKD)

ARPKD is uncommon and occurs primarily in neonates and children. The gene responsible for ARPKD (*PKHD1*) has recently been identified on chromosome 6. Fibrocystin is defective in ARPKD [21, 22]. The occurrence of ADPKD is most common when compared to ARPKD and the mean age of onset is between 30 and 40 years. Both men and women are equally affected [23]. Hence the present study is also focused on PKD1 and PKD2 gene polymorphism in autosomal dominant polycystic kidney disease subjects and control subjects among South Indian population.

Tables 1 and **2** show polymorphism study in PKD1 and PKD2 gene among various populations on both national and international level.

3.3. Pathogenesis and genetics of polycystic kidney disease (PKD)

Abnormalities in gene expression, cell polarity, fluid secretion, apoptosis and extracellular matrix have also been described in PKD [17, 34–36]. ADPKD is one of the most common Mendelian disorders in humans [37, 38] and the most frequent genetic cause of renal failure

Author and year	Gene	Population	Mutation
Sumathy [24]	PKD1	Indian	PKD1 C-T or G-A, SSCP
Nair et al. [25]	ACE,	Nellore, Andhra Pradesh	I/D polymorphism
Elumalai et al. [26]	eNOS, VNTR	South Indian	a/b polymorphism
Veeramuthumari and Isabel [27]*	PKD1	South Indian (Madurai)	Ala/Val (C/T) polymorphism
Veeramuthumari et al. [28]*	PKD2	South Indian (Madurai)	Arg/Pro (G/C) polymorphism

*Current study.

Table 1. National reports of PKD1 and PKD2 gene polymorphism.

Author and Year	Gene	Population	Mutation
Hateboer et al. [29]	PKD2	Spain, Netherlands, UK, Bulgaria, Australia	C-T substitution, deletion, nonsense mutation, frameshift, missense, splice mutation
Koptides et al. [30]	PKD1 & PKD2	Cyprus	Mutation in exon 24, mutation in exon 1
	PKD1 & PKD2	Slovenia	Frameshift/missense mutation; nonsense mutation
Son et al. [31]	PKD1	Devis, USA	CT transversion (SNP)
	PKD1 & 2	US	Mutation
Lee et al. [32]	PKD1	Taiwan	C → A transversion
Galeano et al. [33]	PKD1	Belgium	SNP

Table 2. International reports of PKD1 and PKD2 gene polymorphism.

in adults. ADPKD is a genetically heterogeneous condition [39], which is caused by mutations in one of the three genes: PKD1 on chromosome 16 accounts for 85% of cases, whereas PKD2 on chromosome 4 accounts for 15% and mutations in the PKD3 gene are rare [40]. Hence the present study is focused on PKD1 and PKD2 genes in patients with ADPKD among South Indian (Madurai) population.

3.4. Chromosomal location of PKD1 and PKD2 gene

PKD1 has been mapped to the short arm of the 16th (16p13.3) chromosome, which encodes a protein called polycystin-1. The PKD1 gene is very large in size, consisting of 46 exons distributed over 52 kb of genomic DNA [41]. The gene encodes a 14.1-kb mRNA transcript to be translated into a protein composed of 4302 amino acids transcript with an open reading frame (ORF) of 12,909 bp [42] (**Figure 2**). The PKD2 gene maps to chromosome 4q21–23 (**Figure 3**). The PKD2 gene encodes a protein, polycystin-2, which is composed of 968 amino acids [45]. The interaction of polycystin-1 and polycystin-2 in renal tubules promotes normal development and function of the kidneys [46].

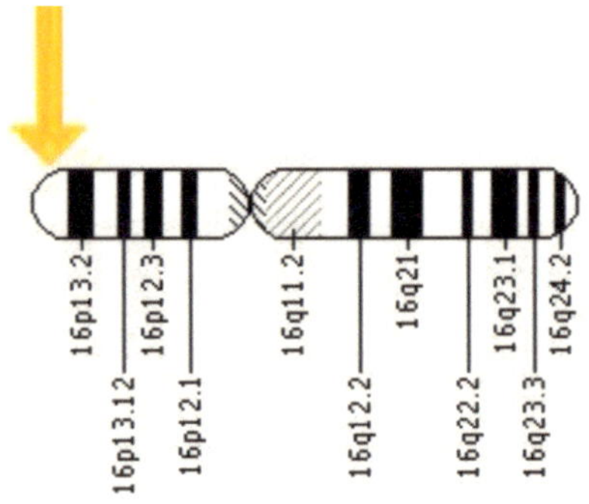

Figure 2. Chromosomal location of PKD1 gene. Source: [43] http://ghr.nlm.nih.gov/gene/PKD1.

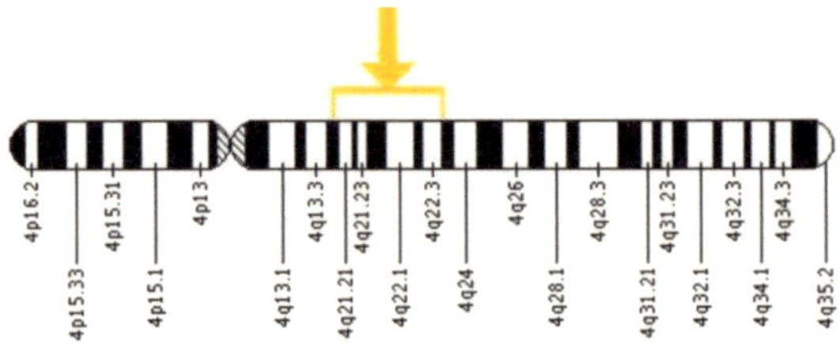

Figure 3. Chromosomal location of PKD2 gene. Source: [44] http://ghr.nlm.nih.gov/gene/PKD2.

3.4.1. *Polycystin-1*

The PKD1 gene codes for polycystin-1 (PC-1) and plays a vital role in cell-cell and cell-matrix interaction [41]. Thus, a defect in polycystin-1 leads to the alteration in the differentiation of epithelial cells and abnormal phenotypic expression of autosomal dominant polycystic kidney disease (ADPKD). The proteins encoded by the PKD1 and PKD2 genes define a new family. The polycystins play an important role in a variety of biological processes including fertilization, ion transduction and mechanosensation. Polycystin-1 is an integral membrane protein, which is predicted to contain an array of distinct protein motifs, including two leucine-rich repeats flanked by cystine-rich domains. Many of these motifs are involved in protein-protein or protein-carbohydrate interaction, which raises the possibility of polycystin-1, as a receptor for a yet unidentified ligand. The carboxyl terminus of polycystin-1 is located in cytoplasm and contains coil-coil domains and mediates the protein-protein interaction as well as several potential sites of phosphorylation. Polycystin-1 is expressed in many tissues, including the kidney, brain, heart, bone and muscles [47]. Foggensteiner et al. [48] have reported that several studies have identified polycystin-1 in the plasma membrane of tubular epithelial cells, in the distal nephron and in the collecting duct. The defect of polycystin-1 might lead to alteration in differentiation of epithelial cells and abnormal phenotypic expression of ADPKD [49].

3.4.2. *Polycystin-2*

Polycystin-2 is also widely expressed in many tissues, particularly the kidney, heart, ovary, testis, vascular smooth muscle and small intestine [47]. In the kidney, polycystin-2 like

http://dx.doi.org/10.5772/intechopen.71201

polycystin-1 is expressed in all nephron segments, with the possible exception of the thin limbs but absent from glomeruli. Several studies have shown that the polycystin-2 channel conducts divalent cations including calcium and that this activity can be stimulated by calcium on the cytosolic side.

3.4.3. Fibrocystin/polyductin

The protein encoded by the *PKHD1* gene has been named polyductin or fibrocystin and is composed of 4074 amino acids [22]. Polyductin/fibrocystin is predicted to be a membrane protein consisting of a large extracellular domain, a single transmembrane segment and a short carboxyl-terminal tail. Polyductin is a novel protein, although it has some similarities to other proteins in the database.

3.5. Mechanism of cyst formation

Cysts will form in these patient's kidneys and several studies suggest that the cells that line these cysts will have lost both functional copies of a polycystin gene [50, 51]. Defects in the genes encoding PC1 or PC2 lead to aberrant gene transcription, cell proliferation and ion secretion, which in turn result in the formation of fluid-filled cysts. These cysts lead to the displacement of the normal renal parenchyma and the formation of a cyst-filled kidney with reduced functional capacity (**Figure 4**).

3.6. ADPKD-associated common complications

Common complications associated with ADPKD are hypertension, hematuria, urinary tract infection, renal calculi, cardiac valve abnormalities, diabetes, hernia of the anterior abdominal wall and cerebral berry aneurysms [29, 53]. Hematuria is the presence of red blood cells (RBCs) in the urine. In microscopic hematuria, the urine appears normal to the naked eye, but examination with a microscope shows a high number of RBCs [54]. Diabetic nephropathy (*neuropatia diabetica*) also known as Kimmelstiel-Wilson syndrome, or nodular diabetic glomerulosclerosis [55] and intercapillary glomerulonephritis, is a progressive kidney disease. Anterior abdominal wall hernias, also known as ventral hernias, are involved in the protrusion of part of the peritoneal sac through a defect in the muscle layers of the anterior abdominal wall [56]. A cerebral or brain aneurysm is a cerebrovascular disorder in which weakness in the wall of a cerebral artery or vein causes a localized dilation or ballooning of the blood vessel [57].

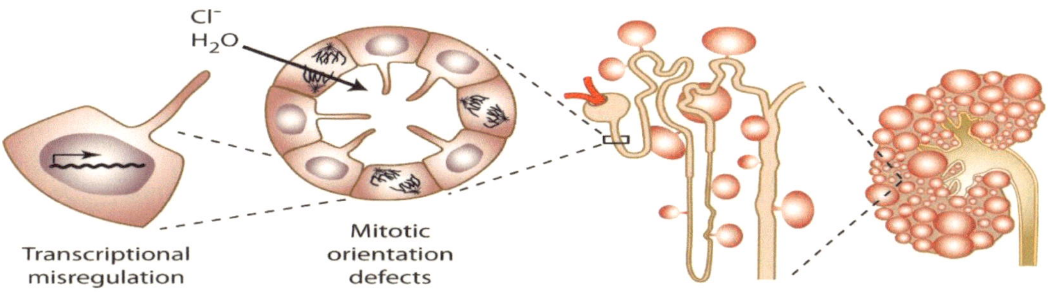

Figure 4. Cyst formation in nephron, kidney and at cellular level [52].

Clinically, PKD is characterized by progressive formation and enlargement of cysts leading to end-stage renal disease (ESRD) in late middle age. Overall, ADPKD accounts for approximately 5–10% of ESRD [58]. Hypertension occurs in 50–75% of patients prior to renal insufficiency and it is thought to accelerate the decline in renal function [59, 60]. Systemic hypertension is also very common, occurring in more than 75% of patients. Increased blood pressure (BP) has been attributed to activation of the renin-angiotensin system, but a primary defect in blood vessels may also exist [61].

3.7. Method of diagnosis and screening

Nowadays, ADPKD is studied by ultrasound, CT or MRI with multiple cysts that are generally visible that increase in size and number with age [62]. ADPKD is typically diagnosed in adults by the detection of bilaterally enlarged polycystic kidneys using transabdominal ultrasound scanning. The diagnosis of ADPKD is established primarily by imaging studies of the kidney [53]. For diagnosis of ADPKD, computer tomography (CT) has been used effectively, which has also revealed multiple cysts in kidneys and left ovary and aneurysm in the brain [53].

3.7.1. Treatment

When renal function, measured by glomerular filtration rate, is persistently poor, dialysis and kidney transplantation could be done. Cotran et al. [63] have stated that a common symptom of kidney stones is a sharp pain in the medial/lateral segments of the lower back. Approximately 50% of afflicted individuals have been shown to develop end-stage renal disease requiring dialysis or kidney transplantation before the age of 60 [8].

3.7.2. Trends in potential therapies and clinical trials

Until now, therapy for ADPKD has been directed toward limiting its complications. Cardiovascular complications, related to hypertension, are a major cause of morbidity and mortality. A major problem in therapeutic interventions in ADPKD is that this is a very slowly evolving condition, and GFR is well maintained until relatively late in the course of the disease at the age of 40. Better understanding of signaling pathways and cellular changes associated with ADPKD has suggested possible therapies to directly inhibit the development or growth of cysts, some of which are now being tested in clinical trials [64]. A stable somatostatin analogue, octreotide, has been shown to be effective at limiting progression in liver and kidney cystic disease in a rat model of PKD [65].

Advanced-stage ADPKD patients frequently receive a renal transplant without removal of the affected cystic kidneys, without side effects. Rapamycin is often used to prevent transplant rejection. The absence of polycystin permits excessive kinase activity in the mTOR pathway and the development of renal cysts [66]. Patients treated with rapamycin have been reported to show a statistically significant reduction in native polycystic kidney size over a period of 24 months compared with patients treated with other antirejection drugs. Other targets for therapy include triptolide, a compound derived from a traditional Chinese herbal therapy, which blocks glycosyl ceramide synthesis [67].

http://dx.doi.org/10.5772/intechopen.71201

4. Methodology to be followed for the discovery of single nucleotide polymorphism in polycystic kidney disease

Genomic DNA preparation: [68, 69].

Reagents required: phosphate buffer saline (PBS), red blood cell (RBC) lysis buffer, cell lysis buffer (CLB), ammonium acetate, isopropyl alcohol, 70% ethanol, TE buffer

Procedure: the blood samples were thawed at room temperature and 300 μl of blood was transferred to centrifuge tubes. Equal volume of PBS was added to it and incubated for 20 min and centrifuged at 3000 rpm for 5 min. The supernatant was removed and the pellet was resuspended in 900 μl of RBC lysis buffer and mixed thoroughly. This was centrifuged at 3000 rpm for 5 min and the supernatant was discarded. To the pellet 600 μl of ice-cold cell, lysis buffer was added and mixed well, and then 200 μl of ammonium acetate was added to the mixture to precipitate the proteins and centrifuged at 3000 rpm for 7 min. The supernatant was separated and 1000 μl of isopropanol was added and the tube was inverted till the DNA was precipitated and centrifuged at 7000 rpm for 2 min. The precipitated genomic DNA was washed with 600 μl of 70% ethanol and allowed to air dry. The DNA was resuspended in TE buffer and stored at −20°C.

Electrophoretic analysis of genomic DNA: the isolated DNA was confirmed by 0.7% agarose gel electrophoresis [68, 69].

Reagents required: Tris-boric acid EDTA buffer (TBE), gel loading dye, ethidium bromide (ETBR).

Equipment required: electrophoresis tank, power pack, voltage (100 V), gel documentation apparatus, UV-transilluminator.

Principle: electrophoresis refers to the separation of macromolecules of different size by application of a constant electric field (100 V) onto the DNA fragments placed in a matrix of polymerized agarose. As the DNA molecule is negatively charged and travels toward the anode, it is loaded at the cathode end. The speed of migration of the fragments has an inverse relation with the size of DNA. The separated fragments are visualized by staining the gels with an intercalating dye (ethidium bromide), which fluoresces under UV light. Acrylamide gels are used for separation of small fragments of DNA (5–500 bp). Agarose gels can resolve DNA fragments varying in size from 200 bp to about 50 kb depending upon the concentration of agarose in the gel.

Procedure: electrophoresis tank was filled with the 1× TBE buffer and the gel was immersed into the tank containing the buffer. Agarose gel (0.7%) was prepared with ethidium bromide and the gel was allowed to run for 1 hour at 80–100 V as pulse voltage. 20 μl of DNA sample was loaded with loading dye (bromophenol blue) in the wells. When bromophenol blue dye reached three fourth of the gel length, the power was shut down, and DNA bands were observed using gel documentation apparatus and photographed.

4.1. Genetic analysis

4.1.1. Polymerase chain reaction (PCR) for PKD1 gene (C/T polymorphism)

Amplification of isolated DNA using the following primers 5′-AGCTGTACGCCCTCACTGG-3′ (forward) and 5′-GTGACAGGTGCCAGGACTC-3′-(reverse). PCR was performed using genomic DNA (50 ng), *Taq* polymerase (1 U), dNTPs (10 mM) and each primers (10 μM) [37, 69, 70].

PCR condition used:

Initial denaturation	94°C	5 min	
Denaturation	94°C	30 s	
Annealing	61°C	30 s	35 cycles
Extension	72°C	30 s	
Final extension	72°C	7 min	

The PCR product (298 bp) was confirmed by 1.8% of agarose gel electrophoresis. The amplified product was subjected to RFLP analysis.

4.1.1.1. Restriction fragment length polymorphism (RFLP)

Amplified PCR product is digested with restriction enzyme *AvaII*, incubated the reaction mixture at 37°C for 3 hours and inactivated by incubation at 64°C for 15 min. The enzyme cuts the sequence if "T" was at position 4058. The digested fragments (298, 225 and 73bp) were confirmed by 1.2% agarose gel [37, 69, 70].

Restriction fragment length polymorphism (RFLP)

Restriction site for *AvaII*	5′....G↓GWCG ....3′
	3′....CCWG↑G....5′

Source: *E. coli* strain that carries the *AvaII* gene from *Anabaena variabilis*

4.1.2. Polymerase chain reaction (PCR) for PKD2 gene (G/C polymorphism)

Amplification of PKD2 gene using the following primers 5′-CGCGCCGGACGCCAGTGACC-3′ (forward) and 5′-GCCGGCCGTTCTGGTTCGT-3′ (reverse). PCR was performed using genomic DNA (50ng), *Taq* polymerase (1U) and dNTPs (10mM) [69, 71].

PCR condition used:

Initial denaturation	94°C	5 min	
Denaturation	94°C	30 s	
Annealing	61°C	30 s	35 cycles
Extension	72°C	30 s	
Final extension	72°C	7 min	

The PCR product (279 bp) is confirmed by 1.8% of agarose gel electrophoresis. The amplified product was subjected to RFLP analysis.

4.1.2.1. Restriction fragment length polymorphism (RFLP)

Amplified product is digested with restriction enzyme *BanII*, incubated the reaction mixture at 37°C for 2 hours and inactivated by incubation at 65°C for 20 min. The enzyme cuts the sequence if "C" was at position 28. The digested segments were confirmed by 1.2% agarose gel [69–71]).

Restriction site for *BanII*:	5′ G RGCY↓ C 3′
	5′ C↑YCGR G 5′

Source: *E. coli* strain that carries the cloned *BanII* gene from *Bacillus aneurinolyticus*.

Sequencing: PKD1 gene (C/T) and PKD2 gene (G/C) single nucleotide polymorphism was sequenced by automated sequencer (Chromous Biotech, Chennai).

Allelic frequency calculation: allelic frequency was calculated by using *Hardy-Weinberg Equilibrium*. The phenotype and genotypic frequencies in sexually reproducing, diploid organisms could be determined by applying simple algebraic expression.

$$p + q = 1 \tag{1}$$

where p is the frequency of dominant allele and q is the frequency of recessive allele.

Statistical analysis:

- Pearson Chi-square (χ^2) test was performed to find the statistical significance of genotypes and the gene frequency between the control group and ADPKD patients.
- Odds ratio (OR) was calculated for allelic frequency.
- Heterozygosity was calculated for the control subject and PKD patients.

5. Identifications of single nucleotide and polymorphisms and discussions

5.1. Genetic analysis

ADPKD is one of the most common genetic diseases in humans, affecting all ethnic groups with a prevalence of 1 in 500 to 1000 individuals [9, 18, 19, 72]. The disease is characterized by the progressive formation and enlargement of fluid-filled cysts in both kidneys due to mutations in PKD1 (85%), PKD2 (15%) and PKD3 (rare) that leads to renal failure [73]. Cyst development involves impairments in a wide range of cellular processes including increased proliferation of the renal epithelial cells, fluid transport defects, alterations in tubular basement membrane, altered cell polarity and increased apoptosis [9, 74].

Genomic DNA was isolated from frozen blood of control and ADPKD patients; it was confirmed by agarose gel electrophoresis (0.7%). After confirming the presence of genomic DNA, most of the prepared gDNA of the 260/280 ratio was found to be 1.8 or 1.9; in a few subjects, the DNA showed 2.0, which might be RNA or protein contamination. To avoid that, RNase, protease was added. Then, it was confirmed and used for PCRanalysis.

5.1.1. Analysis of C/T polymorphism in PKD1 gene

Prepared gDNA when subjected to polymerase chain reaction (PCR), 298bp fragment was obtained. The amplified PCR product was subjected to RFLP analysis using *AvaII* enzyme. When "T" allele was present at position 4058, 225bp and 73bp (homozygous mutant -TT), heterozygous mutant (CT) 298bp, 225bp and 73bp was obtained, and for homozygous normal allele (CC), 298bp fragments were identified **(Figure 5).** The PCR and RLFP products were detected and confirmed by 1.2% agarose gel electrophoresis.

5.2. Genotype and allelic frequency analysis of PKD1 (C/T) gene

The study group comprised 300 ADPKD patients and an equal number of age- and sex-matched control group. Among them, the C/C genotype was observed in 131 (43.67%) control group and in 58 (19.33%) ADPKD patients; C/T genotype in 82 (27.33%) control group and in 99 (33%) ADPKD patients; T/T genotype was found in 87 (29%) control group and in 143 (47.67%) ADPKD patients. The allelic frequency was calculated by using *Hardy-Weinberg equation* ($p + q = 1$) and the study group showed the mutant "T" allele frequency (0.642) to be significantly higher in ADPKD patients than in the control group (0.425) and the normal "C" allele frequency was observed to be significantly decreased in ADPKD patients (0.358) than in the control group (0.575). The significant difference ($P < 0.05$, 9.488, χ^2 calculated value = 14.048) (**Table 3**) was noted both in genotype and in allelic frequency between the ADPKD patients and control group among South Indian (Madurai) population by using chi-square (χ^2) test. This work, which coincides with the work done by Constantinides [70] among Caucasian and Japanese population, also has revealed the association of C/T4058 polymorphism with ADPKD. The PKD1 gene is responsible for causing autosomal dominant polycystic kidney disease and it has been recently cloned and sequenced [75]. ADPKD is reported to be a very

http://dx.doi.org/10.5772/intechopen.71201

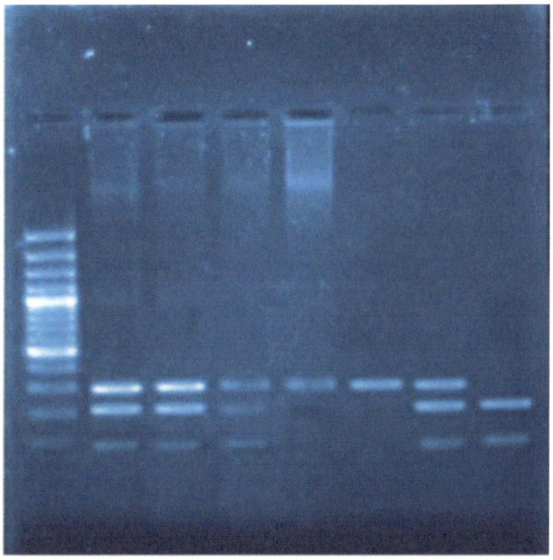

Figure 5. Confirmation of PKD 1 gene polymorphism using 1.2% agarose gel electrophoresis. T/T: homozygous mutant (225, 73 bp); C/T: heterozygous mutant (298bp, 225bp, 73bp) ; C/C: homozygous normal (298bp).

frequent disorder among Caucasian population with an estimated incidence of approximately 1:100. It has been shown to be characterized by genetic heterogeneity and three genes have been implicated in its pathogenesis called PKD1, PKD2 and PKD3 [76, 77].

The study found that the identification of DNA variation at nucleotide position at 12173 of PKD1 gene and C or T allele variation in the second position of amino acid codon at 4058 of polycystin-1 observed in 44 Japanese subjects, leading to suggest that these polymorphic alleles would be useful for linkage analysis only in specific ethnic groups [41]. It has been also reported that the PKD2 gene provides instructions for making a protein called polycystin-2, which is found in the kidneys before birth and in many adult tissues. It is also stated that the polycystin could be regulated by a larger and somewhat similar protein called polycystin-1, which is encoded by PKD1 gene [78].

5.2.1. Analysis of G/C polymorphism in PKD2 gene

Prepared gDNA was subjected to polymerase chain reaction (PCR) and 279bp fragment was amplified. The amplified PCR product is digested with the enzyme *Ban II*. The enzyme acts on the "C" variation but not on the "G" variation. If a "C" allele was present at position 83, 170bp and 109bp were obtained. If it was a homozygous mutant (CC), 170bp and 109bp; heterozygous mutant (GC), 279bp, 170bp and 109bp and homozygous normal (GG), 279bp fragments were identified. One such variation was at position 83 of PKD2, which was occupied by either G or C at exon 1. Hence, the amino acid residue was changed from arginine to proline.

The study also found that *BSP12861* restriction enzyme *also* acts on the "C" variation. This enzyme was added to 10 ADPKD patients of amplified PKD2 gene product (279bp). The results showed to be like *Ban II* restriction digestion gene products. If a "C" allele was present at position 83, 170bp and 109bp were obtained. If it was homozygous mutant (CC), 170bp and 109bp; heterozygous mutant (GC), 279bp, 170bp and 109bp and homozygous normal (GG), 279bp fragments were identified **(Figure 6).** The study was supported by the work of Koptides et al., [30]. Koptides et al. demonstrated that both G/C transversion mutation and six 'Cs" insertion mutation in exon 1 of the PKD2 gene of three separate cysts. This mutation is expected to cause a translation frameshift, leading to the incorporation of 20 novel amino acids before a new stop codon is encountered.

5.3. Genotype and allelic frequency analysis of PKD2 (G/C) gene

The G/G genotype was observed in 137 (45.67%) control group and in 55 (18.33%) ADPKD patients, G/C genotype in 84 (28%) control group and in 93 (31%) ADPKD patients and C/C genotype in 79 (26.33%) control group and in 152 (50.67%) ADPKD patients. The allelic frequency was calculated by using *Hardy-Weinberg equation* ($p + q = 1$) and the study group showed the mutant "C" allele frequency (0.662) to be significantly higher in ADPKD patients than in the control group (0.403) and the normal "G" allele frequency to be significantly decreased in ADPKD patients (0.338) than in the control group (0.597). Significant difference ($P < 0.005$, 14.860, χ^2 calculated value = 20.451) (**Table 4**) was noted in genotype and allelic frequency between the ADPKD patients. G/C polymorphism at position 83 in exon 1 of PKD2 gene among South Indian (Madurai) population with ADPKD revealed the "CC" and "GC" genotype and the frequency of "C" allele was found to be significantly higher in the ADPKD patients compared to the control group. The study has revealed higher frequency of "C" allele and lower frequency of "G" allele in ADPKD patients. These results coincide with the work of Koptides et al., [30], who identified a polymorphism at position 83, which was occupied by either G or C encoding either arginine or proline (R28P).

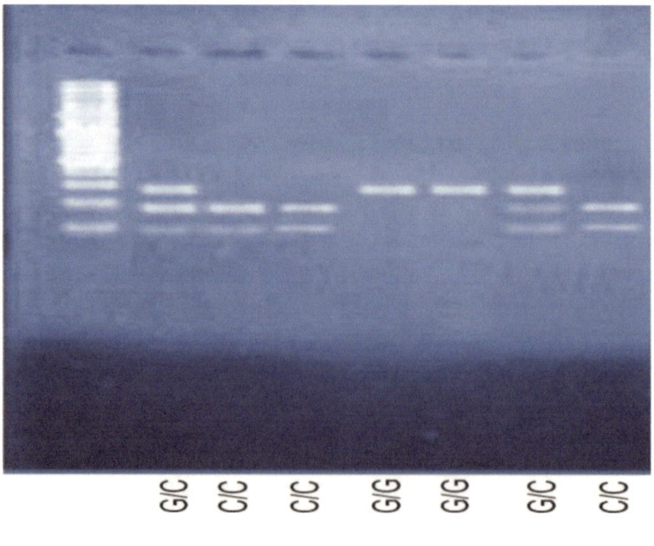

Figure 6. Confirmation of PKD 2 gene polymorphism using 1.2% agarose gel electrophoresis. C/C: homozygous mutant (170 bp, 109 bp); G/C: heterozygous mutant (279 bp, 170, 109); G/G: homozygous normal (279 bp); Lane 1: ladder (100 bp).

	Genotype			Allele frequency		χ^2 value	p value
	T/T	C/T	C/C	T	C		
Control group N = 300	87 (29%)	82 (27.33%)	131 (43.67%)	0.425	0.575	14.16	P < 0.05 9.488
ADPKD patients N = 300	143 (47.67%)	99 (33%)	58 (19.33%)	0.642	0.358	13.93	

T/T: homozygous mutant; /T: heterozygous mutant; C/C: homozygous normal.

Table 3. Comparison of genotype and allelic frequency of PKD1 gene in control group and ADPKD patients among South Indian (Madurai) population.

	Genotype			Allele frequency		χ^2 value	p value
	C/C	G/C	G/G	C	G		
Control group N = 300	79 (26.33%)	84 (28%)	137 (45.67%)	0.403	0.662	20.79	$P < 0.005$, 14.860
ADPKD patients N = 300	152 (50.67%)	93 (31%)	55 (18.33%)	0.597	0.338	20.10	

C/C: homozygous mutant; G/C: heterozygous mutant; G/G–homozygous normal.

Table 4. Comparison of genotype and allelic frequency of PKD2 gene in control group and ADPKD patients among South Indian (Madurai) population.

5.4. PKD1 (C/T) and PKD2 (G/C) SNP sequencing

The PKD1 (C/T) and PKD2 (G/C) single nucleotide polymorphism was also confirmed by sequencing the PCR amplified gene products of PKD1 and PKD2.

PKD1 (C/T) – Ala/Val. 4058 in Exon 45:

Ala

A. 5′-AAG CTG TAC GCC CTC ACT GG-3′—Wild type Allele

Val

5′-AAG CTG TAC GTC CTC ACT GG-3′—Mutant Allele

PKD2 (G/C) – Arg/Pro.28 in Exon 1

Arg

B. 5′-CG CGC CGG ACG CCA CTG ACC-3′—Wild type Allele

Pro

5′-CG CGC CCG ACG CCA CTG ACC-3′—Mutant Allele

Underlined sequence denotes change in allele leads to new amino acid formation, which is known to be polymorphism.

The study coincides with the work of Constantinides et al. [70], Watnick et al. [79] and Koptides et al., [30] in Caucasians, Greek-Cypriot populations. The present study reveals that these mutation/polymorphism leads to evolution of new alleles and formation of new amino acids among South Indian population.

6. Conclusion

Polymorphic DNA markers could be used for presymptomatic and prenatal diagnosis of ADPKD. Breuning et al. [80] and Balcells and Criach [81] recommended that prenatal diagnosis of PKD by chorionic villi sampling and linkage phase of the DNA markers has been established by haplotyping the index family. This testing offers the chance of performing prenatal or preimplantation testing in families with severe cases of the disease. Hence the current study suggests that genetic testing is very important in determining the severity and progression of the disease and could possibly be treated with effective drug and delay the end-stage renal disease (ESRD). Further research of this study is on DNA based on drug design using bioinformatics databases that might help the physicians in providing better treatment for polycystic kidney disease patients.

Author details

Pandiaraj Veeramuthumari[1*] and William Isabel[2]

*Address all correspondence to: muthusdream@gmail.com

1 Department of Zoology, V.V. Vanniaperumal College for Women, Virudhunagar, Tamil Nadu, India

2 Lady Doak College (affiliated by Madurai Kamaraj University), Madurai, India

References

[1] Glodny B, Unterholzner V, Taferner B. Normal kidney size and its influencing factors–A 64-slice MDCT study of 1.040 asymptomatic patients. BMC Urology. 2009;**9**:13-19

[2] Available from: http://www.sugarbp.org/kidneystucture_diabetes.htm

[3] Kriz W, Kaissing B. Structural and Functional Organization of the Kidney. Academic Press; 2008. p. 479-564

[4] Jameson JL, Loscalzo J. Harrison's Nephrology and Acid-Base Disorders. 17th ed. McGraw-Hill Professional; 2010. p. 3

[5] de Hoog JP, Murray S, Chou W. Horseshoe kidney and primary renal carcinoid tumour: A case report of a rare entity. Grand Rounds. 2010;**10**:46-50

[6] Oktem H, Gozil R, Calguner E, et al. Morphometric study of a horseshoe kidney. Medical Principles and Practice. 2008;**17**(1):80-83

[7] Grantham JJ. Polycystic kidney disease: From the bedside to the gene and back. Current Opinion in Nephrology and Hypertension. 2003;**10**:533-542

[8] Harris PC, Torres VE. Autosomal dominant polycystic kidney disease. GeneReviews. 2006;**4**:326-329

[9] Igarashi P, Somlo S. Genetics and pathogenesis of polycystic kidney disease. Journal of the American Society of Nephrology. 2002;**13**:2384-2398

[10] Khonsari RH, Ohazama A, Raouf R, Kawasaki M, Kawasaki K, Porntaveetus T, Ghafoor S, Hammond P, Suttie M, Odri GA, Sandford RN, Wood JN, Sharpe PT. Multiple postnatal craniofacial anomalies are characterized by conditional loss ofpolycystic kidney disease 2 (Pkd2). Human Molecular Genetics. 2013;**22**:1873-1885

[11] Liao M-T, Sung C-C, Hung K-C, C-C W, Lo L, K-C L. Insulin resistance in patients with chronic kidney disease. Journal of Biomedicine & Biotechnology. 2012:1-5

[12] Longo D, Fauci A, Kasper D, Hauser S, Jameson J, Loscalzo J. Harrison's Principles of Internal Medicine. 18th ed. McGraw-Hill Professional; 2011

[13] Webb S, Dobb G. ARF, ATN or AKI? It's now acute kidney injury. Anaesthesia and Intensive Care. 2007;**35**(6):843-844

[14] Available from: http://en.wikipedia.org/wiki/Chronic_kidney_disease; "Chronic Kidney Disease". Medscape

[15] Bacchetta J, Sea JL, Chun RF, Lisse TS. FGF23 inhibits extra-renal synthesis of 1,25-dihydroxyvitamin D in human monocytes. Journal of Bone and Mineral Research. 2012; **28**(1):46-55

[16] Chauhan V, Vaid M. Dyslipidemia in chronic kidney disease: Managing a high-risk combination. Postgraduate Medicine. 2009;**121**(6):54-61

[17] Grantham JJ, Calvet PJ. Polycystein-2, the protein mutated in autosomal dominant polycystic kidney disease (ADPKD), is a Ca^{2+}–Permeable nonselective cation chennel. Proceedings of the National Academy of Sciences of the United States of America. 2001; **98**(3):790-792

[18] Persu A, Stoenoiu T, Messiaen S. Modifier effect of ENOS in autosomal dominant polycystic kidney disease. Human Molecular Genetics. 2002;**11**:229-241

[19] Hoefele J, Mayer K, Scholz M, Klein HG. Novel PKD1 and PKD2 mutations in autosomal dominant polycystic kidney disease (ADPKD). Nephrology, Dialysis, Transplantation. 2011;**26**:2181-2188

[20] Ravind D, Walker R, Gibson R, Forrest S, Richerd R, Friend K, Sheffied L, Kincaid-Smith A, Danks D. Phenotype and genotypes heterogenicity in autosomal dominant polycystic kidney disease. Lancet. 1992;**340**:1330-1333

[21] Onuchic LF, Furu L, Nagasawa Y. PKHD1, the polycystic kidney and hepatic disease 1 gene, encodes a novel large protein containing multiple immunoglobulin-like plexin-transcription-factor domains and parallel beta-helix 1 repeats. American Journal of Human Genetics. 2002;**70**:1305-1317

[22] Ward C, Hogan M, Rossetti S, Walker D, Sneddon T, Wang X, Kubly V, Cunningham J, Bacallao R, Ishibashi M, Milliner D, Torres V, Harris P. The gene mutated in autosomal recessive polycystic kidney disease encodes a large, receptor-like protein. Nature Genetics. 2002;**30**:259-269

[23] Ahmad S, Choi R, Roberts Q, Simpson B, Wallace J. Polycystic kidney disease: The cystematic destruction of renal function. Eukaryon Editor's Corner. 2009. p. 5

[24] Sumathy VJH. Pathogenetic and molecular study of human polycystic kidney population. International Journal of Engineering and Innovative Technology (IJEIT). 2013;**3**(3):20-27

[25] Nair S, Kolla PK, Desai M, Mohan PR, Ramalingam K, Aruna R. Angiotensin-converting enzyme gene polymorphism in autosomal dominant polycystic kidney disease. NJCA. 2014;**3**(2):57-63

[26] Elumalai R, Periasamy S, Ramanathan G, Lakkakula BVKS. Role of endothelial nitric oxide synthase VNTR (intron 4 a/b) polymorphism on the progression of renal disease in autosomal dominant polycystic kidney disease. Journal of Renal Injury Prevention. 2014;**3**(3):69-73

[27] Veeramuthumari P, Isabel W. Identification of C/T genetic marker in autosomal dominant polycystic kidney disease among South Indian population (Madurai). International Journal of Pharma and Bio Sciences. 2013;**2**(6):628-639

[28] Veeramuthumari P, Srividhya K, Isabel W. Evaluation of PKD2 gene (G/C) polymorphism in patients with autosomal dominant polycystic kidney disease among South Indians (Madurai). Journal of Drug Discovery and Therapeutics. 2013;**1**(5):37-41

[29] Hateboer N, Veldhusen B, Peters D, Breuning MH, Dijk MA, Afzal AR, Jeffery S, Saggar AK, Torra R, Dimitrakov D, Matinez I, Sanz S, Krawczak M, Ravine D. Location of mutations within the PKD2 gene influences clinical outcome. Kidney International. 2000;**57**: 1444-1451

[30] Koptides M, Mean R, Demetriou K, Pierides A, Deltas CC. Genetic evidence for a trans-heterozygous model for cystogenesis in autosomal dominant polycystic kidney disease. Human Molecular Genetics. 2000;**9**:447-452

[31] Son D, Kojima I, Inagi R, Matsumoto M, Fujita T, Nangaku M. Chronic hypoxia aggravates injury via suppression of Cu/Zn-SOD: A proteomic analysis. American Journal of Physiology. Renal Physiology. 2008;**294**:F62-F72

[32] Lee Y-J, Chen H-Y, Wong M-L, Hsu W-L, C-M O, Wong M-L. Diagnosis of feline polycystic kidney disease by a combination of ultrasonographic examination and PKD1 gene analysis. Veterinary Record. 2010;**167**:614-617

[33] GaleanoCH, CortesAC, FernansezA, SolerA, Franco-HerreraN, MakundeG, VanderleydenJ, Blair MW. Gene-based single nucleotide polymorphism markers for genetic and association mapping in common bean. BMC Genetics. 2012;**13**(48):1-11

[34] Grantham JJ, Cook LT, Torres VE, Bost JE, Chapman AB, Harris PC, Guay-Woodford LM, Bae KT, Grantham J, Cook L, Wetzel L, et al. Evidence of extraordinary growth in the progressive enlargement of renal cysts. Clinical Journal of the American Society of Nephrology. 2010;**5**(5):889-896

[35] Murcia NS, Richards WG, Yoder BK, Mucenski ML, Dunlap JR, Woychik RP. The Oak Ridge Polycystic Kidney (orpk) disease gene is required for left-right axis determination. Development. 1999;**127**:2347-2355

[36] Wilson PD. Epithelial cell polarity and disease. The American Journal of Physiology. 1997;**272**:434-442

[37] Pei Y, Wang K, Kasenda M, Paterson AD, Chan G, Liang Y, Roscoe J, Brissenden J, Hefferton D, Parfrey P, Somlo S, George Hyslop P. A spectrum of mutation in polycystic kidney disease-2 (PKD2) genes from eight Canadian kindred. Journal of the American Society of Nephrology. 1998;**9**:1853-1860

[38] Tazon-Vega Mireia V. Study of candidate genes affecting the progression of renal disease in autosomal dominant polycystic kidney disease type 1. Nephrology, Dialysis, Transplantation. 2007;**22**:1567-1577

[39] Torra R, Viribay M, Tellaria D, Badenas C, Watson M, Harris P, Darnell A, San Millan JL. Seven novel mutations of the PKD2 gene families with autosomal dominant polycyctic kidney disease. Kidney International. 1999;**56**:28-33

[40] Koptides M, Hadjimichael C, Koupepidou P, Pierides A, Constantinou Deltas C. Germinal and somatic mutations in the PKD2 gene of renal cysts in abnormal dominant polycystic kidney disease. Human Molecular Genetics. 1999;**8**(3):509-513

[41] Hughes J, Ward CJ, Peral B, Aspinwall R, Clark K, San MJ, Gamble V, Harris PC. The polycystic kidney disease 1 (PKD1) gene encodes a novel protein with multiple cell recognition domains. Nature Genetics. 1995;**10**:151-160

[42] Bogdanova N, Markoff A, Gerke V, McCluskey M, Horst J, Dworniczak B. Homologues to the first gene for autosomal dominant polycystic kidney disease are pseudogenes. Genomics. 2002;**74**:333-341

[43] Avialable from: http://ghr.nlm.nih.gov/gene/PKD1

[44] Available from: http://ghr.nlm.nih.gov/gene/PKD2

[45] Torres VE, Harris PC. Autosomal dominant polycystic kidney disease: The last 3 years. Kidney International. 2009;**76**:149-168

[46] Charron A, Nakamura S, Bacallao R, Wandinger-Ness A. Compermised cytoarchitecture and polarised trafficking in autosomal dominant polycystic kidney disease cells. The Journal of Cell Biology. 2000;**149**:111-124

[47] Geng L, Segal Pavlova A, Barros EJ, Lohing C, Lu W, Nigam SK, Frischauf AM, Reeders ST, Zhou J. Distribution and developmentally regulated expression of murine polycystine. The American Journal of Physiology. 1997;**272**:451-459

[48] Foggensteiner L, Beven AP, Thomos R, Coleman R, Boulter C, Bradely J, Klinger K, Sandford R. Cellular and subcellular distribution of polycystin-2, the protein product of PKD gene. American Society of Nephrology. 2009;**11**:814-827

[49] Boletta A, Quian F, Onuchic LF, Cortese M, Courtoy PJ, Soria MR, Devuyst O, Monaco L. Biochemical characterization of bonafied polycystine-1 in vitro and in vivo. American Journal of Kidney Diseases. 2002;**38**:1421-1429

[50] Brasier J, Henske EP. Loss of the polycystic kidney disease (PKD1) region of chromosome 16p13 in renal cyst cells supports a loss of function model for cyst pathogenesis. The Journal of Clinical Investigation. 1997;**99**:194-199

[51] Qian F, Watnick TJ, Onuchic LF, Germino GG. The molecular basis of focal cyst formation in human autosomal dominant polycystic kidney disease type I. Cell. 1996;**87**:979-987

[52] Chapin HC, Caplan MJ. The cell biology of polycystic kidney disease. JCB. 2010;**191**(4): 701-710

[53] Harris PC, Bae KT, Rossetti S. Cyst number but not the rate of cystic growth is associated with the mutated gene in autosomal dominant polycystic kidney disease. Journal of the American Society of Nephrology. 2006;**11**:3013-3019

[54] Hebert DN, Nadasd T, Nadasdy G, Agarwal G, Mauer M, Agarwal AK, Khabiri H, Nagaraja HN. Proposed pathogenesis of idiopathic loin pain-hematuria syndrome. American Journal of Kidney Diseases. 2006;**47**(3):419-427

[55] Gross JL, de Azevedo MJ, Silveiro SP, Canani LH, Caramori LM, Zelmanovitz T. Diabetic nephropathy: Diagnosis, prevention, and treatment. Diabetes Care. 2005;**28**(1):164-176

[56] Hannah CC, Caplan MJ. The cell biology of polycystic kidney disease. The Journal of Cell Biology. 2010;**191**:701-710

[57] Brisman JL, Song JK, Newell DW. Cerebral aneurysms. The New England Journal of Medicine. 2006;**355**(9):928-939

[58] Fick GM, Johnson AM, Strain JD, Kimberling WJ, Kumar S, Manco-Johnson ML, Duley IT, Gabow PA. Characteristics of very early onset autosomal dominant polycystic kidney disease. Journal of the American Society of Nephrology. 1994;**3**:1863-1870

[59] Luft FC. Hypertensive nephrosclerosis—A cause of end-stage renal disease? Nephrology, Dialysis, Transplantation. 2000;**15**(10):1515-1517

[60] Tylicki L, Rutkowski B. Hypertensive nephropathy: Pathogenesis, diagnosis and treatment. Polski Merkuriusz Lekarsk (in Polish). 2003;**14**(80):168-173

[61] Torres VE, Cai Y, Chen X, GQ W, Geng L, Cleghorn KA, Johnson CM, Somlo S. Vascular expression of polycystin-2. Journal of the American Society of Nephrology. 2001;**12**:1-9

[62] Grantham JJ, Chapman AB, Torres VE. Volume progression in autosomal dominant polycystic kidney disease: The major factor determining clinical outcomes. Clinical Journal of the American Society of Nephrology. 2006;**1**:148-157

[63] Cotran RS, Vinay K, Nelson F, Stanley L, Abbas K. Robbins and Cotran Pathologic Basis of Disease. 2005;**72**(1):16, 187-190

[64] Torres VE, Chapman AB, Devuyst O, Gansevoort RT, Grantham JJ, Higashihara E, Perrone RD, Krasa HB, Ouyang J, Czerwiec FS, For the TEMPO 3:4 Trial Investigators. Tolvaptan in patients with autosomal dominant polycystic kidney disease. The New England Journal of Medicine. 2012;**367**:2407-2418

[65] Masyuk TV, Masyuk AI, Torre VE, et al. Octreotide inhibits hepatic cystogenesis in a rodent model of polycystic liver disease by reducing cholangiocyte adenosine 3′,5′-cyclic monophosphate. Gastroenterology. 2007;**132**:1104-1116

[66] Shillingford JM, Murcia NS, Larson CH, Low SH, Hedgepeth R, Brown N, Flask CA, Novick AC, Goldfarb DA, Kramer-Zucker A, Walz G, Piontek KB, Germino GG, Weimbs T. The mTOR pathway is regulated by polycystin-1, and its inhibition reverses renal cystogenesis in polycystic kidney disease. Proceedings of the National Academy of Sciences. 2006;**103**:5466-5471

[67] Natoli TA, Smith LA, Rogers KA, Wang B, Komarnitsky B, Budman Y, Belenky A, Bukanov NO, Dackowski WR, Husson H. Inhibition of glucosylceramide accumulation results in effective blockade of polycystic kidney disease in mouse models. Nature Medicine. 2010;**16**:788-792

[68] Sambrooke J, Russel DW. Molecular Cloning, A Laboratory Manual. 3rd ed. New York: Cold Spring Horbor Laboratory Press, Cold Spring Horbor; 2001

[69] Veeramuthumari P, Isabel W, Kannan K. A study on the level of T3, T4, TSH and the association of A/G polymorphism with CTLA-4 gene in Graves' hyperthyroidism among South Indian population. Indian Journal of Clinical Biochemistry. 2011;**26**(1):66-69

[70] Constantinides R, Xenophontos S, Neophytou P, Nomura S, Pierides A, Constantinou C. New amino acid polymorphism, Ala/Val4058, in exon 45 of the polycystic kidney disease 1 gene: Evolution of alleles. Human Genetics. 1997;**99**:644-647

[71] Reynolds D, Hayashi T, Cai YQ, Veldhuisen B, Watnick T, Lens X, Mochizuki T, Qian F, Maeda Y, Li L, Fossdal R, Coto E, GQ W, Breuning M, Germino G, Peters D, Somlo S. Aberrant splicing in the PKD2 gene as a cause of polycystic kidney disease. Journal of the American Society of Nephrology. 1999;**10**:2342-2351

[72] Hogan MC, Masyuk TV, Page LJ, Kubly VJ, Bergstralh EJ, Li X, Kim B, King BF, Glockner J, Holmes DR III, Rossetti S, Harris PC, Nicholas F, La Russo NF, Torres VE. Randomized clinical trial of long-acting somatostatin for autosomal dominant polycystic kidney and liver disease. Journal of the American Society of Nephrology. 2010;**21**:1052-1061

[73] Brown BJ, Bihoreau MT, Sigrid BK, Iulia T, Obermiller N, Podich D, Suzanna NB, Pamela J, Kaisaki MN, Danoy P, Richard R, Jhon CB, Witzgall R, Lathrep M, Getz N, Dominique. Missense mutation in sterile α motif of novel protein Sam cystin is associated with polycystic kidney in (cyl +) rat. American Society of Nephrology. 2005;**16**:3517-3526

[74] Harris PC, Torres VE. Genetics disease online reviews at gene-test polycystic kidney disease. Annual Review of Medicine. 2009;**60**:321-337

[75] Obeidova L, Elisakova V, Stekrova J, Reiterova J, Merta M, Tesar V, Losan F, Kohoutova M. Novel mutations of PKD genes in the Czech population with autosomal dominant polycystic kidney disease. BMC Medical Genetics. 2014;**15**(41):1-12

[76] Kimberling WJ, Fain PR, Kenyon JB, Goldgar D, Sujansky E, Gabow PA. Linkage heterogeneity of autosomal dominant polycystic kidney disease. The New England Journal of Medicine. 1993;**319**:913-918

[77] Peters DJM, Spruit L, Saris JJ, Ravine D, Sandkuijl LA, Fossdal R, Boersma J, van Eijk R, Norby S, Constantinou-Deltas CD, Pierides A, Brissenden JE, Frants RR, van Ommen GJB and Breuning MH. Chromosome 4 localization of a second gene forautosomal dominant polycystic kidney disease. Nature Genetics. 1993;**5**:359-362

[78] Chang M-Y, Chen HM, Jenq CC, Lee SY, Chen YM, Tian YC, Chen YC, Hung CC, Fang JT, Yang CW, Wu-Chou YH. Novel PKD1 and PKD2 mutations in Taiwanese patients with autosomal dominant polycystic kidney disease. Journal of Human Genetics. 2013;**58**: 720-727

[79] Watnick T, Phakdeekitcharoen B, Johnson A, Gandolph MA, Wang M, Briefel G, Klinger KW, Kimberling W, Gabow P, Germino GG. Mutation detection of PKD1 identifies a novel mutation common to three families with aneurysms and/or very-early-onset disease. American Journal of Human Genetics. 1999;**65**:1561-1571

[80] Breuning MH, Snijdewin FG, Brunner H, Verwest A, Ijdo JW, Saris JJ, Dauwerse JG, Blonden L, Keith T, Callen DF. Map of 16 polymorphic loci on the short arm of chromosome 16 close to the polycystic kidney disease gene (PKD1). Journal of Medical Genetics. 1990;**27**:603-613

[81] Balcells RT, Criach EA. Molecular diagnosis of autosomal dominant polycystic kidney disease. Nefrología. 2011;**31**(1):35-43

Section 5

Clinical Management in CKD

Chapter 12

Fluid Overload in Peritoneal Dialysis

Leonardo Pazarin-Villaseñor,
Francisco Gerardo Yanowsky-Escatell,
Jorge Andrade-Sierra,
Luis Miguel Roman-Pintos and
Alejandra Guillermina Miranda-Diaz

Additional information is available at the end of the chapter

http://dx.doi.org/10.5772/intechopen.69324

Abstract

The prevalence of end-stage renal disease (ESRD) has increased globally to 10% due to diabetes mellitus, hypertension, and stroke. When chronic kidney disease (CKD) maintenance therapy fails, patients require renal replacement therapy (RRT) to survive, such as peritoneal dialysis (PD), hemodialysis, and renal transplantation. The most common therapy in Mexico is PD because it is a feasible, low-cost, and easy-to-perform procedure; however, fluid overload is a frequent condition in patients with this RRT modality. The usual adverse comorbidities in patients with PD are cardiovascular diseases (CVD) associated to atherosclerosis, uremia, inflammation, and oxidative stress. Fluid overload is intimately associated to hypertension, left ventricular hypertrophy, heart failure, and worsening of kidney failure, leading to increased hospital admissions, higher cardiovascular mortality, and reduced life expectancy. Two main pathologies are involved in the deterioration of both heart and kidney functions, namely, cardiorenal syndrome and uremic cardiomyopathy. Along with these phenomena, patients in PD with rapid peritoneal transport have reduced ultrafiltration, increased glucose absorption, and albumin loss in the dialysate, which lead to overhydration, hypertension, dyslipidemia, and malnutrition. This review focuses on the clinical, physiological, and biochemical mechanisms involved in fluid overload of patients with CKD undergoing PD.

Keywords: end-stage renal disease, peritoneal dialysis, fluid overload, cardiorenal syndrome, uremic cardiomyopathy, ultrafiltration failure

1. Introduction

1.1. Chronic kidney disease

The prevalence of chronic degenerative diseases has recently increased due to aging of the society and advances in medical technology [1]. In Mexico, there is a significant increase in the prevalence and incidence of non-transmittable diseases, such as diabetes mellitus (DM), hypertension, and stroke, which raises the prevalence of end-stage renal disease (ESRD) up to 10% globally [2–5].

Chronic kidney disease (CKD) is defined as a severe, irreversible kidney damage, measured by the level of proteinuria and reduced glomerular filtration rate that prevents the kidneys from functioning properly and removing toxins and waste products from the blood [6, 7]. Among the many traditional risk factors for CKD, DM is the leading cause of kidney dysfunction in the developed world. CKD induce vascular damage and therefore a raise in cardiovascular mortality; it is considered an independent risk factor for cardiovascular events, even from the early stages of the disease [8–13].

When CKD maintenance therapy fails, patients will require renal replacement therapy (RRT) to survive; among the alternatives of RRT, there is peritoneal dialysis (PD), hemodialysis (HD), and renal transplantation (TR) [14, 15]. The most common cause of ESRD in the world is type 2 DM (38%) according to the study of Kidney Early Evaluation Program (KEEP) [16–18]. The second most common cause is hypertension, and the combination of DM and hypertension raises the prevalence up to 42% [3, 19]. However, ESRD of unknown origin is one of the most prevalent diagnoses due to a lack of prompt recognition of the disease, and is unclear whether hypertension is a cause or consequence of CKD [20]. Furthermore, a study including 3564 healthy subjects reported a prevalence of deteriorated creatinine clearance <60 mL/min of 37% [21].

The United States Renal Data System (USRDS), in 2013, reported that Mexico, USA, and Portugal had a rate of 63, 58, and 54 patients per million of habitants (ppmh), respectively. The overall prevalence of CKD in adults varies between 6% and 69% [22]. The Registry of Dialysis and Transplant in Jalisco and Morelos has reported an increase of patients who require a RRT in the last decade [23, 24]. In 2013, Mendez et al. reported an incidence of 421 per million and a prevalence of 1653 per million of habitants, which places Mexico in the second country with more ESRD incident cases and the sixth most prevalent [25].

Health systems are taking emergency measures to control the burden of the disease due to the health impact, elevated costs, overall risk of developing CKD, and its consequences. Thanks to the National Kidney Foundation (NKF) that produces clinical practice guidelines through the NKF Kidney Disease Outcomes Quality Initiative (NKF K/DOQI), in 2002, it has been possible to establish an early diagnosis, risk stratification, and well-defined action plans to mitigate the progression of the disease and its cardiovascular complications [26].

1.2. Chronic kidney disease and renal replacement therapy

In Mexico, PD is the most frequent RRT implemented, followed by HD, which has increased rapidly over the last years [5]. The PD is a feasible, low-cost, and easy-to-perform procedure, reason for why in Latin America is gaining popularity. Chile is the more prevalent country with PD as the first-line RRT, and Mexico has the second place in Latin America and eighth place around the world [3, 27]. Hemodialysis is mainly available in social security and private institutions; however, HD is more expensive for governmental institutions, and hence it is not an open resource for all patients with ESDR [28]. Renal transplant is the RRT associated with better long-term survival rates and is considered the best RRT for ESDR patients; immunosuppressive drugs have reduced mortality and improved the viability of the graft [29]. The highest proportion of renal transplantation in the world is in Jalisco, Mexico, according to the USRDS [22]. However, the waiting lists for a RT are increasing exponentially, in spite of the fact that in Mexico the donation of live donors is privileged [5].

Unfortunately, RRT generate high costs and are limited to treating certain populations with social security, leaving the so-called disadvantaged populations in abandonment, generating a high rate of morbidity and mortality in younger populations. In 2005, the Mexican Institute of Social Security (IMSS) reported that treating ESDR represented 21% of the total expenditure of its main program, with only 0.7% of the beneficiaries' investment [22].

HD increase chronic inflammation by different mechanisms. A continuous contact with artificial filter dialysis membranes that induce complement activation, cytokines, and nitric oxide production characterizes HD. There also may be exposure to dialysate contaminants, which cross the dialysis membranes with monocyte stimulation and activation. Another deleterious process contributing inflammation in HD is local or systemic infections through contamination of vascular accesses, such as endovascular catheters, synthetic grafts, and arteriovenous fistulas. Fluid overload also occurs in HD due to extracellular fluid expansion and ventricular growth, which enhances CVD risk [30].

1.3. Peritoneal dialysis and cardiovascular mortality

ESDR is among the leading causes of death worldwide; morbidity and mortality in this group of patients are mainly due to CVD [31]. CVD in patients with PD is associated to traditional risk factors, such as atherosclerosis, DM, and hypertension, in addition to uremia, inflammation, and oxidative stress [12]. Cardiorenal syndrome (CRS) is a manifestation of CVD in patients with ESRD and is manifested by acute and chronic conditions where the primary dysfunction may be renal or cardiac. Among the five categories of CRS, type 4 is characterized by pre-existing CKD that leads to ESRD with progressive worsening of cardiac function [32].

Fluid overload is one of the main characteristics of patients with late CKD. The abnormal state of fluid in the disease correlates with hypertension, left ventricular hypertrophy (LVH), and other adverse cardiovascular sequels [33]. There is evidence that fluid overload is associated with significant increased risk of mortality from all cardiovascular causes in dialysis patients [34], which makes strict volume control imperative to improve the survival of patients undergoing dialysis [35]. A previous study showed the positive relationship between fluid overload with an increased risk of initiating dialysis and decrease in rapid renal function in late CKD, which means that fluid overload is not a feature in CKD, but also a prognostic marker of rapid progression of late CKD [36]. Adverse progression of kidney disease in patients with DM is associated with changes for fluid, thus contributing to fluid overload [37]. There appears to be a complex interaction between DM, fluid overload, and progression of kidney disease [38]. Dialysis procedure by itself plays an important role in the pathogenesis of accelerated atherosclerosis in patients with ESRD [39] (**Figure 1**).of fluid retention in patients undergoing peritoneal dialysis are shown

1.3.1. Cardiorenal syndrome

There is a close relationship between cardiac and renal functions. It is bidirectional and has physical, chemical, and biological implications. Primary disorders of one of these two organs often result in secondary dysfunction or injury to the other [40]. Over the last decade, cardiovascular mortality in patients with CKD has remained strikingly elevated. CKD is a recognized risk factor for the development of CVD [41] and increases 10- to 20-fold the risk of cardiac death compared to non-CKD subjects, after adjusting for age and gender [42]. A glomerular filtration rate (GFR) below 60 mL/min/1.73 m^2 is associated with cardiovascular risk; therefore, patients with CKD should be thoroughly evaluated in the search for cardiovascular risk factors that may require aggressive management [43].

Cardiorenal syndrome is a pathophysiological disturbance of the interaction between the heart and the kidneys caused by acute or chronic dysfunction in one of the two organs, capable of inducing acute or chronic dysfunction in the other organ. In 2008, Ronco et al. proposed five subtypes according to the temporal sequence of organ failure and the clinical context [31]:

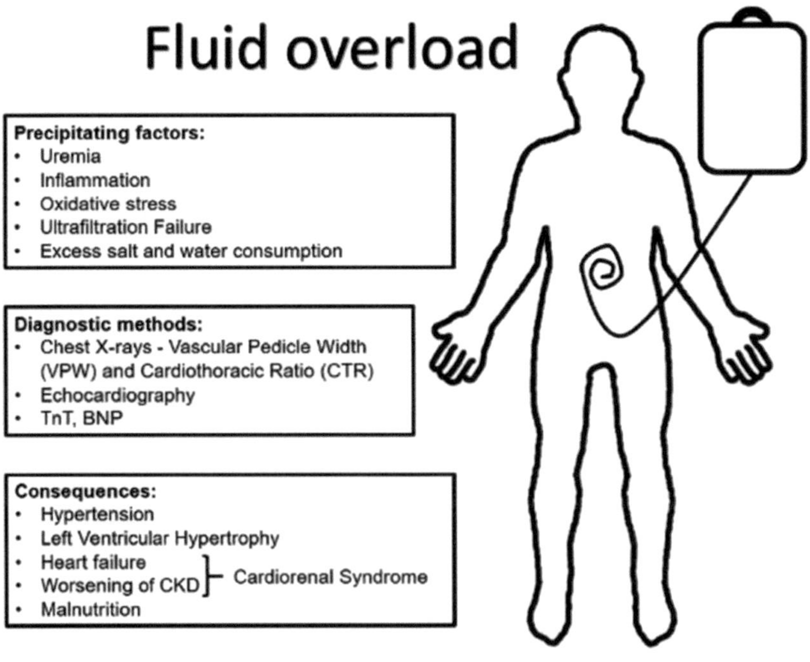

Figure 1. Fluid overload. The mechanisms of fluid retention in patients undergoing peritoneal dialysis are shown schematically.

An acute cardiac disease that leads to acute kidney injury (AKI) [33] or worsening of a chronic kidney failure characterizes acute cardiorenal syndrome or *CRS type 1*. It is also a consequence of low cardiac output due to acute coronary syndrome. When renal function worsens, it is possible to predict significantly higher rates of hospitalization and mortality from acute heart failure [44].

In *CRS type 2*, a chronic heart failure leads to CKD due to a hemodynamic imbalance. It is often manifested as a chronic renal dysfunction associated to chronic heart failure [45]. An episode of AKI that leads to acute heart failure characterizes *CRS type 3*. Retention of uremic solutes and/or volume overload may contribute to cardiac injury. According to experimental data, it is suggested that cardiac dysfunction may be related to activation of the immune system, release of inflammatory mediators, oxidative stress, and cellular apoptosis [46]. Other proposed mechanisms include electrolyte and fluid imbalance, metabolic acidosis, and uremia [47].

Chronic cardiorenal syndrome or *CRS type 4* is defined as a primary CKD that induces heart failure, ventricular hypertrophy, diastolic dysfunction, and/or greater risk of major cardiovascular events. Clinically, it is very difficult to distinguish between *CRS types 2* and *4*, since the first insult is not often recognized [39]. The prototype of *CRS type 4* is polycystic renal disease, an autosomal dominant genetic disease that leaves no doubt of the primary event. Increased fluid retention characterizes *CRS type 4*, found in approximately 70–80% of patients with ESRD [48, 49].

CRS type 5 comprises simultaneous heart and kidney dysfunction due to a systemic disease. Given the broad spectrum of diseases that contribute to this syndrome, there are several pathophysiological mechanisms consequence of the systemic disease: an overwhelming insult leads to the simultaneous development of AKI and acute cardiac dysfunction [50]. Sepsis and drug-induced toxicity are the most common causes leading to *CRS type 5*. It may develop in a patient with previously impaired organ function or when there is no discernible evidence of prior abnormality. The sequence of organ involvement may vary depending upon the acuity and nature of the underlying disorder. Other known systemic diseases that lead to *CRS type 5* are autoimmune disorders, such as lupus, Wegener's granulomatosis, and sarcoidosis. It is difficult to identify the underlying pathophysiological mechanisms in order to develop a diagnostic and therapeutic intervention strategy; thus, to identify the underlying mechanism, it is essential to consider the temporal events that initially lead to this syndrome. *CRS type 5* has the following phases: hyperacute (0–72 h after the diagnosis), acute (3–7 days after), subacute (7–30 days), and chronic (>30 days). Most of the evidence of hyperacute stage comes from clinical trials of sepsis, and patients with cirrhosis support the research from chronic stage. A precipitating event usually contributes to the development of *CRS type 5* in a chronic patient, for example, a spontaneous bacterial peritonitis in a patient with cirrhosis. Therefore, we may find superimposition of acute *CRS type 5* on an indolent chronic process with immediate relevance for intensive care physicians, nephrologists, and cardiologists [51].

Almost 75% of the patients with ESRD have a cardiovascular pathology [31]. Kidney failure worsens the short- and long-term prognosis due to several comorbid cardiovascular conditions. Acute myocardial infarction survival is lower as the deterioration of renal function increases, and the chance for survival is even worst in patients with ESRD and congestive heart failure [52]. CKD patients have 10–20 times higher risk for cardiovascular mortality than healthy subjects; even small reductions in kidney function can induce a significant increase of cardiovascular risk: patients with stage 1–3 of CKD have 25–100 times higher risk of CVD, and stage 5 has a similar kidney and heart morbidity and mortality [31]. Almost half of the patients with ESRD in PD have cardiac arrhythmias (especially atrial fibrillation) [53]. Other risk factors for cardiovascular mortality in PD users are cardiac valvulopathies, water retention, hypertension, DM, vascular calcifications, altered oxidative status, bone mineral disorders, and uremic cardiomyopathy [54].

1.3.2. Uremic cardiomyopathy

Uremic cardiomyopathy (UC) is a suitable example for *CRS type 4*, as it is characterized by cardiac dysfunction leading to fluid overload and hypertension, accentuated by the presence of high levels of myocardial urea [55, 56]. UC is found at early stages of CKD and leads to structural and functional cardiovascular damage as the kidney dysfunction progresses [57, 58]. UC can predict CVD mortality at the beginning of PD [30]. The main feature is LVH, considered as a primary manifestation of UC, but it also induces left ventricular dilation and both systolic and diastolic cardiac dysfunctions [28].

The first-line treatment for UC is conventional HD, since it leads to a reduction in LVH. HD can also reverse systolic dysfunction by improving the left ventricular ejection fraction. The earlier HD is initiated in patients with PD and fluid retention, the more damage to the myocardium induced by UC can be avoided [59]. Angiotensin-converting enzyme inhibitors decrease LVH even in normotensive subjects. Likewise, RT confers remodeling to the myocardium affected by UC in patients with ESRD undergoing PD during short or medium time lapses, although some data are contradictory because of the dyslipidemia, hypertension, and DM associated to immunosuppressants in RT recipients [60].

1.4. Diagnostic methods and cardiovascular disease biomarkers

Chronic intravascular hypervolemia in patients with PD is an important contributor to CVD. There is no simple and reliable method to assess the volume status in patients with PD [61]; ankle edema or elevated jugular venous pressure is not accurate because they can only detect abnormal body water volume. Traditionally, body fluid compartment is measured by dilution methods for solutes or isotopes, but the tests are cumbersome and rarely used in routine clinical practice. More recently, measurement of vascular pedicle width (VPW) and cardiothoracic ratio (CTR) on chest radiographs is a noninvasive surrogate marker of intravascular volume status in critically ill patients [62]. Moreover, temporary changes in fluid balance are reflected in simple chest X-rays. The objective radiographic findings of intravascular volume may be more appropriate for fluid balance than subjective measurements; the VPW is the most sensitive determination. When systematically quantified, sequential chest radiographs provide substantial information to other clinically available data to help handle fluids in patients with water retention [63]. In patients with long-standing PD, CTR is an independent predictor of hospitalization-free patient survival; this radiological parameter can be used for risk stratification of patients undergoing PD [64].

Echocardiography is the most reliable, noninvasive, diagnostic procedure, capable to identify UC-related findings. Its capacity to quantify ventricular mass, ejection fraction, valvular disease, pericardial effusion, or pulmonary arterial hypertension [65] makes it useful to predict the damage extent of ESRD patients with recent RRT [66, 67]. Diastolic dysfunction and LVH have been described in three out of four patients, and systolic dysfunction in half of the patients who undergo initial PD. It is also very common to find aortic and mitral valve alterations, almost in one third of these patients. These findings have repercussion in the prognosis of patients with ESDR who start a PD program [68].

There are several useful biomarkers already evaluated in patients with CKD: troponin (TnT), plasminogen activator inhibitor type 1 (PAI-1), homocysteine, brain natriuretic peptide (BNP), C-reactive protein (CRP), serum amyloid-A protein, ischemia-modified albumin, and advanced glycation products (AGEs) have been shown to correlate with adverse cardiovascular (CV) events in patients with CKD [31].

Troponin T (TnT) and BNP have a good predictive value in this population [69, 70]. They were both elevated in patients with hypervolemia and were able to identify asymptomatic patients with CKD who have 2–5 times increased CV risk. BNP is also a useful marker in patients with left ventricular dysfunction and cardiovascular congestion. Increased levels of TnT represent a strong independent predictor of overall cardiovascular mortality in asymptomatic patients with HD [31]. Renal biomarkers, such as cystatin C (CysC) and neutrophil gelatinase-associated lipcalin (NGAL), have recently been studied as prognostic and diagnostic markers of cardiovascular outcomes in CKD patients [71]. There are increased levels of CysC in atherosclerotic processes and LVH; it has association with the latter, independently of renal function. Researchers found increased levels of NGAL expression in the atherosclerotic plaque of patients with heart failure due to coronary heart disease [31, 72].

1.5. Peritoneal transport

A useful tool for the management of patients in PD is the peritoneal equilibration test (PET). This method has proved to be effective in assessing peritoneal function. In this test, the saturation curves of the solutes in the peritoneum with respect to the plasma are evaluated; thus, it is possible to classify the peritoneal functioning in an easy and reproducible way [73, 74]. PET has been shown to have a prognostic value in patients undergoing PD [75] and allows patients to be classified according to the ratio of solute concentrations in dialysate and plasma (D/P ratio) 4 h after the test. Creatinine, urea, electrolytes, phosphate, and proteins are the commonly tested solutes, and it classifies patients in different types of transporters: (a) high or fast, (b) average high, (c) low average, and (d) low. PET allows the clinician to determine the best dialysis modality for each individual who will undergo continuous ambulatory PD or automated DP (continuous cyclic DP or intermittent nocturnal DP) [76].

Patients with high peritoneal solute transport rates often have inadequate transport of the peritoneal fluid. It is not known whether inadequate transport of fluids is solely due to a rapid drop in osmotic pressure or if the reduction in the efficiency of liquid transport is also a contributing factor. The difference in fluid transport between the abovementioned groups is apparently due to variances in the rate of disappearance of the total osmotic pressure of the dialysate, resulting from the transport velocity of glucose and other small solutes [77]. Although glucose gradient is the main factor influencing the rate of ultrafiltration, other solutes, such as urea, are also important [78]. However, there is a relationship between comorbid states that lead to an elevated mortality and the rapid transport of solutes [79].

Patients in PD with rapid peritoneal transport have reduced ultrafiltration, increased glucose absorption, and albumin loss in the dialysate. This phenomenon induces fluid overload, hypertension, dyslipidemia, and malnutrition, along with increased mortality. In addition, systemic vascular disorders observed in DM, hypertension, atherosclerosis, sepsis, and smoking contribute to survival deterioration in these patients; vascular and endothelial disorders are closely related to malnutrition-inflammation-atherosclerosis syndrome [80]. By its own, this syndrome can explain the high mortality rate observed in patients with rapid peritoneal transport [81].

The rapid transport of solutes at the beginning of PD is closely associated with genetic, inflammatory, and structural factors of the peritoneal membrane [82]. The clinical consequences of these alterations are CVD, metabolic disturbances of glucose and lipids, hypoalbuminemia, and malnutrition. In order to treat adequately patients with rapid solute transport, it is necessary to improve their comorbidities and modify their dialytic solutions with better osmotic substances different from glucose, as well as dialysis modalities that optimize ultrafiltration [60].

1.5.1. Ultrafiltration failure

Peritoneal transport dysfunction is usually associated with ultrafiltration failure (UF) or deficit. Ultrafiltration failure is defined by the Society of Peritoneal Dialysis as the impossibility to maintain a stable dry weight in spite an adequate fluid restriction, and the total ultrafiltration volume is less than 400 mL after two or more hypertonic dialytic exchange with at least 4 h inside the peritoneal cavity using dextrose solution of 3.86% [83]. The prevalence of UF increases with duration of PD, so that 30–50% of patients with PD develop UF, many patients abandon PD due to UF, and dropout increases depending on the type of PD. It has been reported up to 3% of dropouts during the first year and 31% after the next six years [59, 84].

There are four ultrafiltration failure causes:

- Type I, due to an increase of the effective peritoneal surface with increase in solute transport. It appears in the acute phase of peritonitis episodes associated to PD and is characterized by an early recovery after 30 days [85].
- Type II is characterized by a reduced effective peritoneal surface with irreversible peritoneal involvement due to peritoneal adhesions or sclerosing peritonitis secondary to previous surgical scars or repetitive bacterial peritonitis [86].
- Type III is due to the increased rate of peritoneal lymphatic reabsorption [87].
- Type IV, also known as transcellular UF, is the most recently described and illustrated by a cellular dysfunction or disruption of aquaporins in the cellular wall [88].

Some mechanical problems should be discarded if fluid overload is suspected: lost from dialysate fluid due to herniation or history of multiple abdominal surgeries, poorly positioned catheters secondary to migration of the original catheter, inadequate placement during the surgical procedure, and abdominal adhesions from previous surgeries [89].

The functional study of the peritoneal membrane is useful to guide the prescription of PD, predict the response of standard exchanges, and diagnose ultrafiltration disturbances during PD treatment. Knowing the pathophysiological mechanisms can help determine the underlying etiology of UF to ensure prompt actions that can help preserve peritoneal membrane for longer periods [90].

1.6. Salt restriction and volume status

Salt is an ionic component composed of sodium chloride (60% chloride and 40% sodium), with a molar mass of 58,433 g/mol. Sodium is an essential nutrient for the correct functioning of nerves and muscles, as well as water self-regulation and fluid balance. Salt is widely used to preserve processed foods, cooking, and seasoning. Processed foods have higher amounts of salt than natural foods, such as meats, fruits, and vegetables, which have a significant impact on a higher daily intake of sodium derived from the consumption of these foods [91]. Excessive salt intake stimulates thirst and promotes water intake, which contributes to fluid overload and hypertension [92]; therefore, a common strategy for patients with ESRD is salt and water restriction. In patients with PD, the salt balance can be improved by different strategies, among them the reduction in dietary intake, the use of diuretics to increase urinary secretion, and the increase of extraction by peritoneal ultrafiltration. The appropriate salt intake is the first treatment option for proper maintenance of the volume state [93]. The recommendation according to the Cardiovascular and Metabolic Guidelines of the International Society for Peritoneal Dialysis is to reduce intake to <2 g of sodium or <5 g of salt per day [94]. The lack of adherence to these recommendations is an important cause of fluid gain in patients undergoing PD [95].

Although at the beginning of PD excessive ingestion of salt and liquids is not usually a problem due to the preservation of residual renal function, as renal function decreases, it is imperative to advise patients to decrease salt and water intake [96]. The advice of diet salt and water restriction in patients with PD leads to a decrease in body weight of 2.8 ± 0.5 kg and consequently to a reduction of blood pressure from 158.2 ± 17.0/95.7 to 119.7 ± 16.0/77.9 mmHg, in addition, a decrease in CTR from 48.0% ± 5.6% to 42.9% ± 4.5%. The role of salt and water restriction for the management of volume overload is highlighted due to the impact on the maintenance of volume status in patients with PD, which makes it fundamental for the adequate control of volume status [97]. However, some contradictory studies like the one by Fine et al. found that administration of 60 mEq/day of sodium chloride was significantly associated with an increase in blood pressure. The raise in systolic blood pressure was from 135 ± 19 to 144 ± 21 and diastolic blood pressure from 77 ± 8 to 82 ± 12 mmHg, without body weight gain (72 ± 10 to 72 ± 11 kg) in 20 patients undergoing PD enrolled to a double-blinded crossover clinical trial. They concluded that patients tolerate a diet with normal sodium intake and does not lead to volume overload [98]. Nevertheless, salt restriction in these patients has been widely recommended for adequate maintenance of volume status.

There is no gold standard for assessing dietary salt intake in PD patients. The tools used for the evaluation are food diaries, 24-h reminders, consumption frequency questionnaires, and urine analysis for 24 h. The limitations of these tools include variation in day-to-day sodium intake, errors related to memory lapses, patient motivation, false perception of diet, difficulty in measuring salt use, over-/under-collection of urine, among others [99].

Urine 24-h sodium determination does not reflect the current sodium intake in patients with PD, since the elimination of sodium occurs through urine and dialysate. In addition, the removal of sodium from the dialysate depends on the convection through the peritoneal membrane, so it cannot reflect the current sodium intake in these patients [100, 101]. The measurement of total sodium withdrawal during dialysis adequacy assessment might be a simple and effective method of estimating sodium ingestion in patients with PD. Total sodium withdrawal during dialysis adequacy assessment may be a simple and effective method to estimate sodium intake [102]:

$$\text{Sodium intake (mg/dL)} = 15.64 \times \text{total sodium withdrawal (mEq/d)} + 646 \quad (1)$$

For example, a sodium intake of 2000 mg would correspond to a total sodium removal of approximately 87 mEq/d [102].

In a cohort of 305 PD incident patients, Dong et al. reported that low sodium ingestion was significantly associated with nutrient deficiency and poor muscle reserve and an independent predictor for mortality. It is necessary to consider whether salt restriction in the diet would improve outcomes in patients with low calorie and protein intake [100].

A correct nutritional advice can achieve a decrease in salt intake, minimizing processed foods and avoiding salt in food preparation. Certain strategies to reduce salt ingestion can be useful to improve the taste of food, such as substitution with flavor enhancers like pepper, paprika, curry, thyme, and oregano; also changing to salt substitutes, which contain potassium chloride in patients who do not require potassium restriction [103]. An advantage of salt substitutes compared to flavor enhancers is that the former have a higher salty taste, but the disadvantage is the risk of hyperkalemia [104].

Finally, another strategy is to prepare a diet containing 2 g of sodium (88 mM NaCl), by allowing to add 1/3 of tablespoon of salt for each meal during that day. It is worth noting the impact of salt intake on patients with PD. Therefore, under this context, the previously mentioned strategies to maintain a low ingestion of salt in the diet could help to avoid a deficit in the consumption of nutrients and the maintenance of the state of volume.

2. Conclusions

The incidence and prevalence of ESRD are increasing, making the need for PD necessary as a demanding RRT for patients with CKD. The main morbidity and mortality cause in patients with CKD is still primarily due to CVD. It is important to start an early approach to fluid overload by performing and interpreting different assessments, such as echocardiography, PET, UF test, and an adequate food survey for the identification of factors that contribute to poor adherence to dietary recommendations in water and saline intake. Fluid overload is an important cause for hospital admissions; thus, clinicians must have this in mind for the early identification of the causes of cardiac decompensation, besides attending the individual disorders of each patient with PD.

http://dx.doi.org/10.5772/intechopen.69324

Conflict of interest

There are no conflicts of interest.

Author details

Leonardo Pazarin-Villaseñor[1], Francisco Gerardo Yanowsky-Escatell[1], Jorge Andrade-Sierra[1], Luis Miguel Roman-Pintos[2,3] and Alejandra Guillermina Miranda-Diaz[4*]

*Address all correspondence to: kindalex1outlook.com

1 Department of Nephrology, Hospital Civil de Guadalajara "Dr. Juan I. Menchaca" Guadalajara, Jalisco, México

2 Department of Sickness and Health as an Individual Process, Centro Universitario de Tonalá, Universidad de Guadalajara, Guadalajara, Jalisco, México

3 Department of Internal Medicine, Hospital Ángeles del Carmen, Guadalajara, Jalisco, México

4 Department of Physiology, Centro Universitario de Ciencias de la Salud, Universidad de Guadalajara, Guadalajara, Jalisco, México

References

[1] Choi ES, Lee J. Effects of a face-to-face self-management program on knowledge, self-care practice and kidney function in patients with chronic kidney disease before the renal replacement therapy. Journal of Korean Academy of Nursing. 2012;**42**(7):1070-1088

[2] Correa-Rotter R, González-Michaca L. Early detection and prevention of diabetic nephropathy: A challenge calling for mandatory action for Mexico and the developing world. Kidney International. 2005;(98):S69-S75

[3] Parfrey PS, Foley RN. The clinical epidemiology of cardiac disease in chronic renal failure. Journal of the American Society of Nephrology. 1999;**10**:1606-1615

[4] Shastri Sh, Sarnak MJ. Cardiovascular disease and CKD: Core curriculum 2010. American Journal of Kidney Disease. 2010;**56**(2):399-417

[5] Alonso Gómez AM. ¿Qué debe de conocer el nefrólogo de la afectación cardiaca del pacienteen diálisis peritoneal? Nefrología. 2008;**28**(6):105-111

[6] White SL, Chadban SJ, Jan S, Chapmanc JR, Cass A. How can we achieve global equity in provision of renal replacement therapy? Bulletin of the World Health Organization. 2008;**86**:229-237

[7] Jin DC, Han JS. Renal replacement therapy in Korea, 2012. Kidney Research and Clinical Practice. 2014;**33**(1):9-18

[8] Weiner DE, Tighiouart H, Stark PC, et al. Kidney disease as a risk factor for recurrent cardiovascular disease and mortality. American Journal of Kidney Disease. 2004;**44**:198-206

[9] Zhang L, Zuo L, Wang F, et al. Cardiovascular disease in early stages of chronic kidney disease in a Chinese population. Journal of the American Society of Nephrology. 2006;**17**:2617-2621

[10] Chronic Kidney Disease Prognosis Consortium. Association of estimated glomerular filtration rate and albuminuria with all-cause and cardiovascular mortality in general population cohorts: A collaborative meta-analysis. Lancet. 2010;**375**:2073-2081

[11] Van der Velde M, Matsushita K, Coresh J, et al. Lower estimated glomerular filtration rate and higher albuminuria are associated with all-cause and cardiovascular mortality. A collaborative meta-analysis of high-risk population cohorts. Kidney International. 2011;**79**:1341-1352

[12] Clase CM, Gao P, Tobe SW, et al. Estimated glomerular filtration rate and albuminuria as predictors of outcomes in patients with high cardiovascular risk: A cohort study. Annals of Internal Medicine. 2011;**154**:310-318

[13] Fox CS, Matsushita K, Woodward M, Bilo HJ, Chalmers J, et al. Chronic Kidney Disease Prognosis Consortium: Associations of kidney disease measures with mortality and end-stage renal disease in individuals with and without diabetes: a meta-analysis. Lancet. 2012;**380**:1662-1673

[14] Garcia-Garcia G, Briseño-Rentería G, Luquín-Arellano VH, Gao Z, Gill J, Tonelli M. Survival among patients with kidney failure in Jalisco México. Journal of the American Society of Nephrology. 2007;**18**:1922-1927

[15] Kim EJ, Chung CH, Park MY, Choi SJ, Kim JK, Hwang SD. Mortality predictors in patients treated with continuous renal replacement. Korean Journal of Nephrology. 2011;**30**:73-79

[16] Kidney Disease: Improving Global Outcomes (KDIGO) CKD Group. KDIGO 2012 Clinical Practice Guideline for the Evaluation and Management of Chronic Kidney Disease. Summary of Recommendation Statements. Kidney International. 2013;**3**(1):5-14

[17] Cueto-Manzano A, Quintana-Piña E, Correa-Rotter R. Long term CAPD survival and analysis of mortality risk factors: 12-year experience of a single Mexican center. Peritoneal Dialysis International. 2001;**21**:148-153

[18] Cueto-Manzano A, Rojas-Campos E. Status of renal replacement therapy and peritoneal dialysis in Mexico. Peritoneal Dialysis International. 2007;**27**:142-148

[19] Obrador GT, García-García G, Villa AR, et al. Prevalence of Chronic kidney disease in the Kidney early Evaluation Program (KEEP) Mexico and comparison with KEEP US. Kidney International. 2010;**77**(Suppl 116):S2-S8

[20] Vasavada N, Agarwal R. Role of excess volume in the pathophysiology of hypertension in chronic kidney disease. Kidney Int. 2003 Nov;**64**(5):1772-9

[21] Amato D, Alvarez-Aguilar C, Castañeda-Limones R, et al. Prevalence of chronic kidney disease in an urban Mexican Population. Kidney International. 2005;**68**(Suppl 97):S11-S17

[22] The US Renal Data System. Available at: https://www.usrds.org/adr.aspx. Accessed: February 12, 2017

[23] Saran R, Li Y, Robinson B, et al. US Renal Data System 2015 Annual Data Report: Epidemiology of kidney disease in the United States. American Journal of Kidney Diseases. 2016;**67**(3 suppl 1):S1-S434

[24] Guía de Práctica Clínica. Prevención, Diagnóstico y Tratamiento de la Enfermedad Renal Crónica Temprana. México; Secretaría Nacional de Salud; 2009

[25] Mendez DA, Mendez-Bueno F, Tapia YT, Muñoz MA, Aguilar SL. Epidemiologia de la insuficiencia renal crónica en México. Diálisis y Trasplante. 2010;**31**(1):7-11

[26] National Kidney Foundation. K/DOQI Clinical Practice Guidelines for chronic kidney disease: Evaluation, classification and stratification. American Journal of Kidney Disease. 2002;**39**(Suppl 1):S1-S266

[27] Garcia GG, Monteon RF, Garcia BH, et al. Renal replacement therapy among disadvantaged populations in Mexico a report from the REDTJAL. Kidney International. 2005;**68**:s58-s61

[28] Durán-Arenas L, Avila-Palomares PD, Zendejas-Villanueva R, Vargas-Ruiz MM, Tirado-Gómez LL, López-Cervantes M. Direct cost analysis of hemodialysis units. Salud Pública de México. 2011;**53**(4):516-524

[29] Garcia GG, Harden P, Chapman J. El papel global del trasplante renal. Nefrología. 2012;**32**(1);1-6

[30] Clementi A, Virzi GM, Go ChY, Cruz D, Granata A, Vescovo G, et al. Cardiorenal syndrome type 4: A review. CardioRenal Medicine. 2013;**3**:63-70

[31] Ronco C, Haapio M, House AA, Anavekar N, Bellomo R. Cardiorenal syndrome. Journal of the American College of Cardiology. 2008;**52**:1527-1539

[32] Shah BN, Greaves K. The cardiorenal syndrome. International Journal of Nephrology. 2011;**2011**:920195

[33] Wizemann V, Schilling M. Dilemma of assessing volume state—The use and the limitations of a clinical score. Nephrology, Dialysis, Transplantation. 1995;**10**:2114-2117

[34] Paniagua R, Ventura MD, Avila-Díaz M, Hinojosa-Heredia H, Méndez-Durán A, et al. NT-proBNP, fluid volume overload and dialysis modality are independent predictors of mortality in ESRD patients. Nephrology, Dialysis, Transplantation. 2010;**25**:551-557

[35] Ozkahya M, Ok E, Toz H, Asci G, Duman S, et al. Long-term survival rates in haemodialysis patients treated with strict volume control. Nephrology, Dialysis, Transplantation. 2006;**21**:3506-3513

[36] Tsai YC, Tsai JC, Chen SC, Chiu YW, Hwang SJ, Hung CC, Chen TH, Kuo MC, Chen HC. Association of fluid overload with kidney disease progression in advanced CKD: A prospective cohort study. American Journal of Kidney Disease. 2014;**63**(1):68-75

[37] Tucker BJ, Collins RC, Ziegler MG, Blantz RC. Disassociation between glomerular hyperfiltration and extracellular volume in diabetic rats. Kidney International. 1991;**39**: 1176-1183

[38] Forbes JM, Fukami K, Cooper ME. Diabetic nephropathy: Where hemodynamics meets metabolism. Experimental and Clinical Endocrinology and Diabetes. 2007;**115**:69-84

[39] Li PK, Kwan BC, Ko GT, Chow KM, Leung CB, Szeto CC. Treatment of metabolic syndrome in peritoneal dialysis patients. Peritoneal Dialysis International. 2009;**29**(2): S149-S155

[40] Stevenson LW, Nohria A, Mielniczuk L. Torrent or torment from the tubules? Challenge of the cardiorenal connection. Journal of the American College of Cardiology. 2005;**45**(12): 2004-2007

[41] Chertow GM, Normand S-LT, Silva LR, McNeil BJ. Survival after acute myocardial infarction in patients with end-stage renal disease: Results from the cooperative cardiovascular project. American Journal of Kidney Disease. 2000;**35**(6):1044-1051

[42] Herzog CA. Dismal long-term survival of dialysis patients after acute myocardial infarction: can we alter the outcome? Nephrology, Dialysis, Transplantation. 2002;**17**(1):7-10

[43] Clementi A, Virzì GM, Brocca A, de Cal M, Vescovo G, Granata A, Ronco C. Cardiorenal syndrome type 4: Management. Blood Purification. 2013;**36**(3-4):200-209

[44] Damman K, Navis G, Voors AA, Asselbergs FW, Smilde TD, Cleland JG, van Veldhuisen DJ, Hillege HL. Worsening renal function and prognosis in heart failure: Systematic review and meta-analysis. Journal of Cardiac Failure. 2007;**13**:599-608

[45] De Vecchis R, Baldi C. Cardiorenal syndrome type 2: From diagnosis to optimal management. Therapeutics and Clinical Risk Management. 2014;**10**:949-961

[46] Bagshaw SM, Cruz DN. Epidemiology of cardiorenal syndromes. Contributions to Nephrology. 2010;**165**:68-82

[47] Clementi A, Virzì GM, Brocca A, de Cal M, Pastori S, Clementi M, Granata A, Vescovo G, Ronco C. Advances in the pathogenesis of cardiorenal syndrome type 3. Oxidative Medicine and Cellular Longevity. 2015;**2015**:1-8

[48] Cheung AK, Sarnak MJ, Yan G, Berkoben M, Heyka R, Kaufman A, Lewis J, Rocco M, Toto R, Windus D, Ornt D, Levey AS; HEMO Study Group. Cardiac diseases in maintenance hemodialysis patients: Results of the HEMO study. Kidney International. 2004;**65**:2380-2389

[49] Corradi GMVV, Panagiotou A, Gastaldon F, Cruz DN, de Cal M, et al. ADPKD: Prototype of cardiorenal syndrome type 4. International Journal of Nephrology. 2011;**2011**:490795

[50] Mehta RL, Rabb H, Shaw AD, Singbartl K, Ronco C, McCullough PA, Kellum JA. Cardiorenal syndrome type 5: Clinical presentation, pathophysiology and management strategies from the eleventh consensus conference of the Acute Dialysis Quality Initiative (ADQI). Contributions to Nephrology. 2013;**182**:174-194

[51] Ronco C, McCullough PA, Anker SD, Anand I, Aspromonte N, Bagshaw SM, et al. Cardiorenal syndromes: An executive summary from the consensus conference of the Acute Dialysis Quality Initiative (ADQI). Contributions to Nephrology. 2010;**165**:54-67

[52] Schroten NF, Damman K, Valente MA, Smilde TD, van Veldhuisen DJ, Navis G, Gaillard CA, Voors AA, Hillege HL. Long-term changes in renal function and perfusion in heart failure patients with reduced ejection fraction. Clinical Research in Cardiology. 2016;**105**(1):10-16

[53] McCullough PA, Assad H. Diagnosis of cardiovascular disease in patients with chronic kidney disease. Blood Purification. 2012;**33**(1-3):112-118

[54] Cuba M, Batista R. Cardiac calcification in patients with terminal chronic renal insufficiency and kidney transplant patients. Nefrología. 2004;**24**(2):196-197

[55] Chinnappa S, Hothi SS, Tan LB. Is uremic cardiomyopathy a direct consequence of chronic kidney disease? Expert Review of Cardiovascular Therapy. 2014;**12**(2):127-130

[56] Alhaj E, Alhaj N, Rahman I, Niazi T, Berkowitz R, Klapholz M. Uremic cardiomyopathy: An underdiagnosed disease. Congestive Heart Failure. 2013;**19**(4):E40-E45

[57] Kunz K, Dimitrov Y, Muller S, Chantrel F, Hannedouche T. Uraemic cardiomyopathy. Nephrology, Dialysis, Transplantation. 1998;**13**(4):39-44

[58] Riggato C, Parfrey PS. Uraemic Cardiomyopathy. Journal of Clinical and Basic Cardiology. 2001;**4**:93-95

[59] Codognotto M, Piccoli A, Zaninotto M, Mion M, Plebani M, Vertolli U, Tona F, Ruzza L, Barchita A, Boffa GM. Renal dysfunction is a confounder for plasma natriuretic peptides in detecting heart dysfunction in uremic and idiopathic dilated cardiomyopathies. Clinical Chemistry. 2007;**53**(12):2097-2104

[60] Rosales BG, Sotelo CM, Monteon RF, Quirarte JA, Zuñiga G, Cueto-Manzano A. Metabolic and echocardiographic changes during dialysis and after renal transplantation. Nefrología Mexicana. 2002;**23**(1):5-10

[61] Szeto CC, Li PK. Salt and water balance in PD. In: Molony D, Craig J, editors, Evidence-Based Nephrology. Oxford: Wiley Blackwell (BMJ Books); 2009. pp. 488-499

[62] Ely EW, Haponik EF. Using the chest radiograph to determine intravascular volume status: The role of vascular pedicle width. Chest. 2002;**121**(3):942-950

[63] Martin GS, Ely EW, Carroll FE, Bernard GR. Findings on the portable chest radiograph correlate with fluid balance in critically ill patients. Chest. 2002;**122**(6):2087-2095

[64] Gao N, Kwan BC, Chow KM, Chung KY, Leung CB, Li PK, Szeto CC. Longitudinal changes of cardiothoracic ratio and vascular pedicle width as predictors of volume status during one year in Chinese peritoneal dialysis patients. Kidney and Blood Pressure Research. 2009;**32**(1):45-50

[65] Stewart GA, Gansevoort RT, Mark PB, Rooney E, McDonagh TA, Dargie HJ, Stuart R, Rodger C, Jardine AG. Electrocardiographic abnormalities and uremic cardiomyopathy. Kidney International. 2005;**67**(1):217-226

[66] Hung KC, Lee CH, Chen CC, Chu CM, Wang CY, Hsieh IC, Fang JT, Lin FC, Wen MS. Advanced left ventricular diastolic dysfunction in uremic patients with type 2 diabetes on maintenance hemodialysis. Circulation Journal. 2012;**76**(10):2380-2385

[67] Pecoits-Filho R, Berberato SH. Echocardiography in chronic kidney disease: Diagnosticand prognostic implications. Nephron. Clinical Practice. 2010;**114**:c242-c247

[68] Pazarín-Villaseñor L, Reyes LU, León-Flores AM, Miranda-Díaz AG, Andrade-Sierra J. Miocardiopatía urémica y trasporte peritoneal en pacientes incidentes con diálisis peritoneal en el occidente de México. Nefrología. 2016 (in press). http://dx.doi.org/10.1016/j.nefro.2016.11.005

[69] Daniels LB, Maissel AS. Natriuretic peptides. Journal of the American College of Cardiology. 2007;**50**:2357-2368

[70] deFillipi CR, Fink JC, Nass CM, Chen H, Christenson R. N-terminal Pro B –type natriuretic peptide for predicting coronary disease and left ventricular hypertrophy in asymptomatic CKD not requiring dialysis. American Journal of Kidney Disease. 2005;**46**:35-44

[71] Iwanaga Y, Miyazaki S. Heart Failure, chronic kidney disease, and biomarkers—An integrated viewpoint. Circulation Journal. 2010;**74**(7):1274-1282

[72] Ynstead A, Landro L, Uelan T, Dahl CP, Flo TH, Vinge LE, et al. Increased Systemic and Myocardial expression of neutrophil gelatinase-associated lipocalin in clinical and experimental heart failure. European Heart Journal. 2009;**30**(10):1229-1236

[73] Twardowski ZJ, Nolph KDA, Prowant LBF, Moore HL, Nielsen MP. Peritoneal equilibrium test. Peritoneal Dialysis Bulletin. 1987;**7**(3):138-147

[74] Cueto-Manzano AM. Peritoneal dialysis in Mexico. Kidney International. 2003;**63**(83): s90-s92

[75] Scott BK, Walker M, Margetts PJ, Kundhal KK, Rabbat CG. Metanalysis: Peritoneal membrane transport, mortality and technique failure in peritoneal dialysis. Journal of the American Society of Nephrology. 2006;**17**:2591-2598

[76] Chávez Valencia V, Orizaga de la Cruz C, Pazarin Villaseñor HL, Fuentes Ramírez F, Parra Michel R, Aragaki Y, et al. Frequency of peritoneal transport in a population of the Hospital General Regional No. 46, Instituto Mexicano del Seguro Social. Gaceta Médica de México. 2014;**150**(2):186-193

[77] Waniewski J, Debowska M, Lindholm B. Water and solute transport through different types of pores in peritoneal membrane in CAPD patients with ultrafiltration failure. Peritoneal Dialysis International. 2009;**29**(6):664-669

[78] Sobiecka D, Waniewski J, Weryński A, Lindholm B. Peritoneal fluid transport in CAPD patients with different transport rates of small solutes. Peritoneal Dialysis International. 2004;**24**(3):240-251

[79] Cueto-Manzano AM. Rapid solute transport in the peritoneum: Physiologic and clinical consequences. Peritoneal Dialysis International. 2009;**29**(2):s90-s95

[80] Jeznach-Steinhagen A, Słotwiński R, Szczygieł B. Malnutrition, inflammation, atherosclerosis in hemodialysis patients. Roczniki Panstwowego Zakladu Higieny. 2007;**58**(1):83-88

[81] Abe M, Okada K, Maruyama T, Maruyama N, Matsumoto K, Soma M. Relationship between erythropoietin responsiveness, insulin resistance, and malnutrition-inflammation-atherosclerosis (MIA) syndrome in hemodialysis patients with diabetes. International Journal of Artificial Organs. 2011;**34**(1):16-25

[82] Chung SH, Stenvinkel P, Bergström J, Lindholm B. Biocompatibility of new peritoneal dialysis solutions: What can we hope to achieve? Peritoneal Dialysis International. 2000;**20**(5):S57-S67

[83] Teixidó-Planas J, Troya-Saborido MI, Pedreira-Robles G, Del-Rio-Lafuente M, Romero-Gonzalez R, Bonet-Sol J. Measuring peritoneal absorption with the prolonged peritoneal equilibration test from 4 to 8 hours using various glucose concentrations. Perit Dial Int. 2014;**34**(6):605-11

[84] Aguirre AR, Abensur H. Protective measures against ultrafiltration failure in peritoneal dialysis patients; Clinics (São Paulo, Brazil). 2011;**66**(12):2151-2157

[85] Fusshoeller A. Histomorphological and functional changes of the peritoneal membrane during long-term peritoneal dialysis. Pediatric Nephrology. 2008;**23**:19-25

[86] La Milia V, Di Filippo S, Crepaldi M, Del Vecchio L, Dell'Oro C, Andrulli S, Locatelli F. Mini-peritoneal equilibration test: A simple and fast method to assess free water and small solute transport across the peritoneal membrane. Kidney International. 2005;**68**:840-846

[87] Kawaguchi Y, Kawanishi H, Mujais S, Topley N, Oreopoulos DG. Encapsulating peritoneal sclerosis: Definition, etiology, diagnosis, and treatment. International Society for Peritoneal Dialysis Ad Hoc Committee on Ultrafiltration Management in Peritoneal Dialysis. Peritoneal Dialysis International. 2000;**20**:S43-S55

[88] Flessner MF. Peritoneal ultrafiltration: Mechanisms and measures. Contributions to Nephrology. 2006;**150**:28-36

[89] Prasad N, Gupta S. Ultrafiltration failure in peritoneal dialysis: A review. Indian Journal of Peritoneal Dialysis. 2012;**22**(1):15-24

[90] Heimburger O, Waniewski J, Werinski A Tranaeus A, Lindholm B. Peritoneal transport in CAPD patients with permanent loss of ultrafiltration capacity. Kidney International. 1990;**38**:495-506

[91] Ha SK. Dietary salt intake and hypertension. Electrolyte Blood Press. 2014;**12**:7-18

[92] Inal S, Erten Y, Akbulu G, et al. Salt intake and hypervolemia in the development of hypertension in peritoneal dialysis patients. Advances in Peritoneal Dialysis. 2012;**28**:10-15

[93] Biesen WV, Vanholder R, Veys N, Lameire N. Improving salt balance in peritoneal dialysis patients. Peritoneal Dialysis International. 2005;**25**(S3):S73-S75

[94] Wang AY, Brimble KS, Brunier G, et al. ISPD Cardiovascular and Metabolic Guidelines in Adult Peritoneal Dialysis Patients. Part I—Assessment and management of various cardiovascular risk factors. Peritoneal Dialysis International. 2015;**35**:379-387

[95] Tzamaloukas AH, Saddler MC, Murata GH, et al. Symptomatic fluid retention in patients on continuous peritoneal dialysis. Journal of the American Society of Nephrology. 1995;**6**:198-206

[96] Ates K. Salt and wáter in PD. The Turkish contribution. Peritoneal Dialysis International. 2008;**28**(3):224-228

[97] Inal S, Erten Y, Tek N, et al. The effect of dietary salt restriction on hypertension in peritoneal dialysis patients. Turkish Journal of Medical Sciences. 2014;**44**(5):814-819

[98] Fine A, Fontaine B, Ma M. Commonly prescribed salt intake in continuous ambulatory peritoneal dialysis patients is too restrictive: results of a double-blind crossover study. Journal of the American Society of Nephrology. 1997;**8**:1311-1314

[99] McMahon EJ, Campbell KL, Mudge DW, Bauer JD. Achieving salt restriction in chronic kidney disease. International Journal of Nephrology. 2012;**2012**:720429

[100] Dong J, Li Y, Yang Z, Luo J. Low dietary sodium intake increases the death risk in peritoneal dialysis. Clinical Journal of the American Society of Nephrology. 2010;**5**:240-247

[101] Cheng LT, Wang T. Changes in total sodium intake do not lead to proportionate changes in total sodium removal in CAPD patients. Peritoneal Dialysis International. 2006;**26**(2):218-223

[102] Bae SY, Kim SB, Kim SM. Simple method to estimate daily sodium intake during measurement of dialysis adequacy in chronic peritoneal dialysis patients. Clin Nutr. 2016;**35**(1):S191-S192

[103] Haddad N, Shim R, Hebert LA. Nutritional management of water, sodium, potassium, chloride, and magnesium in kidney disease and kidney failure. Nutr Manag Renal Dis Chapter 22: 323-338, 2013

[104] Yip T, Wan W, Hui PC, Lui SL, Lo WL. Severe hiperkalemia in a peritoneal dialysis patients after consuption of salt substitute. Perit Dial Int. 2012;**32**(2):206-208

Subjective Wellbeing Assessment in People with Chronic Kidney Disease Undergoing Hemodialysis

Luís Manuel Mota de Sousa, Ana Vanessa Antunes,
Cristina Rosa Soares Lavareda Baixinho,
Sandy Silva Pedro Severino,
Cristina Maria Alves Marques-Vieira and
Helena Maria Guerreiro José

Additional information is available at the end of the chapter

http://dx.doi.org/10.5772/intechopen.71194

Abstract

The aim of this study was to analyze the relationship between satisfaction with life in general and the sociodemographic and emotional factors and components of quality of life in people with chronic kidney disease undergoing hemodialysis. A cross-sectional and correlational study was performed on a sample of 171 people with chronic kidney disease in two hemodialysis units at a Clinic in Lisbon between May and June 2015. Subjective wellbeing (personal wellbeing index) is positively related with subjective happiness, positive affect, and quality of life and is negatively associated with negative affect. Subjective happiness, negative affect, and the physical component of quality of life influence subjective wellbeing. These conclusions can assist us in understanding that people with chronic kidney disease (CKD) encounter greater feelings of wellbeing, mainly related to pleasant affect (subjective happiness and positive affect).

Keywords: subjective wellbeing, emotion, quality of life, chronic renal insufficiency, renal dialysis

1. Introduction

Due to its prevalence, chronic kidney disease (CKD) has been recognized as an important public health problem [1].

It has high economic implications in health systems and is also an independent risk factor for cardiovascular disease (CVD) [2]. All six stages of CKD [3] are associated with the increased risk of cardiovascular morbidity, premature mortality, and/or decreased quality of life (QoL) [2, 3].

CKD has an estimated prevalence of 11–13%, mostly related with stage 3 [2]. In the United States in 2012, its prevalence in stages 3–4 was about 6.9% (5.5–8.3) [4]. The adjusted prevalence of CKD in stages 1–5 varied between 3.31% (95% confidence interval [95% CI], 3.30–3.33%) in Norway and 17.3% (IC 95%, 16.5–18.1%) in north eastern Germany [5].

Worldwide, there are about 1.9 million people with CKD undergoing renal replacement therapy [6], namely hemodialysis (HD) or peritoneal dialysis. The first is the most common treatment modality [7].

HD is a treatment method usually performed in hospitals or clinics during 3–4 hours, three times a week [8]. This complex treatment has a high impact on the life of people with CKD. It requires several radical lifestyle changes that affect social and psychological functioning [9] as well as cause pain [7]. Therefore, it is considered a long-term treatment with significant side effects on the physical and mental wellbeing [10].

Health is a state of complete physical, mental, and social wellbeing and not merely the absence of disease or infirmity [11].

People with CKD receiving HD treatment can experience emotional instability and psychological distress, financial burdens, inadequate disease knowledge, and less social support, which influences their QoL [12]. CKD directly interferes in functional capacity, independence, and quality of life [13].

QoL and wellbeing as perceived by people with CKD are important measures of patients' health outcomes [12, 14].

As stated by the World Health Organization, subjective wellbeing (SWB) is considered within the research community as an indicator for the evaluation of QoL [14]. It consists of a range of phenomena that include emotional responses, satisfaction domains, and the judgment about global satisfaction with life. The components of SWB are pleasant affect (e.g., joy, contentment, pride, affection, and happiness), unpleasant affect (e.g., guilt and shame, anxiety and worry, anger, stress, and depression), life satisfaction (e.g., desire to change, satisfaction with current life, past, and future), and a satisfaction domain (e.g., work, family, leisure, health, finances, and self) [15].

A study developed in Indonesia using people with CKD undergoing HD showed that subjective wellbeing is directly related with the positive interpretation of the dialysis process. It also showed that people with CKD have happy feelings and are still able to manage negative emotions that arise. The negative feelings experienced by these people with CKD were anger, sadness, hopelessness, boredom, annoyance, and concern. The positive affects experienced were happiness, pleasure, gratefulness, and optimism [16].

Despite being considered as an important indicator for the QoL in people with CKD undergoing HD, SWB is still underexplored by researchers [17]. Therefore, we found it relevant to explore the sociodemographic and emotional factors that influence the cognitive dimension of the subjective wellbeing, that is to say, the satisfaction with life in general. Therefore, our main goal is to analyze the relationship between satisfaction with life in general and the sociodemographic and emotional factors and components of quality of life.

2. Methods

2.1. Study design

A cross-sectional and correlational study [18], developed in two units of the Diaverum Dialysis Clinic in the Lisbon region, Portugal, with people with CKD undergoing HD between May and June 2015.

2.2. Subjects and setting

The inclusion criteria defined for the population were people undergoing HD routinely for at least 6 months and aged 18 years or over. Exclusion criteria were people with cognitive impairment and active psychiatric illness. Information regarding these conditions was obtained through medical records, 253 people with CKD met the eligibility criteria (139 in clinic 1 and 114 in clinic 2).

A simple random sample of 171 people undergoing HD was selected from the dialysis clinics, 93 of clinic 1 and 78 of clinic 2.

2.3. Procedures

Approval was received from the ethics committees of Diaverum (Approval No 1/2015). Both the purpose of the study and the guaranteed confidentiality of data with the right to withdraw without risk to oneself were explained to the people with CKD. Informed consent was therefore obtained from those who met the inclusion criteria and agreed to participate.

Interviews were performed by five trained nurses during the HD session.

One of the researchers met with these nurses to explain the objectives and how to collect the data, followed by a written roadmap to assist in completing the data collection instruments.

Data were collected through a sociodemographic and health information questionnaire (age, gender, nationality, education, occupation, marital status, dialysis sessions length, presence of hypertension, and diabetes), the subjective happiness scale (SHS) [19–21], the satisfaction with life in general (SWLG), the personal wellbeing index (PWI) [22, 23], the Portuguese version of positive and negative affect schedule (PANAS) [24–26], and the 12-item short form health survey (SF-12) [27, 28].

Retrospective license was obtained for the use of SF-12 (license No QM030904).

2.4. Outcomes measurement

The SHS [18] consists of four items; in items two and three, participants are asked to self-characterize themselves compared to their peers in absolute and relative terms. Items one and four correspond to descriptions of happiness and unhappiness. The last item score is reversed. On this scale, respondents are asked to self-characterize within a visual analogue scale with seven positions. The scale is based on two antagonistic statements, which express the level of happiness or lack of it [19, 20]. The Portuguese version in people with CKD shows a single factor with an internal reliability with a Cronbach's α of 0.90 [21].

The PWI [22] consists of seven domains of the overall measure of life satisfaction (satisfaction with standard of living, health, personal development, personal relationships, sense of security, connection to the community, and security for the future). For each statement, the respondents are asked to classify their satisfaction within a scale from zero (extremely dissatisfied) to 10 (very satisfied) with a neutral intermediate position. The PWI is calculated on a rating ranging from zero to 100 (maximum percentage of the scale) [22, 23]. The Portuguese version in people with CKD revealed the existence of a single factor, with an internal reliability with a Cronbach's α of 0.82 [23].

The PANAS [24] scale was adapted and translated for the Portuguese population and consists of two subscales: PA and NA, with 10 items each, in which constructs are assessed on a Likert scale of 1–5. The respondents are asked to classify their emotions (for each of the 20 items) at the present time. The PA dimension is much more present than the higher score, a maximum of 50 points [25]. The study of the Portuguese version of PANAS in people with CKD revealed the same as the original scale, the existence of two factors, internal consistency with Cronbach's α of 0.86 (in the original, $\alpha = 0.88$) for the positive affect and 0.88 (in the original, $\alpha = 0.87$) for the negative affect scale [26].

SF-12 [27] is a health questionnaire developed in the United States of America, validated for several countries, from different continents. It measures the perception of health-related QoL through the use of 12 items with a resumed physical and mental component in which the constructs are evaluated on a Likert type scale from three to five points [27, 28]. The version translated and adapted to Portuguese showed reliability and satisfactory validity [27].

2.5. Data analysis

Data were analyzed with descriptive and inferential statistics using the Statistical Package for Social Sciences (SPSS) 20.0 statistical software. Data obtained by SF12 were analyzed using the Quality Metric Health Outcomes™ Scoring Software 4.5. Descriptive statistics are reported as frequency, percentage, mean, and standard deviations, while inferential procedures included Spearman correlation coefficients and multiple linear regression. A 0.05 level of significance was adopted.

3. Results

The typical characteristics of participants were male (61%), an average age of 60.2 years old (SD = 14.34). About 80.1% had Portuguese nationality and the remaining were from an African country as follows: Cape Verde 14%; São Tomé 3.5%; Angola 1.8%, and Guinea 0.6%. On what concerns the educational level, 3.6% were illiterate, 42.3% had the 4th grade, 18.5% the 6th grade, 14.9% the 9th grade, 11.8% the 12th grade, and 8.9% have completed higher education. Regarding their marital status, 56.5%were married, 26.5% were single, 11.2% widowers, and 5.8% were divorced. About 76.7% were retired, only 23.3% had a regular professional activity. Concerning health data, the subjects were undergoing HD for about 72.17 months (±54.2), 62.1% had hypertension, and 27.1% had diabetes.

Portuguese people with CKD had the higher score for satisfaction with life in general ($p = 0.015$), compared with the remaining population (Cape Verde, São Tomé, Angola, and Guinea).

Table 1 shows both sociodemographic and clinical factors related with CKD, which are associated to satisfaction with life in general/personal wellbeing index.

Satisfaction with life in general/personal wellbeing index has a mean score of 64.7% (±18.2%). Mean scores for the other variables are as follows: subjective happiness 19.9 (±5.9), positive affect 24.9 (±8.5), negative affect 14.2 (±6.1), physical component summary SF-12 41.1% (±9.2%), and mental component summary SF-12 com 47.2 (±10.7%) (**Table 2**).

Table 3 shows that the personal wellbeing index is positively correlated with subjective happiness ($\rho = 0.605$, $p < 0.001$), positive affect ($\rho = 0.328$, $p < 0.001$), physical component summary SF-12($\varrho = 0.470$, $p < 0.001$), and mental component summary SF-12 ($\rho = 0.319$, $p < 0.001$). However, it presents a low negative correlation with the negative affect ($\rho = -0.161$, $p < 0.05$). Higher scores on the personal wellbeing index are associated with higher levels of subjective happiness, positive affect, physical component summary SF-12, and mental component summary SF and lower levels of negative affect.

Subjective happiness shows a significant positive correlation with the positive affect ($\rho = 0.415$, $p < 0.001$), physical component summary SF-12($\rho = 0.326$, $p < 0.001$), and mental component summary SF-12 ($\rho = 0.287$, $p < 0.001$). Nevertheless, it shows a lower negative correlation with the negative affect ($\rho = -0.126$, $p < 0.01$). When subjective happiness values increase, positive affect, physical component summary SF-12, and mental component summary SF also increase. Simultaneously, negative affect values decrease.

Positive affect shows a significant positive correlation with the physical component summary SF-12 ($\rho = 0.190$, $p < 0.01$) and a mental component summary SF-12 ($\rho = 0.166$, $p < 0.01$).

Negative affect shows a significant negative correlation with the mental component summary SF-12 ($\rho = -0.271$, $p < 0.001$).

	Satisfaction with life in general/personal wellbeing index	p-Value
Gender		
Male	64.2 ± 18.0	p = 0.779
Female	64.8 ± 18.1	
Age		
Under 63 years	66.5 ± 17.1	p = 0.060
More than 63 years	62.6 ± 18.9	
Nationality		
Portuguese	70.5 ± 15.9	p = 0.015
Other	63.2 ± 18.3	
Professional activity		
Retired	64.4 ± 19.0	p = 0.364
Active	66.8 ± 15.4	
Marital status		
Single	67.4 ± 18.2	p = 0.134
Married	64.9 ± 17.5	
Other	59.5 ± 18.9	
Arterial hypertension		
No	67.6 ± 18.1	p = 0.177
Yes	62.9 ± 17.9	
Diabetes		
No	66.0 ± 18.4	p = 0.080
Yes	60.1 ± 16.5	
Hemodialysis time		
Less than 5 years	65.7 ± 17.3	p = 0.937
More than 5 yeas	63.4 ± 19.0	

Table 1. Sociodemographic and clinical factors associated to satisfaction with life in general. Lisbon, Portugal (2017).

The physical component summary SF-12 shows a lower positive correlation with the mental component summary SF-12 ($\varrho = 0.181$, $p < 0.01$).

The adjusted R^2 for the model was 46.6% with subjective happiness, negative affect, and physical component summary SF-12 that consistently contributed as best predictors of satisfaction with life in general/personal wellbeing index. The resulting R2 were statistically significant at the $p < 0.00$ and $p < 0.05$ levels.

	Range	Minimum	Maximum	Mean	Standard deviation
1. Satisfaction with life in general/personal wellbeing index	0–100	6.3	100	64.7	18.2
2.Subjective happiness	4–28	4	28	19.9	5.9
3.Positive affect	10–50	10	44	24.9	8.5
4.Negative affect	10–50	10	40	14.2	6.1
5. Physical component summary SF-12	0–100	17.3	63.2	40.1	9.2
6. Mental component summary SF-12	0–100	21.6	66.1	47.2	10.7

Table 2. Mean and standard deviation for the different variables. Lisbon, Portugal (2017).

	1	2	3	4	5	β	t
Constant							1.035
1. Satisfaction with life in general/personal wellbeing index							
2. Subjective happiness	0.605‡					0.426	6.422‡
3. Positive affect	0.328‡	0.415‡				0.,086	1.378
4. Negative affect	−0.161*	−0.126†	0.084			−0.121	−2.006*
5. Physical component summary SF-12	0.470‡	0.326‡	0.190†	0.100		0.310	5.121‡
6. Mental component summary SF-12	0.319‡	0.287‡	0.166†	−0.271‡	0.181†	0.093	1.520
Sample size = 171, Adjusted $R^2 = 0.466$, F = 30.637‡							

*Significance $p < 0.05$,
†Significance $p < 0.01$,
‡Significance $p < 0.001$.

Table 3. Regression for personal wellbeing index with other variables and correlations. Lisbon, Portugal (2017).

Both subjective happiness and physical component summary SF-12 have a positive effect on satisfaction with life in general (respectively, $\beta = 0.426$, $p < 0.001$; $\beta = 0.310$, $p < 0.001$). However, negative affect has a negative effect on satisfaction with life in general ($\beta = -0.121$, $p < 0.05$).

4. Discussion

This study is aimed at examining the relationship between satisfaction with life in general and the components of quality of life, sociodemographic characteristics, and emotional factors.

Our findings are in line with the literature on the effects of HD on the life of people with CKD and factors associated with reduced wellbeing.

On what concerns sociodemographic factors, differences were only found in people with CKD of a different nationality. This may be explained by cultural differences, as people with CKD from foreign countries may experience social integration difficulties.

The economic level of countries generally influences all indicators of health and quality of life; however, the SWB in higher income countries is affected by other factors such as income inequality, social welfare, individualism, democracy and freedom, social capital, and physical health [29]. These data are reinforced by the results of a study, which report that the economic level of people negatively affects the SWB in both low income and high income countries [30].

As already mentioned, there is a scarcity of literature concerning wellbeing in people with CKD. Our study confirmed lower scores for GWLS in people with CKD (64.7 ± 18.2). Similarly, the Australian study with people with end-stage kidney disease got an average PWI of 64.7 ± 19.2 and of 74.8 ± 15.7 for the general population [17]. Lower SWB may cause adverse health behaviors in people with CKD. In a study involving people living with HIV, it was suggested that reduced SWB increased the risk of medication nonadherence [31]. Future studies should explore the relationship between wellbeing, adherence to medication, food, and physical activity levels. This association can allow the development of individualized interventions that promote wellbeing in the hemodialysed population and impact on other domains of the personal and social life of these people.

The mean scores for all domains of QoL for people with CKD were considerably below the general population norms. Similar results were found in an Irish study on the QoL of people with CKD undergoing HD treatment [32].

Our main finding is that happiness, pleasant affect, physical, and mental components of QoL are significantly higher in people undergoing HD who got higher scores for the personal well-being index/satisfaction with life in general. Subjective happiness and physical components of QoL are those that contribute the most for the overall life satisfaction. On the other hand, negative affect has a significant negative association and influences satisfaction with life in general.

The association between quality of life, morbidity, and mortality has already been explored in previous studies [17]. Chida and Steptoe [33] described SWB as a significant and independent variable predicting increased survival times in CKD. Our study shows the importance of evaluating the components of SWB in people with CKD undergoing HD treatment. It allows us to examine the influence of both emotional components (subjective happiness and negative affect) and physical components of QoL, in cognitive dimension of SWB (satisfaction with life in general/personal wellbeing index).

4.1. Limitations

There are some limitations in this study. Our results are based on a cross-sectional design that may limit the discussion of a cause-effect relationship between SWB and the variables.

Also, both clinics involved in the study are in the same region influencing sociodemographic characteristics and preventing the generalization of conclusions. Data collection environment (HD room) can lead to distraction in people with CKD. However, others studies [34, 35] were conducted in the same conditions, which do not seem to affect the results. Questionnaires were self-reported or by interview, so some might have given socially accepted answers that could lead to response bias. Finally, the small sample size might have limited the validity of the results. Therefore, a study with a larger sample might have more statistical meaning in examining associations between variables.

4.2. Implications for practice

Nursing professionals have an important role in the promotion of wellbeing and quality of life. The SWB measured by the PWI is an important element in QoL [17]. This study results suggest that people with CKD with higher levels of subjective happiness and quality of life (mental and physical component) also have higher levels of SWB. Thus, these results may help future interventions related to the wellbeing of people with CKD, aimed at improving nurse training for the identification and monitoring of these dysfunctional behaviors. Nurses will be boosted to optimize patient health outcomes.

Depressive symptoms in people with CKD are associated with decreased quality of life [36] and decreased wellbeing [17]. Dialysis nurses should therefore be encouraged to increase people with CKD's happiness through the integration of laughter yoga [37], the Fordyce's happiness program [38], and the visualization of humor films [39], during dialysis sessions. This intervention will improve both people with CKD's wellbeing and health outcomes, such as quality of life, affect, and depressive symptoms.

5. Conclusion

Our results show that SWB (personal wellbeing index) is positively related with subjective happiness, positive affect, and quality of life and is negatively associated with negative affect. Subjective happiness, negative affect, and the physical component of quality of life influence SWB. These conclusions can assist us in understanding that people with CKD encounter greater feelings of wellbeing, mainly related to pleasant affect (subjective happiness and positive affect).

This study has confirmed that SWB is lower in people with CKD than in the general population, though this is partly explained by the negative affect. However, SWB increases when both subjective happiness perception and quality of life increase. These conclusions can assist us in understanding that people with CKD encounter higher feelings of wellbeing, not only related to pleasant affect (subjective happiness and positive affect) but also to many other aspects of QoL.

Future studies should be performed in people undergoing HD that demonstrate the effect of interventions on cognitive and emotional variables of the SWB, as is the case of the visualization of humor films.

Author details

Luís Manuel Mota de Sousa[1,2]*, Ana Vanessa Antunes[1],
Cristina Rosa Soares Lavareda Baixinho[3], Sandy Silva Pedro Severino[1,2],
Cristina Maria Alves Marques-Vieira[4] and Helena Maria Guerreiro José[5]

*Address all correspondence to: luismmsousa@gmail.com

1 Atlântica Higher School of Health Sciences, Atlântica University, Oeiras, Portugal

2 Curry Cabral Hospital, Central Lisbon Hospital Center, Lisbon, Portugal

3 Nursing School of Lisbon – ESEL, Lisbon, Portugal

4 School of Nursing of Lisbon, Institute of Health Sciences, Catholic University of Portugal, Lisbon, Portugal

5 Polytechnic Health Institute of Multiperfil, Luanda, Angola

References

[1] Du Y, Zhang S, Hu M, Wang Q, Shen H, Zhang Y, Yan D, Li Y, Zhang M, Meng Q. Prevalence of chronic kidney disease markers: Evidence from a three-million married population with fertility desire in rural China. Scientific Reports. 2017 [cited 2017 Aug 18];**7**(1):2710. DOI: 10.1038/s41598-017-02355-2

[2] Hill NR, Fatoba ST, Oke JL, Hirst JA, O'Callaghan CA, Lasserson DS, Hobbs FR. Global prevalence of chronic kidney disease–A systematic review and meta-analysis. PLoS One. 2016 Jul 6 [cited 2017 Aug 18];**11**(7):e0158765. https://doi.org/10.1371/journal.pone.0158765

[3] Inker LA, Astor BC, Fox CH, Isakova T, Lash JP, Peralta CA, Tamura MK, Feldman HI. KDOQI US commentary on the 2012 KDIGO clinical practice guideline for the evaluation and management of CKD. American Journal of Kidney Diseases. 2014 May 31 [cited 2017 Sep 4];**63**(5):713-735. DOI: 10.1053/j.ajkd.2014.01.416 Epub 2014 Mar 16

[4] Murphy D, McCulloch CE, Lin F, Banerjee T, Bragg-Gresham JL, Eberhardt MS, Morgenstern H, Pavkov ME, Saran R, Powe NR, Hsu CY. Trends in prevalence of chronic kidney disease in the United States trends in prevalence of CKD in the United States. Annals of Internal Medicine. 2016 Oct 4 [cited 2017 Aug 18];**165**(7):473-481. DOI: 10.7326/M16-0273 Epub 2016 Aug 2

[5] Brück K, Stel VS, Gambaro G, Hallan S, Völzke H, Ärnlöv J, Kastarinen M, Guessous I, Vinhas J, Stengel B, Brenner H. CKD prevalence varies across the European general population. Journal of the American Society of Nephrology. 2016 Jul 1 [cited 2017 Aug 18];**27**(7):2135-2147. DOI: 10.1681/ASN.2015050542 Epub 2015 Dec 23

[6] Anand S, Bitton A, Gaziano T. The gap between estimated incidence of end-stage renal disease and use of therapy. PLoS One. 2013 Aug 30 [cited 2017 Aug 18];**8**(8):e72860. https://doi.org/10.1371/journal.pone.0072860

[7] Sousa LM, Marques-Vieira CM, Severino SS, Pozo-Rosado JL, José HM. Validation of the brief pain inventory in persons with chronic kidney disease. Aquichan. 2017 Jan [cited 2017 Aug 19];**17**(1):42-52. http://dx.doi.org/10.5294/aqui.2017.17.1.5

[8] Ferguson TW, Tangri N, Rigatto C, Komenda P. Cost-effective treatment modalities for reducing morbidity associated with chronic kidney disease. Expert Review of Pharmacoeconomics & Outcomes Research. 2015 Mar 4 [cited 2017 Aug 19];**15**(2):243-252. DOI: 10.1586/14737167.2015.1012069 Epub 2015 Feb 8

[9] Nabolsi MM, Wardam L, Al-Halabi JO. Quality of life, depression, adherence to treatment and illness perception of patients on haemodialysis. International Journal of Nursing Practice. 2015 Feb 1 [cited 2017 Aug 19];**21**(1):1-10. DOI: 10.1111/ijn.12205 Epub 2013 Oct 11

[10] Mehrabi Y, Ghazavi Z, Shahgholian N. Effect of Fordyce's happiness program on stress, anxiety, and depression among the patients undergoing hemodialysis. Iranian Journal of Nursing and Midwifery Research. 2017 May 1 [cited 2017 Aug 19];**22**(3):190-194. DOI: 10.4103/1735-9066.208162

[11] World Health Organization. WHO Terminology Information System [Online Glossary] [cited 2017 Aug 19]. Available from: http://www.who.int/healthsystems/hss_glossary/en/index5.html

[12] Yu HD, Petrini MA. The HRQoL of Chinese patients undergoing haemodialysis. Journal of Clinical Nursing. 2010 Mar 1 [cited 2017 Aug 19];**19**(5-6):658-665. DOI: 10.1111/j.1365-2702.2009.03071.x

[13] Fassbinder TR, Winkelmann ER, Schneider J, Wendland J, Oliveira OB. Functional capacity and quality of life in patients with chronic kidney disease in pre-dialytic treatment and on hemodialysis–A cross sectional study. Jornal Brasileiro de Nefrologia. 2015 Mar [cited 2017 Aug 19];**37**(1):47-54. DOI: 10.5935/0101-2800.20150008

[14] Weinberg MK, Bennett PN, Cummins RA. Validation of the personal wellbeing index for people with end stage kidney disease. Applied Research in Quality of Life. 2016 Dec 1 [cited 2017 Aug 19];**11**(4):1227-1240. https://doi.org/10.1007/s11482-015-9431-x

[15] Diener E, Suh EM, Lucas RE, Smith HL. Subjective well-being: Three decades of progress. Psychological Bulletin. 1999 [cited 2017 Aug 19];**125**:276-302. Available from: http://web.yonsei.ac.kr/suh/file/Subjective%20Well%20Being_Three%20Decades%20of%20Progress%20-Diener,%20Suh,%20Lucas&Smith.pdf

[16] Setyawati R. Subjective well-being description of patients with chronic kidney disease undergoing hemodialysis. Indigenous Psychology Seminar. 2014 Apr 19 [cited 2017 Aug 19];**1**(1):301-307. Available from: http://digilib.ump.ac.id/files/disk1/27/jhptump-ump-gdl-rrsetyawat-1334-1-38-roro--7.pdf

[17] Bennett PN, Weinberg MK, Bridgman T, Cummins RA. The happiness and subjective well-being of people on haemodialysis. Journal of Renal Care. 2015 Sep 1 [cited 2017 Aug 19];**41**(3):156-161. DOI: 10.1111/jorc.12116 Epub 2015 Mar 26

[18] DVM L. Research design: A contribution to the author. Online Brazilian Journal of Nursing [Internet]. 2011 [cited 2017 Aug 19];**10**(2). Available from: http://www.objnursing.uff.br/index.php/nursing/article/view/3648/html_2

[19] Lyubomirsky S, Lepper HS. A measure of subjective happiness: Preliminary reliability and construct validation. Social Indicators Research. 1999 [cited 2017 Aug 19];**46**(2):137-155. Available from: http://www.cnbc.pt/jpmatos/26.%20lyubomirsky.pdf

[20] Pais-Ribeiro JL. Validação transcultural da Escala de Felicidade Subjectiva de Lyubomirsky e Lepper. Psicol Saúde Doenças [Internet]. 2012 [cited 2017 Aug 19];**13**(2):157-168. Available from: http://www.scielo.mec.pt/scielo.php?script=sci_arttext&pid=S1645-00862012000200003&lng=pt

[21] Sousa LM, Vieira CM, Severino SS, Pozo-Rosado JL, José HM. Validation of the subjective happiness scale in people with chronic kidney disease. Enfermeria Global. 2017 Jul [cited 2017 Aug 19];**16**(3):60-70. Available from: http://revistas.um.es/eglobal/article/view/266571

[22] Ribeiro JP, Cummins R. O bem-estar pessoal: estudo de validação da versão portuguesa da escala. In: Actas do 7° Congresso Nacional de Psicologia da Saúde [Internet]. Lisboa: ISPA; 2008 [cited 2017 Aug 19]. p. 505-508. Available from: http://repositorio-aberto.up.pt/handle/10216/21065

[23] Sousa LMM, Marques-Vieira CMA, Severino SSP, Pozo Rosado JL, MHG J. Validación del Índice de Bien-estar Personal en personas con enfermedad renal crónica. Enfermería nefrológica. 2016 Jun [cited 2017 Aug 19];**19**(2):135-141. Available from: http://scielo.isciii.es/scielo.php?script=sci_arttext&pid=S2254-28842016000200005&lng=es&nrm=iso&tlng=es

[24] Watson D, Clark LA, Tellegen A. Development and validation of brief measures of positive and negative affect: The PANAS scales. Journal of Personality and Social Psychology. 1988 [cited 2017 Aug 19];**54**:1063-1070. http://dx.doi.org/10.1037/0022-3514.54.6.1063

[25] Galinha I, Ribeiro J. Contribuição para o estudo da versão portuguesa da Positive and Negative Affect Schedule (PANAS): II–Estudo psicométrico. Analise Psicologica [Internet]. 2005 [cited 2017 Aug 19];**23**(2):219-227. Available from: http://publicacoes.ispa.pt/index.php/ap/article/viewFile/84/pdf

[26] Sousa LM, Marques-Vieira CM, Severino SS, Rosado JL, José HM. Validation of the positive and negative affect schedule in people with chronic kidney disease. Texto & Contexto–Enfermagem. 2016 [cited 2017 Aug 19];**25**(4) e5610015 (1-8). Available from: http://www.scielo.br/scielo.php?pid=S0104-07072016000400332&script=sci_arttext

[27] Ferreira-Valente MA, Ribeiro JLP, Jensen MP. Contribución adicional para la validación de la versión portuguesa de la Escala de Interferencia del Inventario Breve de Dolor. Clínica y Salud. 2012 [cited 2017 Aug 19];**23**(1):89-96. http://dx.doi.org/10.5093/cl2012a6

[28] Sousa LM, Antunes AV, Marques-Vieira CM, Valentim OS, José HM. Qualidade de vida e pessoa com doença renal crónica: um estudo transversal. In: Missias-Moreira R, Sales

ZN, Nascimento LCG, Valentim OS, editors. Qualidade de vida e condições de saúde de diversas populações. Vol. 2. Curitiba: Editora CRV; 2017 Sep. p. 139-154

[29] Jorm AF, Ryan SM. Cross-national and historical differences in subjective well-being. International Journal of Epidemiology. 2014 Feb 28 [cited 2017 Sep 5];**43**(2):330-340. DOI: 10.1093/ije/dyt188 Epub 2014 Feb 28

[30] Sarracino F. Determinants of subjective well-being in high and low income countries: Do happiness equations differ across countries. The Journal of Socio-Economics. 2013 Feb 11 [cited 2017 Sep 5];**42**(3):51-66. https://doi.org/10.1016/j.socec.2012.11.006

[31] Hutton VE, Misajon R, Collins FE. Subjective wellbeing and 'felt'stigma when living with HIV. Quality of Life Research. 2013 Feb 1 [cited 2017 Sep 1];**22**(1):65-73. DOI: 10.1093/ije/dyt188 Epub 2014 Feb 28

[32] Alshraifeen A, McCreaddie M, Evans JM. Quality of life and well-being of people receiving haemodialysis treatment in Scotland: A cross-sectional survey. International Journal of Nursing Practice. 2014 Oct [cited 2017 Sep 1];**20**(5):518-523. DOI: 10.1111/ijn.12194

[33] Chida Y, Steptoe A. Positive psychological well-being and mortality: A quantitative review of prospective observational studies. Psychosomatic Medicine. 2008 Sep 1 [cited 2017 Sep 1];**70**(7):741-745. DOI: 10.1097/PSY.0b013e31818105ba Epub 2008 Aug 25

[34] Saffari M, Pakpour AH, Naderi MK, Koenig HG, Baldacchino DR, Piper CN. Spiritual coping, religiosity and quality of life: A study on Muslim patients undergoing haemodialysis. Nephrology. 2013 Apr 1 [cited 2017 Sep 1];**18**(4):269-275. DOI: 10.1111/nep.12041

[35] Vitorino LM, Soares RCS, Santos AEO, Lucchetti PALG, Cruz JP, Cortez PJO, Lucchetti G. Two sides of the same coin: The positive and negative impact of spiritual religious coping on quality of life and depression in dialysis patients. Journal of Holistic Nursing. 2017 Aug [cited 2017 Sep 1]. DOI: 10.1177/0898010117725429

[36] Belayev LY, Mor MK, Sevick MA, Shields AM, Rollman BL, Palevsky PM, Arnold RM, Fine MJ, Weisbord SD. Longitudinal associations of depressive symptoms and pain with quality of life in patients receiving chronic hemodialysis. Hemodialysis International. 2015 Apr 1 [cited 2017 Sep 1];**19**(2):216-224. DOI: 10.1111/hdi.12247 Epub 2014 Nov 18

[37] Bennett PN, Parsons T, Ben-Moshe R, Neal M, Weinberg MK, Gilbert K, Ockerby C, Rawson H, Herbu C, Hutchinson AM. Intradialytic laughter yoga therapy for haemodialysis patients: A pre-post intervention feasibility study. BMC Complementary and Alternative Medicine. 2015 Jun 9 [cited 2017 Sep 1];**15**(1):176. DOI: 10.1186/s12906-015-0705-5

[38] Mehrabi Y, Ghazavi Z, Shahgholian N. Effect of Fordyce's happiness program on stress, anxiety, and depression among the patients undergoing hemodialysis. Iranian Journal of Nursing and Midwifery Research. 2017 May 1 [cited 2017 Sep 1];**22**(3):190-194. DOI: 10.4103/1735-9066.208162

[39] Sousa LMM. Ganhos em saúde com a intervenção "humor" em pessoas com doença renal crónica [Gains in Health with "humor" Intervention in People with Chronic Kidney Disease]Doctoral Dissertation in Nursing. Lisbon: Catholic University of Portugal; 2017